THE DNP NURSE *in* Executive Leadership Roles

Edited by
Joyce E. Johnson, PhD, RN, NEA-BC, FAAN
Associate Professor
The Catholic University of America
School of Nursing
Washington, DC

Linda L. Costa, PhD, RN, NEA-BC
Assistant Professor
University of Maryland
School of Nursing
Baltimore, Maryland

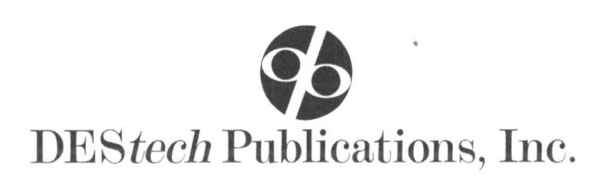

DEStech Publications, Inc.

The DNP Nurse in Executive Leadership Roles

DEStech Publications, Inc.
439 North Duke Street
Lancaster, Pennsylvania 17602 U.S.A.

Copyright © 2019 by DEStech Publications, Inc.
All rights reserved

No part of this publication may be reproduced, stored in a retrieval system, or transmitted, in any form or by any means, electronic, mechanical, photocopying, recording, or otherwise, without the prior written permission of the publisher.

Printed in the United States of America
10 9 8 7 6 5 4 3 2 1

Main entry under title:
 The DNP Nurse in Executive Leadership Roles

A DEStech Publications book
Bibliography: p.
Includes index p. 395

Library of Congress Control Number: 2019940600
ISBN No. 978-1-60595-492-9

HOW TO ORDER THIS BOOK

BY PHONE: 877-500-4337 or 717-290-1660, 9AM–5PM Eastern Time

BY FAX: 717-509-6100

BY MAIL: Order Department
DEStech Publications, Inc.
439 North Duke Street
Lancaster, PA 17602, U.S.A.

BY CREDIT CARD: American Express, VISA, MasterCard, Discover

BY WWW SITE: http://www.destechpub.com

To current and future nurse executives who highly value the Doctor of Nursing Practice degree and to the academicians who equip students with the subject matter knowledge and expertise necessary to enter and succeed in the C-Suite business environment.

—*Joyce E. Johnson and Linda Costa*

Table of Contents

Foreword xiii
Preface xv
Acknowledgments xvii
List of Contributors xix

**Chapter 1. The Evolution of DNP Programs in the
United States** **1**
    K. T. WAXMAN

    Chapter Objectives   1
    Introduction   1
    Current State of DNP Programs Nationally   2
    Differences Between the DNP and the PhD/DNS   3
    The Evolution of Doctoral Education in Nursing   3
    The DNP Essentials and the AONL Nurse Executive
        Competencies   5
    Where Do We Go From Here?   10
    Testimonial #1: My Executive Leadership
        DNP Journey   10
    Testimonial #2: DDNP Executive Testimonial   13
    Chapter Takeaways   14
    Chapter Summary   14
    Chapter Reflection Questions   15
    References   15

**Chapter 2. The DNP Nurse Executive in the
Healthcare Environment** **17**
    LINDA L. COSTA

    Chapter Objectives   17

Introduction   17
Value-Based Care and the DNP Nurse Executive   18
Strategic Agility and the DNP Executive   21
Case Study   23
Adaptive Leadership and the DNP   24
IOM Recommendations and the DNP-prepared
    Nurse Executive   25
C-Suite and the DNP Nurse Executive:
    Performance Expectations   28
Assessment Tools for the DNP executive   31
Transition to DNP Executive Leadership Practice   33
Chapter Takeaways   38
Chapter Summary   38
Chapter Reflection Questions   38
References   39

Chapter 3. The DNP Nurse Leadership Potential: Evolution and Challenges ... 43

ADRIANA PEREZ AMADO, COURTNEY VOSE and KARI A. MASTRO

Chapter Objectives   43
Introduction   43
The Challenge of Changing Educational Requirements
    for Nurse Managers   44
The Evolution of Entry Level Degree Requirements
    of Nursing Leaders   45
Rationale for Degree Progression   50
Evolution to the DNP   53
Building Personal Resilience   56
Emotional Intelligence   57
Behavioral Styles   61
Change in Nursing: The Leadership Mindset
    of the Future   65
Chapter Takeaways   68
Chapter Summary   69
Chapter Reflection Questions   70
References   70

Chapter 4. The Clinical DNP Practice Environment and Leadership Transformation ... 75

NANCY B. LERNER

Chapter Objectives   75
Introduction   75

APN Role Transformation   75
APN Transition to the DNP   76
DNP Role Development   78
Vignette 1: The Role of the DNP in Leadership   79
DNP APN Possibilities in an Aging and Diverse
    Health Care Population   80
Vignette 2   83
Vignette 3   85
Emerging Roles   86
Chapter Takeaways   87
Chapter Summary   88
Chapter Reflection Questions   88
References   88

**Chapter 5. Healthcare System Transformation,
Quadruple Aim, and Quality Improvement 93**
KARI A. MASTRO, JOAN GLEASON-SCOTT
and CHRISTA PREUSTER

Chapter Objectives   93
Introduction   93
The Delivery of Safe, Reliable, and Effective Care   94
The Institute of Health Care Improvement   94
The Evolution of the Quadruple Aim   98
The Role of Patients and Families in Quality and
    Safety Outcomes   113
Future Projections   119
Chapter Takeaways   120
Chapter Summary   120
Chapter Reflection Questions   120
References   121

**Chapter 6. Clinical Research, Quality Improvement,
and the DNP Nurse Executive 125**
PETRA GOODMAN

Chapter Objectives   125
Introduction   125
The DNP Nurse and Clinical Research   126
Collaboration to Increase Research Capacity   128
The DNP Nurse and Quality of Care   133
Quality Improvement Initiative: The National Quality
    Strategy (NQS)   135

Organizations Measuring Health Care Quality   136
Dashboards   148
Quality Improvement Methods   149
Chapter Takeaways   153
Chapter Summary   153
Chapter Reflection Questions   154
References   154

Chapter 7. Health Policy Development, Critical Analysis and the DNP-Prepared Nurse Executive 159

JOYCE E. JOHNSON

Chapter Objectives   159
Introduction   159
Definition of Health Policy   160
The Government and Health Care   161
The Social Compact and the Federalist Model   162
The Impact of Health Politics   163
Health Policy and the Government   164
Defining Characteristics of Public Policy and Policy Analysis   166
Evidenced-Based Analysis   169
The Policy Analysis Process   170
Healthcare Policy and the Role of the DNP-Prepared C-Suite Nurse Executive   186
Chapter Takeaways   187
Chapter Summary   188
Chapter Reflection Questions   188
References   189
Appendix A—Policy Example   193

Chapter 8. Healthcare Finance and the DNP Nurse Executive 217

MARY A. PATERSON

Chapter Objectives   217
Introduction   217
Health System Financing and Regulation   218
Mini-Case #1: Heartland Memorial Hospital   224
Business and Financial Risk in Health Care Organizations   225

Mini-Case #2: Suburban Family Practice
Associates LLC   228
Strategic Financial Management Tools   229
Mini-Case #3: St Alban's Hospital Management
Team   234
Chapter Takeaways   234
Chapter Summary   235
Chapter Reflection Questions   236
References   236
Appendix A   237
Appendix B   238

**Chapter 9. The C-Suite Business Case: The Critical
Role of Business Planning................................241**
JOYCE E. JOHNSON

Chapter Objectives   241
Introduction   241
Business Acumen and the C-Suite DNP-prepared
Nurse Executive   241
Think Like an Entrepreneur   244
Learn How to Write a Winning Business Plan   245
The Business Plan Framework   245
Sample Business Plan—Lourdes Family Clinic   257
Package the Business Plan Professionally   282
Chapter Takeaways   282
Chapter Summary   283
Chapter Reflection Questions   283
References   283

Chapter 10. Informatics for the DNP Nurse Executive.....287
ROSEMARY VENTURA

Chapter Objectives   287
Introduction   287
Essential HIT Skill Set for the DNP-prepared
Nurse Executive   289
The Role of the DNP Nurse Executive in
Technology Selection and Life Cycle   292
Overcoming Challenges in Health Care Technology
Adoption and Utilization   297
Big Data and Analytics   301
Health Care Legislation and the Electronic
Health Record   305

eHealth   307
Future Projections   309
Chapter Takeaways   310
Chapter Summary   310
Chapter Reflection Questions   311
References   311

Chapter 11. Disseminating Knowledge Through Mastering Writing Competency 315

KEVIN RULO

Chapter Objectives   315
Introduction   315
What Writing Is   317
Technical Writing Basics   319
Case Study—Mary Jones   322
Techniques for Writing Improvement:
  A Ten-Point Plan   324
Chapter Takeaways   333
Chapter Summary   333
Chapter Reflection Questions   334
References   335

Chapter 12. C-Suite Soft Skills and the Diverse Workforce. 337

CAROLYN K. ROOT, JEFFREY A. JOHNSON and ROBIN WIKLE

Chapter Objectives   337
Introduction   337
The Leadership "Soft Skills" Toolbox   338
The Workforce in 2020 and Beyond   354
Chapter Takeaways   357
Chapter Summary   357
Case Study: 5G Power Skills   358
Chapter Reflection Questions   361
References   361

Chapter 13. The Executive Leadership Role in Transforming Health Care: Journey into the Executive Suite 365

JEFFREY A. JOHNSON

Chapter Objectives   365
Introduction   365

The C-Suite Agenda   366
Whitewater, Black Swans, Leadership and
    Learning   380
Chapter Takeaways   386
Chapter Summary   386
Chapter Reflection Questions   388
Case Study #1: Trial by Technology   388
Case Study #2: Capturing the Patient's Journey   389
References   390

Index   395

Foreword

This textbook, *The DNP Nurse in Executive Leadership Roles*, could not come at a better time. Many of the 4.2 million nurses in the U.S. are electing to continue their education, with a large number setting their sights on a DNP degree, a credential that contributes to, and certifies, the leadership positions nurses are attaining in acute and ambulatory clinical settings, in the healthcare industry, and in academia.

As G. Rumay Alexander, president of the National League for Nursing, has noted, the DNP and PhD degrees are, for the nursing profession, complementary. We need PhD nurses to generate foundational research and DNP nurses to take the lead in implementing such research as managers and executives. It is in this context, where the present volume excels.

The editors and their contributors, Drs. Joyce Johnson and Linda Costa, have done an outstanding job of creating a book that will be of benefit to nurses during their doctoral training and in their professional practice. With more than 30,000 nurses already enrolled in DNP programs, a text such as this, directed to nurses transitioning to higher levels of responsibility, provides a valuable guide to the theory and application of leadership, which has been determined as essential by the American Association of Colleges of Nursing, as is laid out in the first chapter.

The book offers proven approaches for nurse leaders in working collaboratively with C-Suite colleagues, by analyzing long-term strategies and the ways organizations position themselves for future success. Strategic initiatives are presented in terms of (1) finance, (2) knowledge management, and (3) quality of care, patient safety, and outcomes. In these pages, one will find extensive information on how nursing professionals work most effectively with others in universities, business, and hospitals. Covered here are ways nurse leaders can establish legislative agendas to implement new policies at the local level and to change laws in the political arena. In this respect, the authors are in harmony with Ken Blanchard, who noted that "None of us is as smart as all of us."

This book offers concrete tools, such as data management and analytical resources for performing effectively in the public roles of leadership. At a personal level, it also explains ways nurses can prepare themselves psychologically, emotionally, and intellectually to make contributions as executives. Instructors and students will find in this book the organizational ideas and the ethical ideals that inform and create the role of the nurse as leader.

BOB DENT, DNP, MBA, RN, NEA-BC, CENP, FACHE, FAAN, FAONL
Senior Vice President, Chief Operating and Chief Nursing Officer at Midland Memorial Hospital
Adjunct Faculty at the Texas Tech University School of Nursing and the University of Texas of the Permian Basin School of Nursing
2018 President of the American Organization for Nursing Leadership (formerly the American Organization of Nurse Executives)
Co-author of the AJN award-winning book, Building a Culture of Ownership in Healthcare
Midland, Texas

Preface

Since the 2010 Institute of Medicine report and the American Association of Colleges of Nursing position statement on the doctor of nursing practice (DNP) degree, university schools of nursing have been creating DNP programs worthy of accreditation. Most programs focus on preparing advanced practice nurses for expanded clinical roles, whereas other DNP programs prepare nurse leaders for success in the C-Suite environment as nurse executives.

Written by experienced nurse executives who teach in rigorous academic programs and are executive practice experts, this book offers important insights into the nurse executive role and key management and leadership principles critical for success. Nursing faculty and students will find these principles embedded in quality improvement and evidencebased practice, and advanced by Joint Commission accreditation as well as the Quadruple Aim and Magnet Designation models. The book addresses critical business topics, such as health care policy, informatics, and business planning, and also offers a glimpse into today's C-Suite and the complex contemporary business challenges being navigated by today's health care executives.

We devote this book to both novice and seasoned nurse executives who are advancing their careers as business leaders of the future—the leaders who will help to create the transformational health care environment demanded by consumers and professionals alike.

JOYCE E. JOHNSON
LINDA L. COSTA

Acknowledgments

To our friends, family, and colleagues whose encouragement, support, and patience enabled our vision to become a reality.

To the authors who graciously contributed as subject matter experts in developing the chapters contained in this text.

I would first like to thank Linda Costa for giving me the opportunity to work with her in developing a text dedicated to the advancement of DNP-prepared C-Suite nurse executives. It has been a pleasure developing content that aims to elevate contemporary nurse executive leadership practice and expand traditional healthcare dialogue to describe today's complex, turbulent, and rapidly changing business environment.
My sincere gratitude to my son, Jeff, who has given of his time and expertise to support the development of this work.
—*Joyce E. Johnson*

I would like to thank the nurses who shared their journeys to executive leadership so that future DNPs may follow their paths.
—*Linda L. Costa*

List of Contributors

ADRIANA PEREZ AMADO, PhD(c), MBA, MS-ISD, Ma-HOD, CPLP
Director of Training and Development
New York Presbyterian Hospital
New York, New York

Biography

Adriana Perez Amado, PhD(c), MBA, MS-ISD, Ma-HOD, CPLP, is the Director of Training and Development within Talent Development at New York Presbyterian Hospital (NYP). In this role, she leads the team that creates, develops, and delivers programs that accompany the employees of NYP throughout their life and career. An experienced coach and trainer, she has contributed to the field of learning and development for the past two decades. She has focused on helping people arrive, survive, and thrive at organizations through a combination of high impact orientation programs, partnering with new leaders to help them understand the complexities of leadership, and working one-on-one with others to help them reach their full potential. Always thinking of the best way to meet the learners where they are, she has worked to develop gaming solutions, partners with institutions to deliver learning on demand, and consistently thinks of ways to change the way we learn. Prior to her role at NYP, she held positions in different industries: high-tech telecommunications, financial services, personal goods, and insurance. She has collaborated with the Association for Talent Development (atd); is a pilot CPLP™ and a mindgym coach; is certified in a number of programs and instruments; and is a life-long learner.

LINDA L. COSTA, PhD, RN, NEA-BC
Assistant Professor
University of Maryland
School of Nursing
Baltimore, Maryland

Biography

Linda L. Costa, PhD, RN, NEA-BC, is an Assistant Professor at the University of Maryland School of Nursing (UMB). Her teaching role is primarily in the Doctor of Nursing Practice program. She teaches translation of evidence to practice, leadership in complex adaptive systems, practice leadership of interdisciplinary teams, and implementation science. Dr. Costa earned a Bachelor of Science (BS) degree in Nursing at the University of Maryland and Master of Science (MS) and Doctor of Philosophy (PhD) degrees at The Catholic University of America. She is certified as a Nurse Executive, Advanced, by American Nurses Credentialing Center. Her previous experience in the C-Suite includes Vice President of Nursing and Patient Care Services at Georgetown University Hospital.

JOAN GLEASON-SCOTT, PhD, RN
Administrative Director of Clinical Services
St. Mary Medical Center of Trinity Health System
Langhorne, Pennsylvania

Biography

Joan Gleason-Scott, PhD, RN, is currently the Administrative Director of Clinical Services at St. Mary Medical Center of Trinity Health and Clinical Professor at the University of Pennsylvania. Dr. Gleason Scott's clinical practice was in critical care nursing, with a focus on cardiac care and surgical and trauma units. Throughout her career, she has functioned in various roles, such as Clinical Nurse Specialist in Trauma Nursing at Yale University Medical Center and University Hospital in Newark, New Jersey. She has over twenty-five years of progressive experience in nursing administration and hospital administration, with a focus on quality, safety, and regulatory and accreditation standards. Dr. Gleason Scott directed the licensure and regulatory work for hospitals and ambulatory services at the New Jersey Department of Health. Her quality and safety achievements include the development and implementation of several quality learning collaboratives for medical residents and other clinicians and senior staff, with a focus on measurement of increased knowledge of quality and safety, and translation into successful quality and safety improvement projects. Dr. Gleason Scott has presented at local, state, and national meetings on her work related to health care disparity, culture of safety, health care reform, population health, and administrative health care practice and research. Dr. Gleason Scott received her BSN from Fairleigh Dickenson University, her Master's degree from NYU, and her PhD from the University of Pennsylvania.

PETRA GOODMAN, PhD, MSN, EdM, WHNP, MCCNS, FAANP
COL (Ret), U.S. Army
Associate Professor
Assistant Dean for Research & Faculty Development
School of Nursing
The Catholic University of America
Washington, DC

Biography

Petra Goodman, PhD, MSN, EdM, WHNP, MCCNS, FAANP, Associate Professor, School of Nursing, The Catholic University of America. Primary teaching includes research design, research proposal development, advanced statistics, and management and analysis of large databases. Publications focus on nursing education, clinical issues, evidence-based practice, ethics, leadership, military nursing, military women, and veterans. As a principal investigator or project director, acquired funding in excess of $2,000,000 for multiple studies and projects. Additional experience includes serving as a grant reviewer for two national grant scientific merit review committees and reviewer for four peer-reviewed journals.

JEFFREY A. JOHNSON, MBA, MEng, BS
Director
Strategy/Merger & Acquisition Advisory
Boston, Massachusetts

Biography

Jeffrey A. Johnson, MBA, MEng, BS, Director, Strategy/Merger & Acquisition Advisory, KPMG. Mr. Johnson has contributed as a Senior Manager with Accenture Strategy, and as a Systems Engineer at Northrop Grumman Corporation. Primary focus: assisting Fortune 100 and 500 clients to align technology capabilities (i.e. Cloud, AI, Data Analytics, Liquid Workforce, Agile, and DevOps) with business priorities to drive their short and long term goals. His work extends across multiple industries including communications and high tech, oil and gas, utilities, insurance, banking, and products. His subject matter expertise includes strategic planning, cloud strategy, digital strategies, technology planning, workforce strategy, cost reduction, mergers and acquisitions, divestments, enterprise architecture, and operating / organizational model design.

JOYCE E. JOHNSON, PhD, RN, NEA-BC, FAAN
Associate Professor
The Catholic University of America
School of Nursing
Washington, DC

Biography

Joyce E. Johnson, PhD, RN, NEA-BC, FAAN, is an Associate Professor in the doctoral program at The Catholic University of America School of Nursing doctoral program. Primary teaching focus: Basics of technical writing, policy analysis, health care finance, ethics, scholarship, C-Suite leadership, and dissertation development. Prior to this appointment, Dr. Johnson most recently served as Senior Vice President & Chief Nursing Officer (CNO) at Robert Wood Johnson University Hospital and Associate Dean & Clinical Professor at the Rutgers University School of Nursing in New Brunswick, New Jersey, and as CNO and Hospital Operations Chief at both the Georgetown University Hospital and the Washington Hospital Center in Washington, DC. Numerous articles and books focus on nursing shortage issues, nursing management, information systems technology, patient safety, and quality improvement. Experience includes serving as Associate Editor, Nursing Forum, and as a reviewer for and member of several journal editorial boards. For 13 years founded and published *Nursing Connections*, the first nationally refereed scholarly journal to be published from a practice setting.

NANCY B. LERNER, RN, DNP
Associate Professor
University of Maryland
School of Nursing
Baltimore, Maryland

Biography

Nancy Lerner, RN, DNP, Associate Professor, University of Maryland School of Nursing, has been an educator since 2008 following an extensive administrative career in all aspects of long-term care. Her primary teaching focus involves nursing administration including theory application to health service management, complex adaptive systems, fundamentals of nursing, and both management and DNP practicum experiences. Multiple publications and presentations center on quality in nursing home and assisted living care, nursing assistant training, and job satisfaction in long-term care. Dr. Lerner has also served as an advisor and mentor to both DNP and management and administration students. She serves as a Pathway to Excellence appraiser and has served on multiple committees for nursing related groups.

KARI A. MASTRO, PhD, RN, NEA-BC
Vice President & Chief Nursing Officer
St. Mary Medical Center of Trinity Health System
Langhorne, Pennsylvania

Biography

Kari A. Mastro, PhD, RN, NEA-BC, is the Vice President & Chief Nursing Officer at St. Mary Medical Center of Trinity Health System and visiting Professor at Rutgers, The State University of New Jersey College of Nursing. She has spent her career focused on ensuring that the care provided to patients is of supreme quality regardless of where the care is provided and who is providing that care. She has received many awards for her work and has been recognized for her leadership by the American Nurse Credentialing Center, Certified Nurse Executive Advanced Award; the Hugs for Brady Foundation Humanitarian of the Year and the March of Dimes as Nurse of the Year. Her leadership enabled a team to receive the NDNQI Award for Outstanding Nursing Quality, the Magnet Prize Honors for Innovation, the HRET Community Outreach Award for Improving End-of-Life Care, and the NDNQI Award for Outstanding Nursing Quality in an Academic Medical Center. Dr. Mastro is well published and speaks globally on these topics.

MARY A. PATERSON, PhD, RN
Professor Emerita
The Catholic University of America
School of Nursing
Washington, DC

Biography

Mary Paterson, PhD, RN, Professor Emerita, The Catholic University of America School of Nursing. Dr. Paterson's academic training and experience is in health services and policy analysis with an emphasis on health finance. She holds a PhD in policy analysis from the University of California, Berkeley, an MS in nursing administration from Georgetown University, and a bachelor of science in nursing from The Catholic University of America. Dr. Paterson has 25 years of experience in health policy at the academic, state, federal, and international level. She has also taught health care finance to health care professionals in medical schools, nursing schools, and in professional workshops held in the United States, Russia, the Czech Republic, the Middle East, and Vietnam. She is the author of over 30 publications and a textbook in health care finance for nursing advanced practitioners and interdisciplinary teams. Her areas of research include population health, family and community participation in health care and health policy, international health, and quantitative methods in population health. Dr. Paterson has also served on health system and policy design teams to support health system payment reform in Egypt, Albania, and Iraq for USAID contracts during her service as an international practice manager for ABT Associates, a private policy consulting firm.

Dr. Paterson is currently a professor emerita serving at a school of nursing in an advisory capacity. For the last ten years she served as a tenured full professor at The Catholic University of America School of Nursing, where she designed and taught graduate courses in health care finance, health policy, quantitative methods, and research. She is a fellow of the Institute for Policy Research and Catholic Studies, a member emeritus of the Board of Trustees of the Holy Cross Health System of Maryland, and the former Project Director for the AACN/CDC Academic Partnership Project in Public and Population Health.

CHRISTA PREUSTER, MSN, RN-BC, PMHCNS-BC
Clinical Instructor
Rutgers College of Nursing & Columbia University School of Nursing
New Brunswick, New Jersey

Biography

Christa Preuster, MSN, RN-BC, PMHCNS-BC, is a clinical instructor at Rutgers College of Nursing and at Columbia University School of Nursing. Ms. Preuster has over 20 years of experience in the health care industry. She has published in several peer-reviewed journals and has presented nationally. She has extensive experience as a nurse educator and clinical instructor. Throughout her career, Ms. Preuster has been dedicated to providing patient and family centered care to the children and families with whom she works. In addition to her work as a clinical instructor, she currently works as a pediatric home care nurse. Ms. Preuster earned her BSN from Seton Hall University and her Master of Science, with a focus in nursing education, from William Paterson University. Additionally, she received her postmasters' certificate in Child and Adolescent Psychiatric Mental Health from the University of Medicine and Dentistry of New Jersey. Ms. Preuster is a certified Clinical Nurse Specialist in Child and Adolescent Psychiatric Mental Health.

CAROLYN K. ROOT, PhD
CEO
Alpha UMi LLC
Tarpon Springs, Florida

Biography

Carolyn K. Root, PhD, Chief Executive Officer, Alpha UMi LLC. Primary focus: Entrepreneur, small business growth, new product development, engineering. Recognized expert in underwater acoustics, with papers published in the areas of fluid dynamics and acoustics in technical journals. Experienced in board leadership, consulting at executive levels, managing small to large programs, and directing investment for long term beneficial outcomes. Rotarian since 2011.

KEVIN RULO, PhD, MA, BA
Clinical Assistant Professor of English
Director of the Writing & Rhetoric Program and
Director of the University Writing Center
The Catholic University of America
Washington, DC

Biography

Dr. Kevin Rulo has conducted research in writing and rhetoric studies and has widely published and presented nationally and internationally on a variety of topics related to modernism, theory, and literary studies. As director of the Writing and Rhetoric Program, Dr. Rulo teaches, mentors, and oversees the English Department's doctoral teaching fellows in Writing and Rhetoric and a variety of other writing and literature courses. As Director of the Writing Center, Dr. Rulo strives to strengthen the writing environment of the university and to create a positive atmosphere for the development of writers of all levels.

ROSEMARY VENTURA, DNP, RN-BC
Chief Nursing Informatics Officer
New York-Presbyterian Hospital
New York, New York

Biography

Rosemary Ventura, DNP, RN-BC is the Chief Nursing Informatics Officer at New York-Presbyterian Hospital (NYP) in New York, New York. In this role, she is responsible for leveraging technology and analytics to improve the practice of nursing throughout the NYP enterprise. Dr. Ventura earned a Bachelor of Science in Nursing and Master of Arts in Nursing Informatics from New York University, and a Doctorate of Nursing Practice at Case Western Reserve University in Cleveland, Ohio. She is certified in Nursing Informatics by the American Nurses Credentialing Center. Prior to her role at NYP, she held numerous leadership positions in information technology in multiple organizations throughout New York.

COURTNEY VOSE, DNP, MBA, RN, APRN, NEA-BC
Vice President and Chief Nursing Officer of Nursing and
    Patient Care Services
New York-Presbyterian/Columbia University Medical Center
New York, New York

Biography

Courtney Vose, DNP, MBA, RN, APRN, NEA-BC, is the Vice President and Chief Nursing Officer of Nursing and Patient Care Services at New York-Presbyterian (NYP)/Columbia University Medical Center, NYP/Allen, and the NYP/Ambulatory Care Network. She also holds the title of Clinical Instructor at the Columbia University School of Nursing. She received her Bachelor of Science in Nursing from Indiana University of Pennsylvania. She received her Master of Science in Nursing and became a Certified Registered Nurse Practitioner at Temple University. She has successfully completed the Penn State University Leadership Course and the Wharton Nursing Leaders Program at the University of Pennsylvania. She achieved her Master of Business Administration at DeSales University, where she also recently obtained her Doctor of Nursing Practice in Executive Leadership. She is an active member in the Sigma Theta Tau International Honor Society of Nursing, Delta Mu Delta International Honor Society in Business Administration, and the American Organization for Nursing Leadership (AONL) (formerly the American Organization of Nurse Executives). She is the President Ex-officio and the past Treasurer to the Pennsylvania Eastern Regional Organization of Nurse Leaders, and she completed a 2-year term on the Board of Directors to the Pennsylvania Organization of Nurse Leaders. She was selected as the co-chair for the Education Committee for the New York Organization of Nurse Executives and Leaders, where she also serves Ex-officio on the Board of Directors. She serves as a leadership and research instructor to nurses at numerous universities, including New York University and Columbia University. She was the recipient of the Nightingale of Pennsylvania Nursing Administration Award. She has advanced nursing practice through multiple manuscripts and oral and poster presentations at regional and national meetings.

K. T. WAXMAN, DNP, MBA, RN, CNL, CHSE, CENP, FSSH, FAAN
Associate Professor
Director, Executive Leadership DNP Program
University of San Francisco
San Francisco, California

Biography

Dr. K. T. Waxman is a nurse leader with over 30 years of experience in health care and corporate settings, a tenured Associate Professor at the University of San Francisco, and the Director of the Executive Leader DNP program. She is the Director of the California Simulation Alliance (CSA) at HealthImpact. An internationally known speaker and author, Dr. Waxman is also a past president of the Association of California Nurse Leaders (ACNL) and past board member, serving as Treasurer, for the American

Organization for Nursing Leadership (AONL) (formerly the American Organization of Nurse Executives). She is active in numerous committees for the Society for Simulation in Healthcare (SSH) and serves on the Finance Committee for the International Nursing Association for Clinical Simulation and Learning (INACSL).

Dr. Waxman's work has been published extensively and can be found in the *Journal for Simulation in Healthcare, Clinical Simulation for Nursing, Journal of Nursing Education*, and *Nurse Leader and Creative Nursing* journals, among others. She has authored 3 books on Finance and Budgeting and just completed the second edition of Financial and Business Skills for the DNP, published by Springer. Her book, Healthcare Simulation Program Builder, through HCPro was released last year. She has also authored several chapters in simulation textbooks.

Dr. Waxman received her DNP from the University of San Francisco, with an emphasis on health systems leadership and a concentration in clinical simulation. She holds certifications as Clinical Nurse Leader (CNL), Certification in Executive Nursing Practice (CENP), and Certification as a Simulation Healthcare Educator (CHSE) and is a Fellow in the American Academy of Nursing (FAAN) and the Society for Simulation in Healthcare (FSSH). Dr. Waxman was recently elected as President-elect in the SSH, and her term began in January 2018.

ROBIN WIKLE, MS
Director, Business Development
Alpha UMi LLC
Tarpon Springs, Florida

Biography

Robin Wikle, MS, Director of Business Development, Alpha UMi LLC. Primary focus: national growth of small business, influence at local, state and national levels of government. Experience includes C-suite coaching, major gift fundraising, national hospital CEO mentorship, elected to Pinellas County School Board, has served on numerous boards of civic organizations. Rotarian since 2005.

K. T. WAXMAN

1

The Evolution of DNP Programs in the United States

Chapter Objectives

- Discuss the evolution of DNP programs in the United States.
- Identify differences between the DNP and the PhD degree.
- Articulate various roles the DNP graduate can fill in the rapidly changing health care environment.
- Demonstrate how the American Organization for Nursing Leadership (AONL) Competencies™ (formerly the American Organization of Nurse Executives Competencies™) align with the DNP curriculum.

KEY WORDS: DNP, programs, executive, AONL, competency, leadership

Introduction

In 2004, the American Association of Colleges of Nursing (AACN) endorsed the "Position Statement on the Practice Doctorate in Nursing." This decision was initially made based on research from a task force formed to assess the need for a clinical practice doctorate with specific stakeholders. These stakeholders included education, practice, and research (AACN, 2017). Since 2004, doctor of nursing practice (DNP) programs have skyrocketed around the United States (U.S.) in various forms, such as on ground, online, and hybrid. Some programs are geared to the nurse practitioner (NP) or certified registered nurse anesthetist (CRNA), whereas others are geared towards administration and leadership and, finally, some are focused on the executive leader. As we move into the next decade and our rapidly changing health care environment, the role of the registered nurse (RN), specifically the RN leader, will play a bigger role, leading large scale interprofessional teams and managing quality improvement projects. The DNP degree prepares these RNs for the emerging leadership roles in health care.

Current State of DNP Programs Nationally

On October 25, 2004, the member schools affiliated with the AACN voted to endorse the "Position Statement on the Practice Doctorate in Nursing." This decision called for moving the current level of preparation necessary for advanced nursing practice from the master's degree to the doctorate level by the year 2015. This endorsement was preceded by almost 4 years of research and consensus-building by an AACN task force charged with examining the need for the practice doctorate with a variety of stakeholder groups (AACN, 2017). The DNP degree is a terminal degree in nursing and is a practice doctorate, not a research doctorate. Doctor of nursing practice programs have less content emphasis on theory, metatheory, research methodology, and data analysis than in a research-focus program. Nursing is moving in the direction of other health professions in the transition to the DNP. Medicine (MD), dentistry (DDS), pharmacy (PharmD), psychology (PsyD), physical therapy (DPT), and audiology (AudD) all require or offer practice doctorates to elevate practice and leadership to the highest academic degree.

In 2004, the AACN recommended that the DNP degree be the graduate terminal degree for advanced nursing practice by 2015 (AACN, 2004). Although the first DNP program began at the University of Kentucky in 2001 by Carolyn Williams, PhD, RN, FAAN, many other programs were developed in those early years, with the first cohorts nationwide graduating from 2003 to 2005.

The Commission on Collegiate Nursing Education (CCNE), the leading accrediting agency for baccalaureate- and graduate-degree nursing programs in the US, began accrediting DNP programs in Fall 2008. To date, over 250 DNP programs have been accredited by CCNE (AACN). At the time of this publication, the AACN website (www.aacn.nche.edu/media-relations/fact-sheets/dnp) reports 303 DNP programs are currently enrolling students at schools of nursing nationwide, and an additional 124 new DNP programs are in the planning stages (58 post-baccalaureate and 66 post-master's programs). DNP programs are now available in all 50 states plus the District of Columbia. States with the most programs (10 or more programs) include California, Florida, Illinois, Massachusetts, Minnesota, New York, Ohio, Pennsylvania, and Texas. From 2015 to 2016, the number of students enrolled in DNP programs increased from 21,995 to 25,289. During that same period, the number of DNP graduates increased from 4,100 to 4,855. (AACN, 2017).

Between 2010 and 2016, there were 4,596 doctor of philosophy (PhD) graduates and 19,198 DNP graduates. The Robert Wood Johnson Foundation reports that even though nursing is the largest health profession in the U.S., with more than 3 million RNs, less than 1% of nurses have a doctorate degree in nursing or a related field (Robert Wood Johnson

Table 1.1 Breakdown of Doctoral Graduates Since 2010.
Retrieved from www.campaignforaction.org.

	2010	2011	2012	2013	2014	2015	2016	Total
DNP	1,282	1,595	1,858	2,443	3,065	4,100	4,855	19,198
PhD	532	601	610	628	743	709	773	4,596
Total	1,814	2,196	2,468	3,017	3,808	4,809	5,628	23,794

Foundation, 2017). Table 1.1 shows a breakdown of doctoral graduates since 2010.

The future of nursing campaign's indicator #2, "Double the number of nurses with a doctorate by 2020," has been achieved. As of the end of 2015, there were 21,123 nurses employed with a doctoral degree, which includes PhD, DNP, DNS, and others, with these nurses employed not only in acute care, but also in clinics, in academia, and within the community.

Differences Between the DNP and PhD/DNS

The major difference between the DNP and the PhD/DNS degrees is the focus. The DNP is practice based (whether administrative or clinical focused) and the PhD/DNS are research based (specializing in an area of interest) (Waxman & Maxworthy, 2010). Table 1.2 illustrates other integral differences between the degrees.

The Evolution of Doctoral Education in Nursing

The first nursing-related doctoral program was originated in 1924 at Teacher's College, Columbia University, and was a doctor of education (EdD) degree designed to prepare nurses to teach at the college level (Carpenter & Hudacek, 1996). Doctor of education programs continued into the 1960s and were the mainstay of doctoral education for nursing (Marriner-Tomey, 1990). The first PhD in nursing was offered in 1934 at New York University. But, it wasn't until the 1950s that the PhD in nursing was offered again, and it focused on maternal and child nursing (Carpenter & Hudacek, 1996). Over the next few decades, the PhD became more popular and, in 1960, the doctor of nursing science (DNS) degree was originated at Boston University and focused on "the development of nursing theory for a practice discipline" (Marriner-Tomey, 1990). To that end, the practice doctorate is not a new concept. In 1979, Case Western Reserve created the first nursing doctorate (ND) program, followed by University of Colorado, Rush University, and South Carolina University. (Chism, 2010). There are no ND programs remaining in the U.S., because the DNP has replaced that degree program in many universities.

The first DNP programs emerged in 2001 and were primarily focused

Table 1.2 Breakdown of Doctoral Graduates Since 2010.
Retrieved from www.campaignforaction.org.

	DNP	PhD/DNS
Program of Study	Objectives: • Prepare nurse specialists at the highest level of advanced practice	Objectives: • Prepare nurse researchers
	Competencies: • Based on AACN Essentials of the DNP Degree	Content: • Based on Indicators of Quality in Research Focused Doctoral Programs in Nursing (AACN, 2001)
Students	• Commitment to a practice career • Oriented toward improving outcomes of care	• Commitment to a research career • Oriented toward developing new knowledge
Program faculty	• Practice doctorate and/or experience in area in which teaching • Leadership experience in area of specialty practice • High level of expertise in specialty practice congruent with focus of academic program	• Research doctorate in nursing or related field • Leadership experience in area of sustained research funding • High level of expertise in research congruent with focus of academic program
Resources	• Mentors and/or precepts in leadership positions across a variety of practice settings • Access to diverse practice settings with appropriate resources for areas of practice • Access to financial aid • Access to information and patient care technology resources congruent with areas of study	• Mentors/preceptor in research settings • Access to research settings with appropriate resources • Access to dissertation support dollars • Access to information and research technological resources congruent and program of research
Program assessment and evaluation	Program outcomes: • Health care improvements and contributions via practice, policy change, and practice scholarship • Oversight by the institution's authorized bodies (i.e., graduate school) and regional accreditors • Receives accreditation by specialized nursing accreditor • Graduates are eligible for national certification examination	Program outcomes: • Contributes to health care improvements via the development of new knowledge and other scholarly projects that provide the foundation for the advancement of nursing science • Oversight by the institution's authorized bodies (i.e., graduate school) and regional accreditors

Waxman, K.T., & Maxworthy, J. (2010). American Association of Colleges of Nursing (2006). Doctor of Nursing Practice Roadmap Task Force Report.

on clinical practice. Over the decade, programs focused on non-clinical or administrative practice were created. Focused on the nurse executive, programs such as executive leadership DNP programs launched in 2005 to 2006, with the first programs at Case-Western Reserve and University of San Francisco. Although the original intent of the DNP was focused on the advanced practice registered nurse (APRN), non-clinicians also benefit from the practice doctorate, because leadership is a common thread throughout the DNP essentials. Today, there are many programs with Executive or Leadership in the title. Although some DNP programs cater specifically to the APRN, others focus on the nurse executive leader, or the nonclinician.

The DNP Essentials and the American Organization for Nursing Leadership (AONL) Competencies™

The AACN designed the DNP Essentials in 2006, which provided schools of nursing with outcomes necessary to designing curricula for the programs.

DNP Essentials

In many institutions, APRNs, including nurse practitioners (NPs), clinical nurse specialists, certified nurse-midwives, and CRNAs, are prepared in master's-degree programs that often carry a credit load equivalent to doctoral degrees in the other health professions. The AACN position statement calls for educating APRNs and other nurses seeking top leadership/organizational roles in DNP programs (AACN). Professional organizations in advanced practice, such as the American Association of Nurse Anesthetists and the American Association of Nurse Practitioners, have promoted the DNP as the terminal degree for their profession.

Certified Registered Nurse Anesthetist programs around the country offer either the DNP or the doctor of nurse anesthesia (DNAP), and typical courses in the curriculum include clinical courses. Because the curriculum prepares those students to be leaders in their field, it may include courses such as health policy, medical law, finance, and population health.

Nurse practitioner programs around the country offer either masters or DNP preparation. The National Organization for Nurse Practitioner Faculties (NONPF) published a white paper on "The Doctor of Nursing Practice Nurse Practitioner Clinical Scholar" in 2016. It states that an underlying assumption is that, as the terminal degree for NPs, the primary goal of DNP education is preparation as an independent clinician who provides care within a population focus. The DNP adds the dimension of scholarship that can take on many forms, consistent with the description and definitions of clinical scholarship that are presented in this paper (http://c.ymcdn.com/sites/www.nonpf.org/resource/resmgr/docs/ClinicalScholarFINAL2016.pdf).

The DNP *Essentials* define the curricular elements that must be present in DNP programs. The eight essentials are listed below. Each essential has detail associated with it and can be found at http://www.aacnnursing.org/Portals/42/Publications/DNPEssentials.pdf.

1. Scientific underpinnings for practice
2. Organizational and systems leadership for quality improvement and systems thinking
3. Clinical scholarship and analytical methods for evidence-based practice
4. Information systems/technology and patient care technology for the improvement and transformation of health care
5. Health care policy for advocacy in health care
6. Inter-professional collaboration for improving patient and population health outcomes
7. Clinical prevention and population health for improving the nation's health
8. Advanced nursing practice

DNP essential #2 is focused on leadership: Organizational and systems leadership for quality improvement and systems thinking. Specifically, DNP graduates should be prepared to do the following:

1. Develop and evaluate care delivery approaches that meet the current and future needs of patient populations based on scientific findings in nursing and other clinical sciences, as well as organizational, political, and economic sciences.
2. Ensure accountability for the quality of health care and patient safety for populations with whom they work.
    a. Use advanced communication skills/processes to lead quality improvement and patient safety initiatives in health care systems
    b. Employ principles of business, finance, economics, and health policy to develop and implement effective plans for practice-level and/or system practice initiatives that will improve the quality of care delivery
    c. Develop and/or monitor budgets for practice initiatives
    d. Analyze the cost-effectiveness of practice initiatives accounting for risk and improvement of health care outcomes
    e. Demonstrate sensitivity to diverse organizational cultures and populations, including patients and providers
3. Develop and/or evaluate effective strategies for managing the ethical dilemmas inherent inpatient care, the health care organization, and research (AACN, 2006, pp, 10–11).

Organizational and systems leadership are critical for DNP graduates to improve patient and health care outcomes. Doctoral level knowledge and skills in these areas are consistent with nursing and health care goals to eliminate health disparities and to promote patient safety and excellence in practice. DNP graduates' practice includes not only direct care, but also a focus on the needs of a panel of patients, a target population, a set of populations, or a broad community.

DNP essential #8 is focused on advanced nursing practice. This should not to be confused with advanced practice registered nursing (APN/APRN). Because nurses in leadership or executive roles are not considered to be APRNs (unless they are an APRN), this essential validates that they are advancing nursing practice but not necessarily through clinical practice. Advanced nursing practice is defined as any form of nursing intervention that influences health care outcomes for individuals or populations, including the direct care of individual patients, management of care for individuals and populations, administration of nursing and health care organizations, and development and implementation of health policy (AACN, 2015). The practice doctorate is designed as just that, practice in the form of various settings, both clinical and administrative.

The American Organization of Nurse Executive Competencies™

The American Organization for Nursing Leadership (AONL) supports the DNP. In 2007, the AONL published a position paper supporting the DNP as a terminal degree option for practice-focused nursing. In 2005, the organization created Nurse Executive Competencies (AONL-NEC) to provide a framework for nurse leaders. Using this framework, faculty can direct students in both the clinical and non-clinical programs to crosswalk the competency with fundamental concepts of economics, including interpreting financial statements, learning how to manage financial resources, and ensuring the use of accurate charging mechanisms (Waxman, Roussel, Herrin-Griffith, & D'Alfonso, 2017).

Many academic institutions around the country have embedded the competencies into their graduate curricula for both master's and doctoral programs. One example of the application in academia includes the University of San Francisco School of Nursing and Health Professions Executive Leader Doctor of Nursing Practice Program (ELDNP), in which the AONL-NEC have been incorporated into the curriculum (Waxman *et al.*, 2017).

During 2006 to 2009, a collaboration with additional professional associations, including the American College of Healthcare Executives (ACHE), the American College of Physician Executives (ACPE), the Healthcare Financial Management Association (HFMA), the Healthcare Information and Management Systems Society (HIMSS), and the Medical

Group Management Association (MGMA), formed the Healthcare Leadership Alliance (HLA). Using the AONL competency model as a base, these groups jointly developed and published the HLA Competency Directory (Waxman *et al.*, 2017). These leadership competencies are well aligned with the DNP essentials and provide a framework for curriculum development in the executive programs. It is clear that, in the rapidly changing health care environment, more leaders are needed across the continuum, and preparing leaders at the DNP and Executive DNP level is a perfect fit to assume these positions and roles.

Specific to the AONL-NECs; Competency #5: Business skills. This competency is also very much aligned with the DNP essential #2. Components of this competency include developing and managing budgets, interpreting financial statements, managing financial resources, negotiating contracts, conducting SWOT and gap analyses, and defending the business case for nursing. These are all critical skills that the DNP candidate must have to graduate and will then apply to practice. Whether clinical or nonclinical, these skills are important as DNP graduates need to be able to "talk the talk" of the finance team and clearly articulate their needs from a financial and return on investment (ROI) perspective.

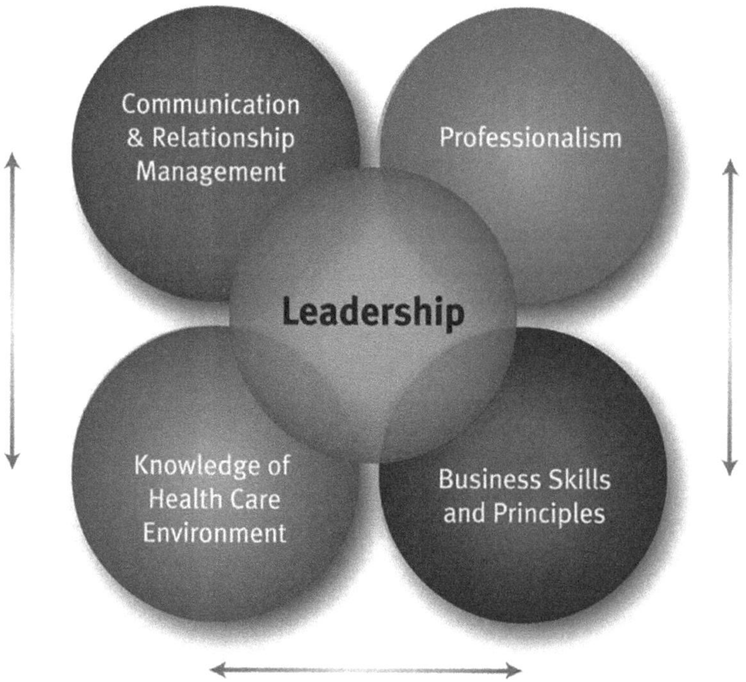

Figure 1.1. *AONL Nurse Executive Competencies. Reprinted with permission from the American Organization for Nursing Leadership (AONL) (formerly the American Organization of Nurse Executives)* © *2018.*

The DNP Curriculum

The DNP leader curriculum focuses heavily on organizational and systems leadership, inter-professional collaboration, and information technology. The DNP leader emerges with skills to manage and operate as a key component in new models of health care, promoting change and advancing delivery of evidence-based, patient-centered care. Nurse managed health care centers and medical homes may be led by the DNP APRN, taking on a team-based approach to health care delivery, and may help to alleviate the strain on the primary care provider shortage (Hammatt & Nies, 2015).

The DNP program prepares the graduate to do the following: (essential 2.2.b, c, d) (b) Employ principles of business, finance, economics, and health policy to develop and implement effective plans for practice-level and/or system-wide practice initiatives that will improve the quality of care delivery; (c) Develop and/or monitor budgets for practice initiatives; and (d) Analyze the cost-effectiveness of practice initiatives accounting for risk and improvement of health care outcomes. Examples of cost-effectiveness are quantifying performance improvement projects such as decreasing readmissions, infections, falls, and medication errors.

As we prepare our students for their DNP degrees and as DNPs move into the workforce with higher level executive roles, it is imperative that we are able to articulate nursing's value and quantify quality, because nursing is at the front line of patient care. Having good business skills will enable the DNP to not only negotiate for what he or she wants for patients and his or her organization, but also for himself or herself and a respective career. Business planning is a process that DNPs will increasingly use as the business of providing health care expands to meet the demands of health care reform (Waxman & Barter, 2017). Whether we are clinical or non-clinical DNPs, we are prepared to build the business case for change and articulate our needs with clear ROI opportunities. These ROIs can be manifested in terms of financial or other ways, such as patient satisfaction, HCAHPS scores, retention, infection rates, and falls. Nurse leaders moving into roles that require a DNP degree must demonstrate knowledge and skills that will help them be successful in advanced nursing practice.

As we prepare DNPs to practice in the complex health care system, business skills are essential. Financial management, strategic management, and overall business acumen are critical for success. Being able to "talk the talk" regarding finance and business can be one of our biggest strengths. The DNP essentials and the AONL-NEC are in perfect alignment with the competencies and skills needed for the future of health care and emerging/existing leadership roles. The changing demands of this nation's complex health care environment require the highest level of scientific knowledge and practice expertise to ensure quality patient outcomes. The Institute of Medicine, The Joint Commission, Robert Wood Johnson Foundation, and other authorities have called for reconceptualizing educational programs that prepare today's health professionals. These programs are designed to prepare "experts in specialized advanced nursing practice" (AACN, 2006).

Some of the many factors building momentum for change in nursing education at the graduate level include shortages of doctorally-prepared nursing faculty and increasing educational expectations for the preparation of other members of the health care team. (AACN). Although most DNP programs do not prepare graduates as faculty, some programs offer elective courses to help prepare graduates to engage as academicians and many schools are hiring DNPs to teach.

Where Do We Go From Here?

In a study competed by Embree, Meek, and Ebright (2017), chief nurse executives identified and ranked the following categories for skills needed in leadership positions specific to the DNP: Leadership, Implementation science/evaluation and translation of evidence into practice methods; Business; Information and technology management and policy/ethics/law. These are all in alignment with the DNP essentials.

The distinctions of the DNP degree and the roles of those who hold the degree are embedded in aspects of practice: practice that increases nursing's presence in health care leadership, practice that improves our health care system through the application of evidence, and practice that leads teams of professionals toward improved health and health outcomes for our population (Udlis & Mancusco, 2016).

Over the last ten years, organizations, formal and informal, have developed to address the DNP specifically. The Doctors of Nursing Practice, Inc. (www.doctorsofnursingpractice.org) has proven to be a virtual venue for DNP students and graduates to frankly discuss their projects and views. The website also has a repository of DNP projects and resources. Annually, they host a national conference with topics of interest to the DNP, and attendees consist of academia, service, administrators, and clinicians.

The DNP curriculum can prepare masters-prepared nurses for executive leader positions. Two DNP nurse leader graduates have contributed testimonials by discussing their journeys to their DNPs and the opportunities the programs have afforded them.

Testimonial #1: My Executive Leadership DNP Journey

Executive Leadership DNP graduate Dr. Marcia Lysaght
Marcia Lysaght, DNP, RN, CENP
Chief Nurse Executive, Miami VA Healthcare System

My first nursing job was as a nursing assistant and I quickly realized that my future career would be in nursing. I pursued my nursing degree while working full time and raising a family and through hard work, resilience and commitment to lifelong learning, I achieved my goal of becoming a Chief Nurse Executive of a healthcare system, a role that I have fulfilled for the past eight years.

As a daughter of an advanced practice nurse, I recognized and appreciated the importance of advanced education and the impact it had on improved patient outcomes. It's with that knowledge, that I set my educational goal of achieving a terminal degree in nursing. As I achieved professional growth and success I often explored the option of returning to school to achieve my educational goal, but was unable to identify a program that I believe best fit my needs and my future professional goals. I knew my passion was leadership and I evaluated several PhD programs, and found that none fully aligned with me achieving my future endeavor. As a nurse executive, leading an integrated and complex health system, the need to promote evidenced based practice and scholarly inquiry at all levels of nursing, with the goals of promoting health, and quality patient outcomes, the ability to translate research into practice was paramount in achieving those goals. I knew prior DNP programs that I evaluated had a clinical focus which was not the right fit for me. Determined to return to school and obtain my doctoral degree, I again researched doctoral degree nursing programs and identified two programs that best fit my current and future professional needs and goals. I evaluated the programs based on rigor and quality of instruction and professors and enrolled in the University of San Francisco Executive leadership Doctor in Nursing Practice Program. One of the key determinants of selecting this program was the alignment of the program's objectives with the American Organization of Nurse Executive (AONE) Core Competencies of the Nurse Executive.

As a chief nurse executive, my passion is translating research into practice, to improve patient care and outcomes, hence the reason for selecting the DNP versus the PhD. Understanding the need for leadership at all levels of nursing, specializing in healthcare leadership was the option selected because in my professional role, I recognize the need to promote quality patient care outcomes while managing cost. At the onset, my expectations of the program were to gain knowledge that would allow me to effectively promote and support scholarly and evidenced based practice at my facility, enhanced my ability to further develop as a nurse leader, and assist me in developing future nurse leaders. However, from my initial course work, I quickly recognized that the knowledge acquired far exceeded my expectations. The classroom and experiential learning assisted me to think differently, and to become a better thought leader, and to more effective lead organizational change. I was able to immediately apply the knowledgely and information gleaned to my role as a Chief Nurse Executive.

Some areas where I have been able to excel include leading people, leading change, business acumen, and achieving results-driven outcomes at the organizational level. The professional growth and development boosted my confidence level as an astute healthcare executive. I expected the program to better prepare me to succeed in the rapidly changing and complex role of the healthcare environment, but what I learned far exceeded my expectation in terms of applicability to my current role.

Throughout the program I experienced tremendous professional and leadership growth, which I immediately applied in my role of Chief Nurse Executive at a healthcare system. While enrolled in the program, I was able to utilize the skills and knowledge gleaned in strategic planning and project management to co-lead a national strategic planning endeavor as well as develop a strategic plan for nursing services at the largest integrated healthcare system in the United States. In addition, I implemented a project that has vastly contributed to improved nurse retention, job satisfaction, competence and confidence in new nursing graduates as well as attain my original goal of promoting scholarly work and evidence-based practice at my organization as well as advancing nursing leadership at all levels of the organization.

As a new graduate DNP, I have a renewed passion to be a lifelong learner and aspire to advance the role of the nursing profession at the state, local, and national level. New employment opportunities have surpassed my expectations and include roles beyond the role of nursing leadership. I have had the opportunity to function in the role of the Chief Executive Officer (CEO) at my organization on numerous occasions during the absence of the CEO, for which the DNP program well prepared me.

As a full-time healthcare executive, attending the program was challenging and rigorous as I anticipated. It required hard work, dedication, and resilience to persevere through to completion. However, the knowledge and wisdom gained, and the doors of opportunities that have opened for me far outweigh the expended effort and resources. Although my passion is and has always been focused in nursing leadership, I feel uniquely positioned to assume new roles such as the Chief Operating Officer or the Chief Executive Officer in a healthcare setting, and I look forward to a whole new world with a future of endless possibilities.

My eight plus years as a chief nurse executive has allowed me to gain valuable knowledge and expertise over time and this has led to my success. I have implemented large-scale projects from development through implementation but have repeatedly faced unexpected challenges that led to delay in time or increased in cost. This in part was because of challenges I experienced in effectively managing all aspects of large scale projects simultaneously. In the DNP program, I acquired expert project management skills which I immediately put to work in developing and implementing a nurse residency program. Using the project management principles and skills acquired, I was able to effectively lead my team through development, implementation and sustainment of a nurse residency program which resulted in a successful Commission on Collegiate Nursing Education (CCNE) Post-Baccalaureate Nurse Residency Accreditation site visit.

Putting my newly acquired project management skills into practice was exciting because for the first time in my career, I felt confident in my ability to lead and sustain a successful large scale project launch. I was also able to impart knowledge and provide mentorship to members of the implementation team. Through staff education and empowerment, less oversight was required which allowed me to focus on other competing priorities.

The DNP program that I experienced was modeled after the American Organization for Nursing Leadership (AONL) Nurse Executive Competencies. Through my many years as a healthcare executive, I found these leadership competencies to be essential for successful nurse executive practice. Through the stellar education and academic preparation, I obtained certification in executive nursing practice (CENP) from AONL on my first examination attempt.

Testimonial #2: DNP Executive Testimonial

Sherrill Sorensen, DNP, MHL, RN, CENP
Chief Nursing Executive/Chief Operating Officer
St. Mary's Medical Center, San Francisco
Executive Leadership DNP graduate, 2012

The passion I had for quality and safety at the bedside led me into nursing leadership roles. I felt that as a nursing leader, I could have more influence and ability to ensure evidence-based practice.

I sought out a Master's Degree to help me in this work and completed a Master's in Health Law. I had a better understanding of patient safety from the perspective of the Legal Disciplines. At this same time, I had progressed to a role as a Chief Nurse and Chief Operating Officer at a small hospital in a large health system.

Working in a complex role in a very complex health system, I felt unprepared for executive leadership with my current educational background. It seemed logical and necessary to have doctoral education to develop into the leader I wanted to become. I talked with colleagues regarding the work they were doing as PhD nurses in executive roles and they felt this same gap. As I was exploring master's level programs in nursing leadership as my next step, I became aware of a new program that seemed to fill the gap in education and executive practice.

I applied and was accepted into the University of San Francisco's inaugural class for the Doctorate of Nursing Practice in Executive Leadership. The cohort model, program courses, faculty expertise and focus on the Jesuit mission of USF are key factors that have helped me be successful as the student in an academic executive leadership program and a practicing nurse executive.

The cohort model allowed me to connect with colleagues expertly practicing in a wide variety of settings across the country who had insight and experience from which I could learn. The cohort group enabled me to be successful in a rigorous program where I continued in my processional work setting while meeting the academic requirements to successfully progress through the program. Even today, I remain in close contact with my fellow students who continually provide me with insight and recommendations to address problems I encounter in my work and offer encouragement as a nurse executive.

The richness and depth in the EL-DNP program has helped me as I continue in my work. For example, I would not have thought that project management and entrepreneurship would be useful to a CNO—yet I find myself often applying and actively using these in practice. Contemporaneous leaders brought real world insight and expertise to me as a student and this was invaluable. Few venues offer this kind of connection and learning.

I often work with organizations in transition, chaos and change. I am able to lead and achieve outcomes in these settings because of the course work, faculty knowledge, guest lecturers and cohort collegiality that were part of the EL-DNP program. These voices continue with me every day as I work to do my part to Change the World.

Chapter Takeaways

1. The DNP degree is the fastest growing terminal degree in the nursing profession out-pacing the PhD degree 4:1.
2. The major difference between the DNP and the PhD degrees is the focus: the DNP is practice-based (administrative or clinical) and the PhD is research based (specializing in an area of research interest).
3. Some of the factors building momentum for change in graduate level nursing education include the shortage of doctorally-prepared nursing faculty and increasing expectations for the preparation of other members of the healthcare team.

Chapter Summary

The DNP is a practice doctorate that can prepare nurse leaders to perform at a higher level, leading interprofessional teams along the continuum. Now, more than ever, we need nurse leaders. With less than 1% of all U.S. nurses holding a doctoral degree, there is not only a need, but also room for all of us, PhDs, EdDs, and DNPs. We should not look at this as a competition. We need nurse researchers to conduct the research and we need practice doctorate graduates to translate that research and implement the evidence-based practice into practice areas. Think about the skill set a chief nursing officer or any nurse leader needs and which degree or program would best serve this role. In reviewing Table 1.2, making the decision as to which degree to obtain and selecting the best-fit option for an individual personal career is critical. Health care organizations need nurses with all types of doctoral degrees to create and maintain a high-quality organization. The DNP curriculum prepares nurse leaders to effectively lead. Remember if we are not at the table, we may be on the menu!

Chapter Reflection Questions

1. How do you feel about the CNO being required to have a doctoral degree? Should it be a PhD or DNP? Why?
2. There is controversy around DNPs being called "doctor." How would you respond to a physician who tells you, as the CNO, that all DNPs in the hospital should not use Dr. in front of their name?
3. Identify and discuss various roles in a health care organization that would require a DNP degree.
4. With nursing being the only health care profession that does not require a doctoral degree, (think about PT, OT, Pharm), what steps do we need to take as a profession to move to the mandatory doctorate?

References

American Association of Colleges of Nursing (AACN). (2018). *Fact sheet: The doctor of nursing practice (DNP)*. Retrieved from http://www.aacnnursing.org/News-Information/Fact-Sheets/DNP-Fact-Sheet.

American Association of Colleges of Nursing (2006). *Doctor of nursing practice roadmap task force report*. Retrieved from http://tobgne.org/download/AACN%20DNP%20Task%20Force%20Report%208-9-06.pdf.

American Association of Colleges of Nursing (2015). *The Doctor of Nursing Practice: Current Issues and Clarifying Recommendations Report from the Task Force on the Implementation of the DNP*. August 2015

American Organization of Nurse Executives (AONE). (2015). *Nurse executive competencies*. Retrieved from http://www.aone.org/resources/nec.pdf .

Carpenter, R., & Hudacek, S. (1996). *On doctoral education in nursing: The voice of the students*. New York, NY: National League for Nursing Press.

Chism, L. (2010). *The doctor of nursing practice.* (1st ed.). Burlington, MA: Jones and Bartlett Learning.

Embree, J. L., Meek, J., & Ebright P. (2017). Voices of chief nursing executives informing a doctor of nursing practice program, *Journal of Professional Nursing.* http://dx.doi.org/10.1016/j.profnurs.2017.07.008

Hammatt, J. s., Nies, M. A. (2015). DNP's: What can we expect? *Nurse Leader, 13*(6), 64–67.

Marshall, Elaine S. (2011). *Transformational leadership in nursing: from expert clinician to influential leader.* New York, NY: Springer Pub. Co.

Marriner-Tomey, A. (1990). Historical development of doctoral programs from the middle-ages to nursing education today. *Nursing and Health Care. (11)*3, 132–137.

National Organization of Nurse Practitioner Faculties. (2016). The doctor of nursing practice nurse practitioner clinical scholar. Retrieved from http://c.ymcdn.com/sites/www.nonpf.org/resource/resmgr/docs/ClinicalScholarFINAL2016.pdf.

Robert Wood Johnson Foundation (2017). Future of nursing scholars. Retrieved from http://futureofnursingscholars.org/ .

Udlis, K., & Mancuso, J. (2016). Perceptions of the role of the doctor of nursing practice-prepared nurse: clarity or confusion. *Journal of Professional Nursing, 31*:274–283.

Waxman, K. T., Roussel, L., Herrin-Griffith, D., & D'Alfonso, J. (2017). The AONE nurse executive competencies: 12 years later. *Nurse Leader, 15*(2), 120–126.

Waxman, K. T., & Maxworthy, J. (2010). The doctorate of nursing practice degree and the nurse executive: The perfect combination. *Nurse Leader, 8*(2), 31–33.

Waxman, K. T., & Barter, M. (2017). The nurse entrepreneur in practice settings: Building a business case. In K. T. Waxman (Ed.). *Finance and business skills for the doctor of nursing practice.* (pp 241–259). New York, NY: Springer Publishers.

LINDA L. COSTA

2

The DNP Nurse Executive in the Healthcare Environment

Chapter Objectives

- Describe models of practice and payment for value-based care.
- Discuss the value of strategic agility in today's health care environment.
- Describe the adaptive leadership model's use in designing effective interventions.
- Assess the current state of nurses' participation in health care as full partners.
- Analyze the value of involving multiple disciplines in developing a culture of health.

KEY WORDS: Value-based care, strategic agility, adaptive leadership, culture of health

Introduction

The Institute of Medicine (IOM) (2011) landmark report "The Future of Nursing: Leading Change, Advancing Health" dedicated a chapter to transforming leadership, which was based on the IOM belief that nurses needed to develop leadership competencies to be full partners with other health professionals in the redesign and reform of the American healthcare system. Today, as millions more Americans have become eligible for care under the Patient Protection and Affordable Care Act (ACA), there have been two important changes in the healthcare environment: (1) The movement from volume to value-based care and (2) a new focus on population health that have increased the need for executive-level nurses.

Work in the C-Suite requires translation of strategic initiatives into operational tactics that enable the completion of organizational work. In this work, the C-Suite nurse executive is naturally positioned between the governance board and the clinical staff. The DNP nurse executive—educated in translation and implementation—has unique knowledge that will support the work of the entire executive team. In addition to this knowledge, the C-Suite DNP nurse executive must have the ability to use strategic agility (SA) for planning, accelerating change, using adaptive leadership, and leading interprofessional (IP) teams.

This chapter explores the skills and competencies that will empower current and future DNP executive leaders to manage the business of health care and to thrive in the C-Suite as full partners on an executive team that works in the complex, expanded health care system. The chapter begins with a brief review of the ACA impact and care delivery innovations, followed by executive skill requisites, and the IOM recommendations for building a "Culture of Health." The chapter concludes with three self-assessment strategies.

Value-Based Care and the DNP Nurse Executive

In November 2011, the final regulatory details were completed for the ACA (Medicare Learning Network, 2016). Demands on the health care system became significant as approximately 32 million additional Americans were able to acquire health insurance (IOM, 2011). Federal and state efforts to reform the health care system and meet the needs of the larger insured population explored a number of innovations in care delivery. Aligned with the ACA were payment incentives that moved the system from volume to value-based care. It is important for the DNP executive to understand models of care and the financial risks and rewards of each. The American Organization for Nursing Leadership (AONL) (formerly the American Organization of Nurse Executives) requires financial management skills that include the use of business models for health care organizations and the application of fundamental concepts of economics (AONE, 2015).

Two new but different value-based care models, accountable care organizations (ACOs) and patient centered medical homes (PCMHs), support the movement away from episodic care and toward value-based care. Revisions to the ACA have encouraged health care providers and hospitals to coordinate care for Medicare Fee-For-Service clients through ACOs. These ACOs offer incentives for providers to treat individuals across care settings, including primary care, hospitals, and long-term care facilities. The Medicare Shared Savings Program rewards the ACOs that lower health care costs while also meeting performance criteria for quality of care. Provider participation in an ACO is voluntary and must be approved by Centers for Medicare and Medicaid Services (CMS). An ACO agrees to be held accountable for the care experience of a population of assigned Medicare beneficiaries. An ACO is eligible to participate in the Shared Savings Program if it has at least 5,000 assigned Medicare Fee-for Service beneficiaries (Medicare Learning Network, 2016).

Each ACO establishes a governing body that represents ACO participants. The ACO is responsible for routine self-assessment, monitoring, and reporting of the care it delivers. When an application to be an ACO is approved, the agreement with CMS covers a period of at least 3 years. The regulations establish the quality performance measures and a method for linking quality and financial performance data that set a high bar for the delivery of coordinated, patient-centered care by the ACO. The regulations emphasize continuous improvement with the three-part aim of better care for individuals, better health for populations, and lower growth in expenditures. The ACOs must have procedures and processes that promote evidence-based medicine, beneficiary engagement, and coordination of care. An ACO that meets the program's quality performance standards receives a share of the savings if its assigned beneficiary expenditures are below its own specific benchmark. The ACOs can also choose to participate in a two-sided performance-based risk model that is accountable for sharing losses and requires an ACO to repay Medicare for a portion of losses. This level of agreement allows the ACO to acquire a higher reward, which is a share of the savings it generates.

The ACO can include any number of providers including primary care, specialists, and hospitals, as compared to a PCMH. This care model is managed by a primary care provider, who leads a clinical team that oversees the care of each patient in a practice and provides enhanced care coordination across the health care system. A medical practice may identify itself as a PCMH without an official certification, although many become certified by a national accrediting body. There are five core attributes of PCMH, as defined by the Agency for Healthcare Research and Quality (2018).

1. *Comprehensive Care*. The PCMH is designed to meet a patient's physical and mental health care needs through a team-based approach to care.
2. *Patient-Centered Care*. The PCMH delivers primary care that is oriented toward the whole person. This includes collaborating with patients and families through an understanding of and respect for culture, unique needs, preferences, and value.
3. *Accessible Services*. The PCMH seeks to make primary care accessible. Wait times are minimal, and there are expanded office hours and after-hours access to providers through communication methods such as telephone or email.
4. *Coordinated Care*. Patient care is coordinated across all encounters with the health care system, such as specialty care, hospitals, home health care, and community services, and there is an emphasis on efficient care transitions.
5. *Quality and Safety*. The model is committed to providing high-quality care through the use of clinical decision-support tools, evidence-based care, performance measurement, and population health management. Sharing quality data and quality improvement activities contributes to a systems-level commitment to quality.

The practice implements the PCMH framework incrementally. The Patient-Centered Primary Care Collaborative (PCPCC) recommends that practices begin their practice transformation in partnership with patients and family caregivers and with a self-assessment of assets and gaps in the five core attributes (PCPCC, 2018). Developing a strategic plan provides direction to the practice.

Once established, the practice's financial incentives are based on performance on specific quality measures that result in better access to care, more coordinated patient care, and improved outcomes. Practices that do well with quality and efficiency measures share in the savings they create. In this model, the consumer benefits from coordinated care, easier appointments, and more time with the care providers.

Quality Payment Program

The Medicare Access and CHIP Reauthorization Act of 2015 (MACRA) ended the Sustainable Growth Rate (SGR) formula, which would have significantly cut payment rates for clinicians participating in Medicare (MACRA, 2016). The MACRA regulation requires CMS to implement an incentive program, the Quality Payment Program, which provides two paths for participation through The Merit-based Incentive Payment System (MIPS) or the Advanced Alternative Program (Advanced APMS) (Quality Payment Program, 2018). The MIPS-eligible clinicians include physicians, physician assistants, nurse practitioners, clinical nurse specialists, and certified registered nurse anesthetists. In later years, eligibility for clinicians will be extended to other professions such as physical therapists and clinical social workers. To be eligible for MIPS payments, clinicians must bill more than $30,000 a year and provide care to more than 100 Medicare patients per year. The components for the MIPS performance for Year 2 (2018) are depicted below in Figure 2.1.

As stated in MACRA Final Rule (2016), a PCMH must be recognized by a nationally accredited organization. These organizations include the following:

- The National Committee for Quality Assurance (NCQA)
- The Joint Commission Designation
- The Utilization Review Accreditation Commission (URAC)
- The Accreditation Association for Ambulatory Health Care

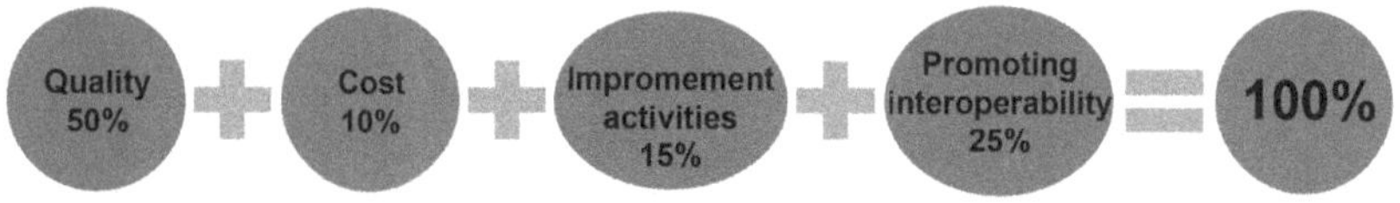

Figure 2.1. *MIPS Payment Structure 2018.*

In MIPS, a PCMH with recognition from one of these accredited bodies automatically earns full credit—or the highest potential score—toward the Improvement Activities performance category (Merit-Based Incentive Payment System and Alternative Payment Model Incentive, 2016). In the 2017 transitional year, the Improvement Activities category was weighted at 15% of the total MIPS score. This meant that PCMH accreditation would earn a MIPS eligible clinician or group 15 points toward the total MIPS score.

Simple documentation is required for a submission to the MIPS Improvement Activities category. However, if recognized as a PCMH, the recognition materials from NCQA or another accreditation body must be available for a potential audit. The CMS specifies that either of the following documents would provide the required support for an audit:

1. Documented implementation of patient-centered medical home activities and improvements that pertain to care coordination, patient-centeredness, or comprehensiveness of care, among others, or
2. Documented recognition as a patient-centered medical home from accredited body, combined with continual improvement.

The movement toward population health is challenging health care executive leaders to identify innovative methods of care delivery that will transform healthcare. Hospitals, primary care practices, and long-term care facilities that develop a continuum of care will be best prepared for future reimbursement models. In this evolving financial milieu, DNP nurse executives must be competent in financial management and must understand the intricacies of healthcare economics and policy across the entire of continuum of care.

Strategic Agility and the DNP Executive

The DNP nurse executive, with both clinical expertise and health care delivery system knowledge, is the ideal professional in the C-Suite to lead initiatives that develop high quality transitional care programs. Shirey (2015) defined "strategic agility" (SA) as the ability to adjust and adapt strategic direction in core businesses to create new, high value business models. Shirey linked the importance of SA to leadership competency and stated that SA differs from strategic management in moving beyond strategic planning to the anticipation of changing market conditions. Three critical SA capabilities include strategic sensitivity, resource fluidity, and collective commitment (Shirey, 2015). Strategic sensitivity includes superior foresight, the ability to sense the signposts of change, and collective commitment. Resource fluidity includes the ability to reconfigure and redeploy resources to engage with market opportunities. Collective commitment is the ability of senior leaders to make fast, unified decisions.

Hwang and Christenson (2008) used the term "disruptive innovation" (DI) as a method for studying what work needs to be done and not trying to improve a service, but designing it according to customer's needs. As health care moves from sick care to a wellness focus, the industry is moving from episodes of care to a health continuum with seamless borders. Disruptive innovation techniques include developing a customer-centered innovation map that includes mapping the route a customer travels to receive services (Bettencourt & Ulwick, 2008). Mind-mapping provides a picture of the interconnections of systems and subsystems built from the center. The scope of the complex system, synthesis of evidence supporting the change, and contingent and alternative approaches to resolutions can be demonstrated interactively along with critical intersections that affect change. Mind-mapping software can be used to create a system map that can be manipulated during team meetings to provide an interactive picture for brainstorming.

Kotter's (2014a) accelerate model focused on SA and addressed the limitations of management driven hierarchies and the need to foster dual operating systems that can capitalize on market opportunities. Kotter identified eight accelerators that in sequence drive change:

1. Create a sense of urgency about the opportunity
2. Build and evolve a guiding coalition of people across the organization
3. Form a change vision and strategic initiatives
4. Enlist a volunteer army
5. Enable action by removing barriers
6. Generate and celebrate short-term wins
7. Sustain acceleration
8. Institute change infusing it into the culture of the organization. Leadership is about setting direction.

Creating a sense of urgency involves recognizing strategic threats and working with a large a group of individuals to seize a "big opportunity" that is rational, data-based, and compelling to those inside the organization. The process involves gathering individuals from across the organization who are excited to move the opportunity forward as the guiding coalition (GC), changing the vision and strategic initiatives to what is needed to "look like" to capitalize on the opportunity, recruiting members of the GC who are ready to work, removing barriers that block quick actions, developing a method to identify barriers and remove them, celebrating movement forward by recognizing short goals reached along the way, and keeping the initiative in the front of other's minds by sharing data on progress. Organizations typically celebrate with items that represent the opportunity symbolically, such as buttons with the acronym for the campaign. Relentless energy is expended to keep moving forward with the initiative, sustain acceleration, and integrate it into the systems and the hierarchy processes. This in turn infuses the change into the culture of the organization.

Case Study

A large urban medical center has a low compliance with on-time first case starts. The culture is to be ready in the preoperative area by 0730, but this time is supposed to be the time the patient is actually in the operating room (OR). The lead DNP-Certified Registered Nurse Anesthetist (CRNA) and the OR Director see a "big opportunity" to manage start times. The impact of late starts is the backup of the OR schedule and cases being canceled that are scheduled later in the day, which in turn lead to low patient satisfaction and potential revenue losses.

1. *Big Opportunity*: First case on-time starts will reach 50% each day for the next six months. Zero cases will be canceled due to late start first cases.
2. *Guiding coalition*: There is no formal committee addressing on-time starts. A volunteer task force was formed. Volunteers from across the organization were solicited by the lead CRNA and OR Director to join the task force.
3. *Form a change vision and strategic initiatives.* Strategic initiatives include the following: Define on-time starts, gather accurate data about on-time starts, and determine the root cause/reasons for delays.
4. *Enlist a volunteer army.* Twelve volunteers are selected representing the main OR, the postanesthesia care unit (PACU), pre-operative testing, surgery floors, general surgeon, anesthesiologist, respiratory therapy, information technology (IT) analyst, and central sterile processing. The task force is led by the Lead DNP-CRNA.
5. *Enable action by removing barriers.* Barriers were defined as lack of cohesive communication among the surgery team; a vertical hierarchy in the OR; lack of concern among key stakeholders, e.g., Chief of Surgery; and possible inaccurate data.
6. *Generate and celebrate short-term wins.* The OR system was programmed by an IT analyst to redefine first case starts based on the new definition developed by the task force. "On-Time" start for a surgical case was defined as the physical presence of the patient in the OR with anesthesia either at or before the booked start time for the case. determined by the schedule. On-time case starts data were displayed on the board as personnel entered the OR for each of the 18 rooms.
7. *Sustain acceleration.* Data on delays were shared among key stakehold-

ers. The top three causes of delays were surgeons being responsible 50% of the time, followed by anesthesia 10% and preoperative issues 6%.
8. *Institute change infusing it into the culture of the organization.* Leadership is about setting direction. The Chief of Surgery instituted late start criteria that included defining a late start as any surgeon who was late for first cases on three or more occasions within a month. Any surgeon meeting the criteria lost the ability to schedule first cases during the following month. Data were shared weekly at the OR multidisciplinary team meetings.

Adaptive Leadership and the DNP

When Kendall-Gallagher and Breslin (2013) proposed that nurses with a DNP degree had a critical role in transforming health care, they selected Heifetz's (1994) model of adaptive leadership as the underpinning for their curriculum that could develop the leadership competencies described in DNP essential #2 (Organizational and Systems Leadership for Quality Improvement and Systems Thinking (American Association of Colleges of Nursing 2006). Heifetz (1994) suggested that it was critical for leaders to distinguish technical from adaptive changes. Technical changes are easy to identify, often lend themselves to quick easy solutions, and are generally well received. Adaptive changes must be addressed through changes in individual priorities, beliefs, and loyalties. For example, fixing a computer is a technical change that someone knows how to complete.

An example of an adaptive change could be redesigning a patient care delivery system. Well-designed interventions provide context that connects an individual's interpretation to the larger purpose or task so that individuals realize that their perspectives are relevant to group collective efforts (Heifetz, 1994). Adaptive challenges require changes in numerous places that often cross organizational boundaries. Solutions require experimentation and new discoveries and can require a long time for implementation.

Heifetz, Grashow, and Linsky (2009) identified adaptive leadership as an iterative process with three key activities: (1) observing events and patterns; (2) interpreting what a person observes with multiple hypotheses; and (3) designing inventions based on observations to identify adaptive challenges. Heifetz (1994) suggested that adaptive leaders need to get "on the balcony" as the first step of designing effective interventions to interpret a situation. Table 2.1 lists the seven steps for designing effective interventions.

Heifetz *et al.* (2009) consider each of these seven steps as a skill, and they recommend that adaptive leaders rank each of their skills on scale from 1 to 10, identify their strengths, and then focus their development activities on the steps that need strengthening.

Table 2.1 Designing Effective Interventions.

Strategy	Tactic
1. Get on the balcony	Watch for patterns while you observe what is going on around you.
2. Determine the ripeness of the issue in the system	Determine if there is an urgency to deal with the issue. Is the issue widespread or located within a subsystem.
3. Ask, who am I in this picture	How experienced are you in the groups, what role do you usually play.
4. Think hard about your framing	Communicate your intervention in a way that group members understand what you have in mind.
5. Hold steady	Once you have made the intervention, the idea is theirs.
6. Analyze the factions that emerge	Who is engaged; who is resistant to the idea.
7. Keep the work at the center of people's attention	Avoiding adaptive work is a common response. Use allies, and others who lead in the system to help keep the work as a focus.

Heifetz, Grashow, & Linsky, 2009.

IOM Recommendations and the DNP-Prepared Nurse Executive

In 2008, the Robert Wood Johnson Foundation (RWJF) approached the IOM to begin a collaboration that would transform the nursing profession and prepare it to meet the challenges of the ACA. The report, *The Future of Nursing: Leading Change, Advancing Health*, was completed in 2011. The underlying premise is that nursing must respond to new opportunities to provide health care to large populations. The four key messages in the report include the following:

1. Nurses should practice to the full extent of their education and training.
2. Nurses should achieve higher levels of education and training through an improved education system that promotes seamless academic progression.
3. Nurses should be full partners, with physicians and other health professionals, in redesigning health care in the United States.
4. Effective workforce planning and policy-making require better data collection and an improved information infrastructure.

The third key message focused on transforming leadership so that nurses could practice as full partners equal to physicians and other health care providers. To be a full partner requires that nurses are ready to assume top leadership roles and have leadership competencies, which require mutual respect and interprofessional (IP) collaboration (IOM, 2011). In 2016, the U.S. Department of Veterans Affairs (VA) permitted full practice authority to three roles of advanced practice registered nurses (APRNs), including certified nurse practitioners, clinical nurse specialists, and nurse-midwives. CRNAs were excluded until the VA could identify evidence for their inclusion (The Future of Nursing: Campaign for Action, 2018).

The RWJF has invested $300 million over 10 years in nursing because the foundation believes that nursing is critical to improving health care (Lavizzo-Mourey, 2012). One of the programs funded by RWJF was the Interdisciplinary Nursing Quality Research Initiative (INQRI). Nurse researchers collaborated with a co-principal investigator from another discipline in interdisciplinary team research. The goals of the nurse-directed research were increasing the rigor of the research and strengthening results to improve care through partnership with other disciplines. The program funded 40 interdisciplinary teams. Although many projects focused on nurses' contributions to quality care and processes, the final round of funding focused on dissemination, the study of processes that lead to widespread use of evidence-based practices, and implementation methods that promote the uptake of EBP and improve health care quality (Naylor *et al.*, 2013).

Dissemination and implementation are critical for quality improvement that increases adoption and spread. The education of DNP nurses focuses on these important components of knowledge translation to expand the use of EBP in practice settings. Understanding the complex environment of health care is an important competency for DNP students. Complexity science is a collection of concepts, frameworks, and theories that provide a new language, thought pattern, and a model for understanding and thinking about the complex world today that is full of illogical patterns. The DNP-prepared executive uses quantum leadership principles as an underpinning to practice. These include nonlinear processes, center-out decisionmaking, complexity-based models, and value-driven action (Porter O'Grady & Malloch, 2018).

After the release of the IOM report, the next step was implementing the recommendations through The Future of Nursing: Campaign for Action (2018). The RWJF and American Association of Retired Persons partnered to launch this campaign, which is focused at the national and state level. Members of 51 State Action Coalitions, including all states and the District of Columbia, perform the work. The State Coalitions create an agenda focused on the IOM report recommendations and join the movement to build a "culture of health."

Culture of Health

The RWJF explored the key role of nurses in building a culture of health, which is broadly defined as "one in which good health and well-being flourish across geographic, demographic, and social sectors; fostering healthy equitable communities guides public and private decision making; and everyone has the opportunity to make choices that lead to healthy lifestyles" (RWJF, 2017). The DNP-prepared nurse is in a position to lead health care systems that support this guiding framework, which is aligned with the goals of *The Future of Nursing: Leading Change, Advancing Health* (2011).

Hassmiller (2017), Senior Advisor for Nursing at RWJF, noted that, "Residents in every county in Maryland should have the same opportunity. If residents of all counties in Maryland had the same opportunities for health, there would be 197,000 fewer adult smokers, 118,000 fewer adults who are obese, and 73,000 fewer children living in poverty." In building a culture of health, professionals go beyond the bounds of medicine, nursing, pharmacy, and dentistry to involve business, housing, recreation, and parks.

DNP students can obtain important information about their communities by using databases such as those supported by RWJF that provide evidence summaries and ratings for policies, programs, and systems changes that can improve health. An example is http://www.countyhealthrankings.org/. This site provides search capability for local health information including quality of health, social and economic factors, and physical environment by state and county. This public information can be used for health care strategic planning to address community needs specific to the population served by the health systems.

Professional Practice Environment

In addition to the community, the executive leader must be cognizant of the professional practice environment. The Triple Aim, proposed by Berwick, focuses on improving health of populations, enhancing the patient experience of care, and reducing the per capita cost of care. After finding widespread burnout and dissatisfaction in health care workers, Bodenheimer and Sinsky (2014) proposed moving from the triple aim to the quadruple aim, which would also focus on improving the work life of health care providers. The authors cited rising societal expectations, particularly in primary care practices, and stated that the well-being of the care team is a prerequisite for the success of the Quadruple Aim. An organizational culture that supports professional practice of health care workers ensures unity of purpose and organizational alignment (Ives-Erickson, 2012). An illustration of a professional practice model can be found in Johns Hopkins Professional Practice Model (JHPPM) (Dang, Rohde, & Suflita, 2017). The editor's note that a change in organizational culture requires changes in local practice culture. The JHPPM is built upon five themes: We Achieve, We Care, We Empower, We Excel, and We Influence.

Interdisciplinary Teams

The role of interdisciplinary teamwork in professional practice is crucial, because these teams provide core underpinnings for professional practice, which is team based. Mitchell *et al.* (2012) defined team-based care as "the provision of health services to individuals, families, and/or their communities by at least two health providers who work collaboratively with patients and their caregivers-to the extent preferred by each patient-to accomplish shared goals within and across settings to achieve coordinated, high-quality care." (p. 5). In 2011, a report entitled "Core Competencies for Interprofessional Collaborative Practice and Team-Based Competencies, Building a Shared Foundation for Education and Clinical Practice" captured action strategies that support implementation of IP education competencies (IEC, 2011). Foundational teamwork is built around the provision of patient-centered care. To support care, an informatics platform is needed to enhance communication and coordination. Evidence-based practice and quality improvement processes are additional foundational components that support team-based work. Core competency domains for IP collaborative practice were defined by the expert panel as values and ethics, IP communication, roles/responsibilities for collaborative practice, and IP teamwork and team-based care (2011). Each competency domain has a general competency statement followed by defined competencies within the domain, as shown in Table 2.2.

The expert panel report provides the DNP student/practitioner with a template for developing and supporting IP teams in healthcare.

In 2015, the RWJF convened a committee to examine changes in the field of nursing since the original report, *The Future of Nursing* (IOM, 2015). The focus was analysis of the recommendation to remove barriers to practice and care, those that hamper nurses to practice to the full extent of their education and training. Although steps have been taken at the federal and state levels, barriers to APRNs who wish to expand their scope of practice remain. The committee recommended that the campaign work with other professions, policy makers, and the nursing community to build common ground for removing restrictions and to increase IP collaboration that will improve health care practice and patient care. The report concluded that no single profession working alone can meet the complex needs of communities and that nurses should continue to develop skills in leadership and innovation.

C-Suite and the DNP Nurse Executive: Performance Expectations

In health care systems, translation of strategic imperatives to operational tactics is the role of C-Suite executives. Senior executives are positioned

Table 2.2 Interprofessional (IP) Collaborative Practice Competency (IEC, 2011).

Values and Ethics for IP Practice	Work with individuals of other professions to maintain a climate of mutual respect and shared values	1. Place the interests of patients and populations at the center of IP health care delivery. 2. Recognize and respect the unique cultures, values, roles/responsibilities and expertise of other health professions
Roles/Responsibilities for Collaborative Practice	Use the knowledge of one's own role and those of other professions to appropriately assess and address the healthcare needs of the patients and populations served.	1. Use the full scope of knowledge, skills, and abilities of available health professionals and healthcare workers to provide care that is safe, timely, efficient, effective, and equitable.
IP Communication Practices	Communicate with patients, families, communities, and other health professionals in a responsive and responsible manner that supports a team approach to the maintenance of health and the treatment of disease	1. Choose effective communication tools and techniques, including information systems and communication technologies, to facilitate discussions and interactions that enhance team function
IP Teamwork and Team Based Practice	Apply relationship-building values and the principles of team dynamics to perform effectively in different team roles to plan and deliver patient/population-centered care that is safe, timely, efficient, effective, and equitable.	1. Share accountability with other professions, patients, and communities for outcomes relevant to prevention and health care. 2. Use process improvement strategies to increase the effectiveness of interprofessional teamwork and team-based care.

(IEC, 2011).

between the governing board and operations. Porter O'Grady and Malloch (2018) identify the central role of C-Suite leaders as follows: (1) Linking between governing board and staff, (2) Creating a positive context for worker relationships, and (3) Building the infrastructure for decisions and actions. From the quantum leadership perspective, the C-Suite executive is interested in the effectiveness of the decision-making system and actions and not the specific decisions and actions that are the responsibility of first and mid-leaders in the organization (Porter O'Grady & Malloch, 2018).

The DNP C-Suite executive brings to the role in-depth clinical knowledge of health system operations and quality improvement knowledge. Leadership in CNO roles is expanding in large systems to a Systems CNO (S-CNO). At this level, strategies for a nursing platform are built among several systems. Young, Lindstrom, Rosenberger, Gidroz, and Albu (2015) described the structure and focus of a Nursing Leadership Council built for Trinity Health (TH), a system with 47 hospitals. The Path to Commitment (PC) model provided the underpinning for the work of the Council. The PC model recognizes that individuals move through stages when committing to change that include awareness and understanding the need for change, belief in the change, understanding the need, and finally commitment when individuals see their role in moving the change forward. The Council members needed to transform their perspective from identifying their role as a CNO in their setting to a role commitment as an active member in the Leadership Council. Young *et al.* (2015) reported on the strategic directions and goals accomplished from each of three strategic priority teams. One team spearheaded moving from 1:1 monitoring for patients at risk for falls to central telemonitoring and ended with a vendor contract for the system including using a standardized toolkit with policies and procedures across the system.

Scoping initiatives such as those described by TH require the DNP executive develop a "blue ocean strategy." This is created when an organization develops an innovation that simultaneously creates value while decreasing costs. Welch and Edmondson (2012) suggested that this strategy should be applied to the foundation of accountable care to optimize health care delivery. The business of health care is extremely complex and changing, and the DNP executive must combine practice knowledge with business skills to build a culture of health in his or her health systems and community.

Barry and Winter (2015) questioned if the DNP should be the degree of choice for chief nurse executives (CNEs). The DNP with a specialty in health systems leadership clearly is prepared to move into a CNE position. CNEs need advanced business planning and strategic planning skills to lead transformational change in U.S. healthcare delivery (Barry & Winter, 2015). The shifting of the payment models in health care with a move toward value challenges the evidence-based knowledge and translational skill of the DNP CNE. Disch, Dreher, Davidson, Sinioris, and Wainio (2011) focused on the role of the CNE as critical to ensure patient safety and quality.

The National Center for HealthCare Leadership together with RWJF examined the role of senior leadership in promoting quality and safety in eight hospitals that were ranked in the first or second quintile of the Solucient Top 100 (Disch *et al.*, 2011). The most frequently cited competence for the CNO was communication and, more specifically, communicating goals and how to accomplish them, followed by strategic thinking or vision. Disch *et al.* (2011) noted two unexpected findings from the study. First was the predominance of sports analogies that are used in quality and safety, including terms such as champions, huddles, scorecards, and dashboards. This can be viewed as establishing a sense of a team. The second finding, which was not as positive, was termed the "quality burden." This is the burden on employees who try to work toward quality goals without clearly understanding the purpose and priority of initiatives and often without adequate resources.

Shirey and Hites (2015) discussed the need to shift from "busyness" to strategic work. Busyness is defined as individual internalized pressure created by a situation with a shortage of time to accomplish value-added work. Factors contributing to busyness include the environment, the culture of the organization (beliefs and norms), and interpersonal or intrapersonal demands. Leaders engaged with unfocused acceleration must evaluate non-value added work and engage in fewer meetings and fewer projects. Other employees can be key resources in identifying what can be stopped as a "spring cleaning" (Shirey & Hites, 2015). Deimplementation is a strategy to identify non-value added work to make room for new initiatives (Harvey & McInnes, 2015). Decisions about effective and ineffective practice should focus on value and, more specifically, patient safety and quality.

Assessment Tools for the DNP Executive

Collaborative Leadership Assessment

A leadership self-assessment can be beneficial in identifying strengths and weakness for the emerging DNP leader. A particularly valuable assessment is the Collaborative Leadership Assessment (Turning Point turnpt@u.washingon.edu) funded by RWJF. Six self-assessment topics include Assessing the Environment, Creating Clarity: Visioning and Mobilizing, Building Trust, Sharing Power and Influence, Developing People and Self-Reflection. The assessment and rating scale provide a score that identifies the area as a strength or area of potential growth. This self-assessment activity is valuable for DNPs who want to build a personal learning plan for their development as collaborative leaders. The assessment can be accessed at https://www3.marshfieldclinic.org/proxy///spf-ch7-collaborative-leadership-self-assessment-tools.1.pdf.

Emotional Intelligence Assessment

Emotional intelligence (EI) is a predictor of leadership success. Goldman and Boyatzis (2017) define EI by four domains and 12 competencies. These domains include self-awareness, self-management, social awareness, and relationship management. The twelve competencies are organized under specific domains. Under self-awareness is a single competency of emotional self-awareness. Under self-management are the competencies that include emotional self-control, adaptability, achievement orientation, and positive outlook.

The domain of social awareness includes two competencies, empathy and organizational awareness. The fourth domain, relationship management, has the greatest number of competencies including influence, coach and mentor, conflict management, teamwork, and inspirational leadership. Emotionally intelligent leaders learn to develop a balance of competencies across the domains. An initial assessment can help the DNP leader determine areas for future development. Several tools are available for assessment. Weisinger's (1998) book *Emotional Intelligence at Work* contains a self-assessment tool that is useful for leadership work with aspiring executives and those in practice. The 45-item self-assessment included in the book is divided into two parts, with Part 1 focusing on increasing personal emotional intelligence and Part 2 on using emotional intelligence in relations with others.

Online tools are also available for no cost. The following free tools are identified by the Harvard Extension School (2017) as favorite assessment tools:

1. *Psychology Today*—146 questions. The test is comprehensive, asking questions in multiple ways to ensure accuracy of the assessment. It takes about 45 minutes to complete. https://www.psychologytoday.com/us/test/3203

2. *Mind Tools*—15 questions. This one is quick and easy, but it will provide a baseline understanding of EI. https://www.mindtools.com/pages/article/ei-quiz.htm

3. *Institute For Health And Human Potential*—17 questions. This research company is dedicated to helping organizations leverage the science of emotional intelligence. They understand a great deal about what it takes to perform under pressure. https://www.ihhp.com/free-eq-quiz/

Manage Your Energy—Personal Assessment

Schwartz and McCarthy (2007) discuss energy as a limited personal resource and define a core problem in organizational work as working longer hours with time as a finite resource. Energy comes from four wells in humans: body, emotions, mind, and spirit. Take a personal energy assessment to learn if adjustments are needed by finding the overall energy score. Each of the four wells is assessed separately. The authors (Schwartz & McCarthy, 2007) provide information and examples of addressing each of the four wells to build personal energy. The DNP executive can use self-assessment as a way to serve as a role model for healthier behaviors among colleagues. http://www.lubnaa.com/files/ManageYourEnergyNotYourTime.pdf

Transition to DNP Executive Leadership Practice

Laura J. Wood, DNP, MS, RN, NEA-BC
Senior Vice President, Patient Care Operations & CNO
Sporing Carpenter Chair for Nursing
RWJF Executive Nurse Fellow Alumna '12
Boston Children's Hospital
Boston, MA 02115

I entered the professional nursing workforce in the late 1970s and was fortunate to secure employment within three leading academic and pediatric care delivery settings during the first two decades of my career. I was guided by more tenured colleagues and encouraged by leaders who inspired me to pursue new clinical and operational leadership roles. Despite the direct support of many, I experienced many long-standing practices in nursing that today are better appreciated as system-level challenges that pose threats to workforce stability, engagement, patient care outcomes, and operational effectiveness including:

- frequent nurse staffing shortages
- large patient assignments
- immature measurement capabilities to effectively capture and value the full scope of practice
- premature advancement to nursing leadership roles fueled by workforce shortages
- excessively large spans of control throughout all areas of nursing
- 24 × 7 accountability for the well-being of registered nurses and team members
- safety and quality vulnerabilities impacting patients and care givers

Following a decade of experience serving in direct patient care, clinical education, as well as front-line and senior level nursing leadership roles, I enrolled in an organizational development and clinical psychology PhD program. To accomplish this, I transitioned from a senior leadership role reporting to the Vice President of Nursing to a direct patient care role to reduce competing professional demands. The economics of full-time nursing doctoral studies were challenging post completion of both bachelors and master of science degrees in nursing given both were demanding and required a full-time academic commitment. Additionally, I struggled to determine how a research-focused doctorate was relevant to my personal goals to improve systems of care to the benefit of patients and families as well as to the health of the work environment. Because there were no alternative doctoral education pathways at the time in the late 1980s, the utility of this degree within traditional nursing academic and practice settings was limited. I ultimately reentered the workforce in a senior nursing leadership role in lieu of completing a PhD degree for family and personal reasons. This was the first in a series of values clarification exercises that affirmed my desire to improve systems of care rather than serve as a researcher as a platform to advance the improvement of health and healthcare and to strengthen the health of the work environment.

Over the next five years, by then the mid-1990s, I was asked to lead a health-system level performance improvement initiative in collaboration with an external national consultancy with a reporting relationship directly to the CEO and CFO. There were significant and growing cost improvement pressures mounting. Likewise, there was a desire to accelerate the integration of information system capabilities developed in the 1980s but not yet implemented and scaled. This work effort ultimately spanned more the 25 inpatient and ambulatory design teams with an aim to measurably improve the cost and quality position of the organization over a multi-year horizon. My participation in this initiative also provided me with C-Suite level mentorship outside of nursing for the first time. Additionally, it provided me a broader appreciation for the workflow and interdependencies of key operational areas beyond nursing and clinical departments including scheduling, registration, billing, collection, and clinical documentation as well as many other non-patient care related areas.

In an effort to apply these learnings toward a broader goal to meaningfully improve health system performance, I next pursued employment within a large, multi-national information systems organization where I worked from the late 1990s thru 2013. Inspired by the potential to better integrate people, process. and technology, I held progressive leadership roles in the professional services division of this company to support the implementation and optimization of information systems. Over the last eight years, I served as Vice President, Clinical Solutions. with the opportunity to engage with both senior leaders and front-line clinicians in hundreds of hospitals and health systems throughout the US and internationally. During this time, I gained a view of the vast challenges and distinct priorities spanning rural, community, urban. and academic health systems and collaborated with nursing and C-Suite leaders. I also came to recognize the distinct skills I had acquired over three decades and began to set new personal and professional goals. I hypothesized how I might ultimately apply what I had learned, pursue a practice doctorate in nursing given such an option now existed, and established a path forward with the support of many generous mentors.

During what was nearly three-year journey from the point of application to graduation with a DNP degree, I was greatly supported by the program director, senior faculty, my advisor, and members of my capstone committee who challenged me to integrate novel clinical and leadership experiences. I was fortunate to be awarded a leadership mentorship fellowship to support a long-held interest in clinical innovation and to be connected to preeminent leaders in healthcare safety and quality. I actively sought guidance from national nursing leaders serving in both practice and academic nursing settings at the highest levels in nursing to evaluate postdoctoral fellowships. Some individuals were long-standing friends and colleagues. Others were new relationships. The same week I graduated from my DNP program, I successfully completed the interview process to be named a Robert Wood Johnson Foundation Executive Nurse Fellow, becoming one of twenty senior nurse leaders accepted to this rigorous three-year nursing leadership development program. Over these three years, I came to better appreciate gaps in my leadership profiles as well as a range of personal capabilities I had not always appreciated. I began to recognize the potential to contribute more broadly to nursing and to the improvement of systems of care.

Later in 2012, a national search opened that would require relocation to another part of the country for the position of Senior Vice President, Patient Care Operations and Chief Nursing Officer, at what is widely considered the leading children's hospital. I did not initially consider being an applicant, but upon personal reflection and through conversation with family and trusted professional colleagues, I decided this might be a compelling and unique opportunity to return to my roots as a pediatric nurse as the leader of the discipline of nursing. I wanted to apply the accrued lessons from 35 years of professional nursing practice in a new setting and was grateful for the tremendous support I had been given to prepare me for the responsibilities of the role. I challenged myself to accept the potential that I might not be selected but would most certainly learn from the process. Following a multi-phase search process, I was offered the position. I remain tremendously humbled to serve with so many exceptional colleagues in a setting that frequently defines the standards of practice for many.

Now nearly six years into my tenure in this role, I recognize how the course content, academic rigor, and leadership lessons fostered throughout my DNP education prepared me to translate key DNP program elements as outlined within the white paper authored by The American Association of Colleges of Nurses (AACN), The Essentials of Doctoral Education for Advanced Nursing Practice. These elements include: organizational and systems leadership, clinical scholarship, information technology leadership, health care policy and advocacy, inter-professional collaboration, population health management, and advanced nursing practice. I have received many questions related to my transition to this role, my service on boards within my hospital's system of care and other national advisory boards, and am often asked to comment on the relevance of the DNP degree for those mid-way or later in their professional career trajectory. I offer the following reflections:

How did your DNP degree completion contribute to your ability to transition from a health care industry business setting to serve as the leader of the discipline of nursing and patient care operations in a leading academic and research-intensive children's health care system?

From my perspective, I did not navigate a "transition" back into nursing and health care. I have always viewed my core professional identity as that of registered nurse and thus never conceptualized my transition from hospital to industry employment as anything other than a change of setting. I pursued employment in a health care information technology (HIT) professional services setting a quarter of a century ago at a time when only billing, lab, and pharmacy systems were automated. At an early phase of my career as a staff nurse and front-line manager, I found the extensive use of costly and unreliable manual processes to be stifling in terms of the time consuming and non-value-added steps required. I also noted how dependent patient safety was on a single individual in the system, and thus potentially dangerous to patients and caregivers. I have long been inspired by the opportunity to reduce and eliminate preventable harm and waste within complex systems by optimizing how people, process and technology are integrated.

My DNP degree contributed to my ability to lead at the highest levels within my organization and to contribute professionally externally. Key areas of ongoing focus include:

- Advocacy related to both state and national health and nursing policies such as mandatory nurse staffing ratios, telehealth, and advanced practice registered nurse (APRN) scope of practice. Related service for past six years as National Co-Chair, Nursing Informatics Working Group (NWIG), American Medical Informatics Association (AMIA) public policy group.
- Leadership related to new national and state-wide care delivery models—contributor to launch of new Medicaid Accountable Care Organization (ACO) with 80,000 covered lives in support of population health and improved health equity both regionally and at state level.
- Advancement of new information technology tools and strategies to enhance safety, quality, and regulatory priorities as well as promoting greater access to care via the patient/family portal, medication and breast milk scanning, and tools to support mobility.
- Participated as senior nursing and patient care leader in the inaugural Interprofessional Education program with external foundation funding to reshape team training and education.
- Shaped the support of both evidence-based practice and nursing science fellowship preparation led by DNP and PhD prepared leadership within the organization.
- One of two named senior hospital leaders guiding health equity index and key nursing diversity and equity initiatives.

The 2010 Institute of Medicine (IOM) report entitled The Future of Nursing *stressed the importance of executive nurse leaders contributing their voices at senior leadership tables as full voting members. Do you serve on boards, advocate for this practice, and to what degree did your DNP preparation prepare you for this service?*

- Appointment and contributions as a full voting member of the hospital's Board of Trustees; several hospital board subcommittees including Finance, Audit and Compliance, and Patient Care Assessment Committee (Safety and Quality); board of affiliated private practice physicians and APRNs; board member of Innovation and Digital Health Accelerator (IDHA); and the ACO related integrated care organization board.
- Appointed member of numerous national advisory boards including: Hospital Advisory Council, Harvard Medical School Center for Bioethics; Nursing Advisory Board, Johns Hopkins School of Nursing; Chief Nursing Officer Advisory Council, Press Ganey; Nursing Executive Council, The Beryl Institute; and, Nursing Advisory Council, The Joint Commission.
- Contributor, American Hospital Association (AHA) annual meeting panel. Nurse Leaders in the Boardroom. Panel Presentation—Three CEO & CNO Dyads. American Hospital Association, National Meeting, Washington, DC. May, 2014.
- My DNP education facilitated my ability to provide meaningful contributions as a board member. Most specifically, the coursework I completed related to complex adaptive systems frequently contributes to my ability to consider how parts of the system interrelate with one another. Through my role as Senior Vice President, Patient Care Operations, and Chief Nursing Officer, I have accountability for nearly 6,000 employees spanning all of the clinical disciplines. These individuals are employed throughout the care continuum; thus, I can often offer insights related to both daily operations and broader strategy.

To what extent is DNP preparation relevant for those nurse leaders at a mid-point or later in their professional career trajectory?

I found DNP coursework and the experience of completing the required Capstone project and quality improvement initiative highly relevant and beneficial to my work as a senior nursing and patient care executive. It was affirming to take stock of what I already knew and easily apply within my daily leadership practices. Likewise, I am certain the new skills and content gains have prepared me to lead in the very challenging and dynamic environment that characterizes health care delivery today.

Chapter Takeaways

1. The DNP graduate is equipped to lead at the executive level as a practice expert in translation and implementation.
2. Scanning the health care environment for upcoming changes or reading the signposts is a critical skill.
3. In the fast-paced environment, developing competencies in strategic agility (SA), accelerating change. and modeling adaptive leadership ensure recognition as a valued member of the C-Suite.
4. Self-assessment and reflection are required as one moves and adjusts to executive positions throughout health systems.

Chapter Summary

It is important for the DNP leader to consider the frame of leadership provided by John Donahoe, President of eBay: "Leadership is a journey, not a destination. It is a marathon, not a sprint. It is a process, not an outcome." The changes in healthcare stimulated by the ACA in conjunction with the IOM *The Future of Nursing* report provide a pathway for DNP leaders to emerge as major players in shaping a new focus on a culture of health that provides innovations across the entire population. DNP C-Suite leaders have developed a strong knowledge base in translation and implementation and will lead others in the C-Suite in evaluation of strategic initiatives, ensuring collective commitment. Gone are the days of the five-year strategic plan. The new world reality calls for SA and reading the signposts of continuous change. The DNP leader lives on the edge of complexity exploring new possibilities through experimentation and valuing the contribution of health care teams.

Chapter Reflection Questions

1. When implementing change, what components of John Kotter's accelerate model do you believe are most important to use and which are most difficult if you apply to a current or prior work situation.
2. Think about adaptive versus technical changes. What steps would you take to identify what type of change is required?
3. In building a culture of health, how would you incorporate information about your practice community into a strategic plan?
4. For nurses to practice to the full extent of their license, what type of resources could you tap into to help move forward this initiative?

References

Agency for Healthcare Research and Quality. (2018). *Tools for implementing the PCMH*. Retrieved from https://pcmh.ahrq.gov/page/tools-implementing-pcmh.

American Association of Colleges of Nursing. (2006). *The essentials of doctoral education for advanced nursing practice*. Washington, DC: American Association of Colleges of Nursing. Retrieved from http://www.aacn.nche.edu/dnp/Essentials.pdf.

American Organization of Nurse Executives (AONE). (2015). *Nurse executive competencies*. Retrieved from http://www.aone.org/resources/nec.pdf.

Barry, J., & Winter, J. (2015). Health system chief nurse executive: Is a DNP the degree of choice? *Journal of Nursing Administration, 45*, 527–528.

Bettencourt, L. A., & Ulwick, A. W. (2008). The customer-center innovation map. *Harvard Business Review, 5*, 109–114.

Bodenheimer, T., & Sinsky, C. (2014). From triple to quadruple aim: Care of the patient requires care of the provider. *Ann Fam Med, 12*, 573–576.

Dang, D., Rohde, J., & Suflita, J. (Eds.). (2017). Johns Hopkins professional practice model: Strategies to advance nursing excellence. Indianapolis, IN: Sigma Theta Tau International.

Disch, J., Dreher, M., Davidson, P., Sinioris, M., & Wainio, J. A. (2011). The role of the chief nurse officer in ensuring patient safety and quality. *Journal of Nursing Administration, 41*(4), 179–185.

Goldman, D., & Boyatzis, R. (2017). *Emotional intelligence has 12 elements. Which do you need to work on*? Retrieved from https://hbr.org/2017/02/emotional-intelligence-has-12-elements-which-do-you-need-to-work-on.

Harvey, G., & McInnes, E. (2015). Divesting in ineffective and inappropriate practice: The neglected side of evidence-based health care. *Worldviews of Evidence-Based Nursing. 12*, 309–312.

Harvard Extension School. (2017). *Assessing your emotional intelligence: 4 tools we love*. Retrieved from https://www.extension.harvard.edu/professional-development/blog/assessing-your-emotional-intelligence-4-tools-we-love.

Hassmiller, S. B. (2017). The role of nurses in building a culture of health. Presented at the Maryland Action Coalition retreat and Leadership Summit, University of Maryland, Baltimore, MD.

Heifetz, R. A. (1994). *Leadership without easy answers*. Cambridge, England: Belknap Press of Harvard University Press.

Heifetz, R., Grashow, A., & Linsky, M. (2009). *The practice of adaptive leadership: Tools and tactics for changing your organization and the world*. Boston, MA: Harvard Business Press.

Huang, J., & Christenson, C. M. (2008). Disruptive innovation in health care delivery: A framework for business-model innovation. *Health Affairs, 27*(5), 1329–1335.

Interprofessional Education Collaborative (IEC). (2011). *Core competencies for interprofessional collaborative practice: Report of an expert panel, 2011*. Retrieved from http://www.uky.edu/cihe/sites/www.uky.edu.cihe/files/Core%20Competencies%20for%20IP%20Practice%202011.pdf.

Institute of Medicine. (2011). *The future of nursing: Leading change, advancing health.* Washington, DC: The National Academies Press.

Institute of Medicine. (2015). Assessing progress on the IOM report The Future of Nursing. Retrieved from http://www.nationalacademies.org/hmd/~/media/Files/Report%20Files/2015/AssessingFON_releaseslides/Nursing-Report-in-brief.pdf.

Ives Erickson, J. (2012). 200 years of nursing—A chief nurse's reflection on practice, theory, policy, education, and research. *Journal of Nursing Administration, 42*(1), 9–11.

Kendall-Gallagher, D., & Breslin, E. (2013). Developing DNP students as adaptive leaders: A key strategy in transforming health care. *Journal of Professional Nursing, 29*, 259–263.

Kim, C., & Mauborgne, R. (2004). Blue ocean strategy. *Harvard Business Review, 82*(10), 76–84.

Kotter, J. P. (2014a). *Accelerate: Building strategic agility for a faster-moving world.* Boston, MA: Harvard Business Review Press.

Kotter, J. P. (2014b). *Discussion guide.* Retrieved from https://www.kotterinc.com/wp-content/uploads/background photos/Accelerate_Discussion_Guide.pdf.

Lavizzo-Mourey, R. (2012). The nurse education imperative. *AACN Advanced Critical Care, 23*, 117–119.

Medicare Learning Network. (2016). Summary of the June 2015 Final Rule Provisions for Accountable Care Organizations (ACOs) under the Medicare Shared Savings Program.*Patient Protection and Affordable Care Act; HHS Notice of Benefit and Payment Parameters for 2018; Amendments to Special Enrollment Periods and the Consumer Operated and Oriented Plan Program.* 81 FR 94058. Retrieved from https://www.federalregister.gov/documents/2016/12/22/2016-30433/patient-protection-and-affordable-care-act-hhs-notice-of-benefit-and-payment-parameters-for-2018.

Merit-Based Incentive Payment System and Alternative Payment Model Incentive under the Physician Fee Schedule, and Criteria for Physician-Focused Payment Models. (MACRA) (2016). FR Document:2016-25240 Citation:81 FR 7700.

Mitchell, P. M., Wynia, R., Golden, B,. McNellis, S., Okun, C. E.,. Webb, V., Rohrbach, and. Von Kohorn, I. (2012). *Core principles & values of effective team-based health care. Discussion Paper.* Washington, DC: Institute of Medicine. Retrieved from www.iom.edu/tbc.

Naylor, M. D., Lustig, A., Kelley, H. J., Volpe, E. M. Melichar, L., & Pauly, M. V. (2103). Introduction: The interdisciplinary nursing quality research initiative. *Medical Care, 51*, S1–5.

Porter-O'Grady, T., & Malloch, K. (2018). *Quantum leadership: Creating sustainable value in healthcare.* (5th Ed.) Burlington, MA: Jones and Bartlett Learning.

Patient-Centered Primary Care Collaborative. (2018). *Defining the medical home. A patientcentered philosophy that drives primary care excellence.* Retrieved from https://www.pcpcc.org/about/medical-home.

Quality Payment Program. (2018). *MIPS overview.* Retrieved from https://qpp.cms.gov/mips/overview.

Robert Wood Johnson Foundation. (2017). *Campaign for actions*. Retrieved from https://campaignforaction.org/.

Robert Wood Johnson Foundation (2018). *A culture of health*. Retrieved from https://www.cultureofhealth.org/.

Schwartz, T., & McCarthy, (2007). Manage your energy, not your time. *Harvard Business Review, 10*, 2–9.

Shirey, M. R. (2015). Strategic agility for nursing leadership. *Journal of Nursing Administration, 45*(6), 305–308.

Shirey, M. R., & Hites, L. (2015). Orchestrating energy for shifting busyness to strategic work. *Journal of Nursing Administration, 45*(3), 124–127.

The Future of Nursing: Campaign for Action (2018). Removing barriers to practice and care. Retrieved from https://campaignforaction.org/wp-content/uploads/2018/02/APRN-Practice-two-pager-2-9-18.pdf.

Welch, S., & Edmondson, B. (2012). Applying blue ocean strategy to the foundation of accountable care. *American Journal of Medical Quality, 27*(3), 256–257.

Weisinger, H. (1998). *Emotional intelligence at work*. San Francisco, CA: John Wiley & Sons, Inc.

Young, J., Lindstrom, G., Rosenberger, S. Gidroz, A. M., & Albu, A. (2015). Leading nursing into the future: Development of a strategic nursing platform on a system level. *Nursing Administration Quarterly, 39*(3), 239–246.

ADRIANA PEREZ AMADO
COURTNEY VOSE
KARI A. MASTRO

3

The DNP Nurse Leadership Potential: Evolution and Challenges

Chapter Objectives

- Identify the classic stages of large-scale change as defined by Lewin and Lippitt.
- Describe the conditions required for successful large-scale change initiatives.
- Understand the empirical research that became the driving force behind advanced education for nurses.
- Learn about the development experience of other nursing leaders.
- Identify the skills and attributes that nurses will need to become effective change agents in the health care industry.
- Understand the career limitations of the imposter syndrome.
- Describe the potential challenges that lie ahead for the nursing profession as the DNP becomes the expected standard in graduate education for nurses executives.

KEY WORDS: Advanced Practice Nurse; Doctor of Nursing Practice; Evidence-Based Practice; Nurse Manager; change; imposter syndrome; resiliency

Introduction

Ongoing discussion continues within the nursing profession as the doctor of nursing practice (DNP) becomes the minimum requirement for entry into the practice of front line nursing leadership. Research has demonstrated a relationship between bachelor of science in nursing (BSN) prepared nurses and improved outcomes in patient mortality and nursing quality indicators, although the nascent impact of doctorally prepared nurse leaders in health care is yet to be examined.

In this chapter, we examine the challenge of the changing educational requirements in the nursing profession, the empirical research that has driven changes in nursing education, the skills and attributes needed by nurses who will assume roles as change agents and top leaders in health care, the reflections of nursing leaders on their personal journeys to higher education and progressive leadership, and some of the challenges that lie ahead as the DNP degree becomes the standard requirement for nurse executives.

The Challenge of Changing Educational Requirements for Nurse Managers

> Leaders are fascinated by the future. You are a leader if and only if you are restless for change, impatient for progress and deeply dissatisfied with status quo. Because in your head, you can see a better future. The friction between 'what is' and 'what could be' burns you, stirs you up, propels you. This is leadership.—*Marcus Buckingham*

The transition from the BSN degree as the entry level into nursing practice to the DNP degree represents a significant, large-scale change for the nursing profession. This process of change can be clarified by revisiting Lewin's seminal work on change. Lewin depicted the change process as three steps of unfreezing, changing, and refreezing (Mitchell, 2013). Lewin is credited with developing the concept of planned change as compared to unintentional or accidental change (Stichler, 2011). Lippitt advanced Lewin's theory by adding more emphasis on the critical role and responsibility of leaders as change agents, who plan, integrate, and sustain change over time (Stichler, 2011).

Lippitt's seven steps of change included the following: (a) diagnosing the problem; (b) assessing the motivation and capacity for change; (c) assessing the resources and motivation of the change agent including the change agent's commitment to change, power and stamina; (d) developing action plans and tactics; (e) establishing the roles of change agents such as champion, cheerleader, expert, facilitator; (f) maintaining and sustaining the change through communication, feedback and group coordination; and (g) gradually withdrawing from the helping relationship as the change becomes integrated into the organizational culture (Kritsonis, 2004–2005). See Figure 3.1.

Lippitt and colleagues state that changes are more likely to be stable and better rooted if they spread organically to neighboring systems or to subparts of the system independently affected (Kritsonis, 2004–2005).

Thus, for nursing, the move to higher educational standards at the doctoral level reflects a major change process for the profession that will

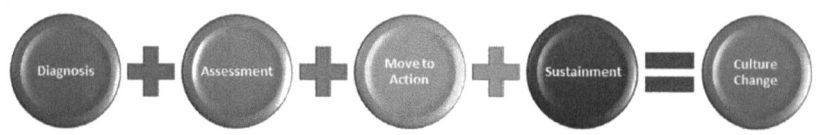

Figure 3.1. *This figure depicts the key concepts of Lippitt's theory. (Lippitt, Watson, & Westley, 1958)*

require strong leadership, learning, resilience, and adaptation. Dr. Hope Johnson, Director of Perioperative and Endoscopy Services, Lehigh Valley Health Network/Cedar Crest, explained how she has adjusted to the changes in her role as she advanced her nursing degree:

> My experience as a front-line manager of peri-operative and endoscopy nursing has provided me the opportunity to experience both the clinical and financial sides of nursing. Recognizing the impact surgery has on a health care organization aided my decision making related to the research I would conduct during my doctoral program. I felt this realm was unexplored by nursing and required the additional perspective a nurse could provide. While in my doctoral program, the United States was in the middle of a Presidential Term. During this term, alterations to our health care payment system were presented under the direction of the Affordable Care Act. Strategy became imperative in the healthcare sector. It was becoming apparent that the traditional cookie-cutter approach to surgery was no longer going to solidify surgical volumes for institutions. Hospitals needed to take a different perspective when drawing in and maintaining volumes.
>
> The scholarly project that emerged from my research focused on the concept of a disruptive innovation within surgical services, the focused factory. Operating Rooms focusing on one specialty or service line were more able to focus on the service and consumer piece of health care. Setting themselves apart from competition could become drivers for market share. While studying the phenomenon of disruptive innovation, which had long been established in the field of technology, I began to focus on its ability to lower cost.
>
> Nursing is accustomed to change. Primary nursing, team nursing, and patient-centered care are among the care delivery models utilized over the years. It is our ability to be nimble and recognize when we need to modify our delivery that supports our success. Throughout my research, this idea of challenging the status quo was found to be meaningful. After the research was completed and the paper was written, this was a theme I could then continue to apply to my practice within operations and management. As I indicated earlier, nursing has an opportunity to become involved in financial conversations and decisions. Having the ability to provide relevance in the conversation surrounding finance and more than clinical has been an important growth strategy for me in my career. Reaching outside the comfort zone of diagnoses, surgical intervention, and education were paramount to this growth. I would challenge any nurse looking to pursue a higher level of education to reach into an area of health care that is outside of their comfort zone; stretch yourself to learn, grow, and develop as a well-rounded nursing leader that has more than just clinical expertise.

The Evolution of Entry Level Degree Requirements of Nursing Leaders

Leadership and learning are indispensable to each other.—*John F. Kennedy*

The historical debate about the entry-level degree requirement for nursing is decades old. By 2003, research by Aiken, Clarke, Cheung, Sloane, and Silber supported the BSN as the entry-level degree requirement, because quality and safety outcomes related to patient care were found to be positively associated with the higher educational level of nurses (Aiken, Clarke, Cheung, Sloane, and Silber, 2003). In March 2005, the American Organization for Nursing Leadership (AONL) (formerly the American Organization of Nurse Executives) released a statement that called for all registered nurses (RNs) to be educated in BSN programs. The AONL based this statement on the need for RNs to be prepared for their increasingly challenging and complex roles in health care. By 2010, the Tri-Council for Nursing—which included the AONL, American Nurses Association (ANA), American Association of Colleges of Nursing (AACN), and National League for Nursing (NLN)—called for all RNs to advance their education to the baccalaureate degree and beyond, because advanced education was required to support the urgent improvements in quality and safety outcomes across the health care industry. The Tri-Council declaration, entitled "Education Advancement of Registered Nurses," asserted that the nation's health would be further in danger without an increasingly educated nursing workforce (Tri-Council for Nursing, 2010).

Later in 2010, The Robert Wood Foundation (RWJF) and the Institute of Medicine (IOM) released their groundbreaking report entitled *The Future of Nursing: Leading Change, Advancing Health* (IOM, 2010). This report emphasized the critical role of nurses in ensuring the highest quality patient- and family-centered care, advancing healthcare, and leading change in the current health care industry, in which patient care had become more complex and more community-oriented (IOM, 2010). The IOM framed this seminal report as a burning platform with a specific charge for nurses who provide the majority of patient assessments, evaluations, and care for patients in hospitals, nursing homes, clinics, schools, places of business, and ambulatory settings (IOM, 2010).

Going beyond the patient-oriented work of nurses in hospitals, ambulatory centers, and the community, the IOM advocated for the greater involvement of nurses in leadership positions in hospital governance that develop hospital policy and lead decision-making in health care organizations. For nurses to have a voice in these top leadership positions, they must be viewed as academic equals at all levels of their organizations. Therefore, the IOM recommended that nursing leaders must advance their educational requirements, as follows (IOM, 2010):

1. Nurses should achieve higher levels education and training through an improved education system that promotes seamless academic progression.
2. Nurses should be full partners, with physicians and other health professionals, in redesigning health care in the United States.

The IOM's national focus on advanced education for nurses built upon the work of two nursing organizations, the AACN "Task Force to Revise Quality Indicators for Doctoral Education" and the American Nurses Credentialing Center (ANCC) Journey to Magnet Excellence®. The AACN 2004 position statement called for transformational change in the education required for professional nurses who will practice at the most advanced levels of nursing—including nursing leadership (AACN, 2004). The ANCC required Magnet® hospitals to establish educational objectives for nurses to achieve an 80% rate of a BSN-prepared workforce and, based on findings from the empirical literature, to require that all nurse managers and nurse leaders have a BSN or higher degree (ANCC, 2018).

As shown in Table 3.1, the recommendations of the major nursing organizations reflect the national transition toward advanced education for nursing.

Dr. Nicole Hartman, DNP, MBA, RN, NEA-BC, Magnet® Program Director, NewYorkPresbyterian/Columbia University Medical Center, offered some reflections on the importance of her academic journey in becoming a DNP nurse leader:

> I was five when my dad slipped off a ladder and fell down the stairs of our two-story foyer. I wasn't sure what to do, but I knew I had to do something, so I followed my instincts. I laid my tiny five-year-old-self down on the floor in my basement next to my six-foot-three inch dad and waited. First, we just rested and then we started moving our toes, our feet, our legs, our hands, our arms and then finally sat up. My dad was lucky that day, he wasn't hurt. But, I was even luckier, I found my calling. I wanted to be a nurse. It was from then on that my course was laid and my journey began.
>
> Fast forward about 30 years and I was ready to tackle one of the biggest journeys in my professional career, my DNP. Just as I knew I wanted to be a nurse when I was a young child, I knew I wanted to get a doctorate in nursing when I was a young nurse. I wanted to help as many clinical nurses as possible and a role as a doctoral prepared nurse leader would allow that. My DNP in nursing administration opened up my eyes to the possibilities nurse leaders have to move nursing forward in health care today. I am prepared to sit at the executive healthcare table and have dialogue with other health care leaders that will position clinical nurses to provide high quality care. Establishing relationships with other health care executives assures that I am a respected member of a multidisciplinary health care leadership team that is focused on clinical outcomes. The focus on business acumen in my DNP program assures I can lead clinical nurses to establish business plans that emphasize the needs of patients, while monitoring the fiscal needs of an organization. The skills I learned during my DNP program allow me to guide clinical nurses through the challenges faced in healthcare today.
>
> As I reflect on my journey in professional nursing, I often think of that day with my dad. He isn't here today to call me Dr. Hartman, but it is because of that moment when I was five that I find myself poised to lead clinical nurses today."

Table 3.1 Recommendations for Nursing Entry Level Degree Requirements.

Professional Organization	Position	Entry Level and Leader Degree Recommendations
AONL	• Believes in the academic progression of nurses. • Member of Tri-Council for Nursing, which has called for all registered nurses (RNs) to advance their education in the interest of enhancing quality and safety across heath care settings. The Tri-Council consensus statement says that more nurses with bachelor of science in nursing (BSN) and higher degrees are needed in all settings. The Tri-Council encourages academic articulation agreements. • The AONL Nurse Executive Competencies (2015) should form the foundation for all graduate nurse leader education and curriculum development. • Nurse leaders should be minimally prepared at the baccalaureate or master degree level. • Nurse leaders at the highest levels of executive leadership are encouraged to seek educational preparation at the doctoral level.	*Entry Level:* None *Nurse Leaders:* Minimally baccalaureate or master degree level *Nurse Executives:* Doctoral level
ANA	• Longstanding position that baccalaureate education should be the standard entry into professional practice. • Member of Tri-Council for Nursing, which has called for all RNs to advance their education in the interest of enhancing quality and safety across heath care settings. The Tri-Council consensus statement says that more nurses with BSN and higher degrees are needed in all settings. The Tri-Council encourages academic articulation agreements. • The DNP prepares nurses for multiple roles including health policy development, leadership, and administration.	*Entry Level:* BSN *Nurse Leaders:* Recommend master degree or doctoral degree *Nurse Executives:* Recommend master degree or doctoral degree
AACN	• Recognizes the BSN degree as the minimum education for professional nursing practice. • Member of Tri-Council for Nursing, which has called for all RNs to advance their education in the interest of enhancing quality and safety across heath care settings. The Tri-Council consensus statement says that more nurses with BSN and higher degrees are needed in all settings. The Tri-Council encourages academic articulation agreements. • The DNP prepares nurse leaders at the highest levels of nursing practice to improve patient outcomes and translate research into practice. Calls for education of advanced practice registered nurses (APRNs) and other nurses seeking top leadership roles in doctor of nursing practice (DNP) programs.	*Entry Level:* BSN *Nurse Leaders:* Master degree *Nurse Executives:* DNP degree

(continued)

Table 3.1 (continued) Recommendations for Nursing Entry Level Degree Requirements.

Professional Organization	Position	Entry Level and Leader Degree Recommendations
NLN	• Promote academic progression of nurses. • Recognizes that the diversity offered by multiple points of entry and the variety of progression options available provide an environment for a diverse workforce, lifelong learning and academic progression. • Member of Tri-Council for Nursing, which has called for all RNs to advance their education in the interest of enhancing quality and safety across heath care settings. The Tri-Council consensus statement says that more nurses with BSN and higher degrees are needed in all settings. The Tri-Council encourages academic articulation agreements.	*Entry Level*: Support three points of entry *Nurse Leaders*: Promote master level *Nurse Executives*: Continue to advance nursing degree
IOM	• Nurses should achieve higher levels of education and training through an improved education system that promotes seamless academic progression. • Double the number of nurses with a doctorate by 2020.	*Entry Level*: Increase the proportion of nurses with a BSN degree from 50% to 80% by 2020 *Nurse Leaders*: Graduate degree
ANCC	• Requirements for Magnet® hospitals to establish education objectives for nurses to achieve an 80% BSN prepared workforce. • Encourages academic progression of all nurses, especially nurse leaders.	*Entry Level*: Educational objectives to increase proportion of nurses with a BSN degree to 80% *Nurse Leaders*: Academic progression *Nurse Executives*: Academic progression

Rationale for Degree Progression

> Let us never consider ourselves finished nurses . . . we must be learning all of our lives. —*Florence Nightingale*

As stated, degree progression for nurses is being driven by the growing body of evidence on the positive association between higher educational degrees and better patient outcomes. Seminal research conducted by Aiken *et al.* (2003) found that the educational levels of hospital nurses, specifically within the surgical specialty, reduced patient mortality (Aiken *et al.*, 2003). The research included a cross-sectional analysis of outcomes data for 232,342 general, orthopedic, and vascular surgery patients discharged from 168 non-federal adult general hospitals and administrative and survey data on the educational composition of the nursing workforce (Aiken *et al.*, 2003). The study concluded that hospitals with higher proportions of nurses educated at the BSN level or higher had lower mortality and failure-to-rescue rates for surgical patients.

In the Aiken study, three hospital characteristics were used as control variables: (1) hospital size defined as < 100 beds, 100–250 beds, and > 250 beds; (2) teaching status defined as those without postgraduate medical students or fellows, those with 1:4 or smaller trainee-to-bed ratios, and those with ratios higher than 1:4 considered major teaching hospitals; and (3) high technology defined as facilities with open-heart surgery, major organ transplantation, or both (Aiken *et al.*, 2003). A 10% increase in the proportion of nurses in hospitals with a BSN degree was associated with a 5% decrease in both the likelihood of patients dying within 30 days of admission and the odds of failure-to-rescue (Aiken *et al.*, 2003). This study, the first analysis that provided empirical evidence that linked educational levels to quality outcomes, has been a driving force for advanced educational requirements for nurses.

Given the national movement toward advanced education for nurses, Altmann (2011) conducted a literature review to assess nurses' attitudes about returning to college. Altmann identified four societal influences that supported the importance of continuing education for nurses:

1. Many nurses are still practicing with an associate's degree in nursing or a nursing diploma and few continue their education.
2. Research has shown that there are improved patient outcomes in hospitals which employ more highly educated nurses.
3. A poor economy during a nursing shortage means high demand and less incentive for nurses to return to college for higher education.
4. The worsening faculty shortage means an increased need for nurses to advance their education.

Altmann analyzed 15 studies that evaluated RN attitudes, motives/reasons, perceptions of influences/incentive, constraints/barriers, and benefits of participation in continuing education. Altmann also reviewed 13 studies that included variables of interest related to continuing formal education for nurses. Across all the studies, design methods were similar, with surveys the most frequently used data collection method. The only published questionnaire used in multiple studies was the Adult Attitudes Toward Continuing Education Scale, which was not specifically designed for use with nurses (Altmann, 2011). The quantitative studies used convenience samples, and the qualitative studies used purposive sampling. Sample size ranged varied from 77 to 770 respondents, with one exception of a notable national study in Canada (n = 2,838). Response rates varied from 11% to 91% (Altmann, 2011).

Altmann's analysis concluded that the barriers and motivators to continuing formal education can be classified as personal, professional, and academic. Motivators included increased self-confidence, autonomy, quality care, improved clinical judgment, career advancement into nursing leadership or advanced practice nursing, and personal growth. Barriers included cost, lack of support, and curricular issues. Altmann concluded that there were sufficient motivators for younger, non-BSN prepared RNs to continue their education to more advanced levels.

The critical importance of advanced education for nurses was highlighted in a 2012 editorial, "The Nurse Education Imperative," by Dr. Risa Lavizzo-Mourey, President and CEO, RWJF. Lavizzo-Mourey, a physician, linked the work of the RWJF to the IOM in the Future of Nursing's Campaign for Action. Lavizzo-Mourey discussed her personal encounters with nursing, the hiring preference of some organizations for BSN-prepared RNs, and options to consider for monetizing the return on investment. Lavizzo-Mourey said, "We cannot wait to take action; failing to grow a better educated nursing workforce risks disastrous results. This is particularly important in light of the aging workforce as well as the coming expansion of health insurance coverage." (Lavizzo-Mourey, 2012, p. 61).

In 2013, McHugh, *et al.*, conducted research on mortality in Magnet® hospitals, which assessed whether and why these hospitals had lower risk adjusted mortality and failure-to-rescue when compared to non-Magnet® hospitals. The analysis linked patient, nurse, and hospital data from 56 Magnet hospitals and 508 non-Magnet adult, general hospitals in California, Florida, Pennsylvania, and New Jersey, four of the largest states with hospitals similar in characteristics to hospitals nationally (McHugh *et al.*, 2013).

Patient data were obtained from discharge databases and were limited to patients between the ages of 21 to 85 years who were undergoing general, orthopedic, or vascular surgery. Nursing related measures, collected with surveys, included information about staffing, work environment, and levels of education. The nurse work environment was measured with the Practice Environment Scale of the Nursing Work Index (PES-NWI), which includes subscale items related to (1) nurse participation in hospital affairs; (2) nursing foundations for quality; (3) nurse manager ability, leadership, and support of staff; (4) staffing and resource adequacy; and (5) collegial nurse-physician relationships. Hospital data were obtained from the 2006–2007 American Hospital Association annual hospital survey.

Differences in the odds of mortality and failure-to-rescue for surgical patients were estimated via logistic regression models (McHugh *et al.*, 2013). The results showed that patients treated in Magnet hospitals had a 14% lower odds of mortality and 12% lower odds of failure-to-rescue (McHugh *et al.*, 2013). "Magnet® hospitals had significantly better work environments and higher proportions of nurses (0.46 versus 0.39; p < 0.001) with bachelor's degrees and specialty certification. These nursing factors explained much of the Magnet® hospital effect on patient outcomes," McHugh *et al.* said (2013, p. 382).

A reflection from Dr. Cynthia A. Cappel, DNP, RN-BC, NE-BC, Vice President for Education, Lehigh Valley Health Network, highlights her passion for nursing and her thirst for higher education as she continues to lead clinical nurses:

> But you are smart enough to be a doctor! Those are the words my father spoke as I shared my career plans. As my biggest supporter, it was not that he saw nursing as a poor career choice, he just didn't feel like his first-born child needed to 'settle' for nursing when she could become anything, at least in his adoring eyes. I have often thought about the perceptions of others as I progressed through my nursing career. Did they share the underlying views of my father?
>
> For me, nursing is a profession for the best and the brightest. It is a career choice for leaders, critical thinkers, decision-makers, and scholars. It takes tremendous compassion, coupled with expert communication skills. It is the soft touch, the stern order, the nagging intuition, and the comic relief. It is knowing what everyone around you needs, and delivering on those needs. It is remembering your own self-care so that you can keep caring for the needs of others. It is not a profession for the faint of heart. It takes courage and stamina to support patients and families in their moments of greatest need. It takes tremendous knowledge and skills to navigate the ever-changing, complex world of healthcare.
>
> Thanks to a great nurse leader, Chief Nursing Officer (CNO), and mentor, I had the opportunity to put this passion for the profession of nursing into action. I was charged with advancing the "Future of Nursing" recommendations for a large academic health system. It was the culmination of all that I believed nursing to be—leadership, academic progression, courageous decision-making, an unending zeal for quality improvement, and lifelong learning. This was meaningful work that brought great satisfaction to me, and rejuvenated my career of almost 30 years. However, there was an inconsistency in my message and my actions. Could I be true to the essence of this work when my formal academic progression ended 19 years ago? What

about the idea of authentic leadership, personal and professional accountability? I knew what I needed to do.

And once again, great nursing mentors, peers, and colleagues supported my journey to a DNP. I found a cohort of brilliant nurses who shared a belief in lifelong learning, setting an example as nurse leaders, and developing expertise to advance the profession that has been so good to us. So on a cold day in January 2017, my father was there to see me become the doctor he always dreamed I would be.

Earning a DNP has been pivotal to my career advancement, resulting in two promotions, most recently to vice president for education. Advancing my education has enhanced my leadership skills, strengthened my commitment to the profession, and afforded me the opportunity to affect system level change. In my role, I oversee interprofessional education for an eight-hospital health system. I continue to support lifelong learning across all the healthcare professions, as well as academic progression, leadership, and enhancing quality patient care. I am . . . smart enough to be a doctor. In fact, I am helping to educate them: those in medicine and nursing.

Evolution to the DNP

> It is not the strongest of the species that survive, nor the most intelligent, but the one most responsive to change.—*Charles Darwin*

In the 1960s, advanced practice roles for nurses were introduced to help solve the growing shortage of primary care in rural and underserved areas. Advanced practice nurses (APNs) offered a less expensive alternative to providing these populations with primary care by professionals trained to be generalists with a breadth of knowledge and the ability to provide a large number of services. Since the inclusion of APNs in primary care, the role has expanded into other areas of health care, such as acute care, intensive care, emergency services, anesthesia, and clinical leadership.

In 2004, the AACN developed a definition and scope of practice position statement for advanced nursing practice that defined this practice as "any form of nursing intervention that influences health care outcomes for individuals or populations, including direct care of individual patients, management of care for individuals and populations, administration of nursing and health care organizations, and the development and implementation of health policy" (AACN, 2004, p.4). Nursing has been flexible in meeting the needs of acute and critically patients, primary care, outpatient services, physician partners, and hospitals and in adjusting their service model to meet these changing demands. This flexibility has served the nursing profession by (1) creating more job opportunities, (2) advancing the practice and reputation of nursing, (3) keeping bedside nurses interested by advancing their degrees in critical and acute care, and (4) serving the health care community and patient needs better.

The DNP is now one of two terminal professional degrees in nursing. The curriculum for the DNP degree builds upon the traditional master's programs by providing education in evidence-based practice, quality improvement, and systems leadership. The DNP degree was established to prepare nursing professionals as APNs or C-Suite health care executives in their organizations. Currently, APNs include mastered-prepared nurse practitioners (NPs), certified registered nurse anesthetists (CRNAs), certified nurse midwives (CNMs), clinical nurse specialists (CNSs), and clinical nurse leaders (CNLs). Nurse anesthetists are now required to achieve either a DNP or a doctor of nurse anesthesia practice (DNAP).

With these changes, nursing is evolving quickly in the direction of other health professions toward the transition to the DNP. Medicine (MD), dentistry (DDS), pharmacy (PharmD), psychology (PsyD), physical therapy (DPT), and audiology (AudD) all require or offer practice doctorates. Doctor of nursing practice programs are growing exponentially, whereas doctor of philosophy (PhD) programs in nursing are stable, because interest in earning a clinical doctorate in advanced nursing practice ranks highly among nurses at all stages of their professional careers. In June 2017, the AACN indicated that there were 303 DNP programs in 50 states plus the District of Columbia, with an additional 124 programs in various planning stages (see Figure 3.2). Although these DNP programs may differ in focus and curriculum, the majority of DNP programs share one common denominator: a focus on clinical leadership.

Currently, there are few academic requirements or recommendations from professional organizations for nurse managers at levels between clinical nurse and chief nursing officer (CNO) or chief nursing executive (CNE). According to AONL, nurse managers are defined as leaders with 24-hour accountability and responsibility for a direct care unit or units, and they are the liaison between administration's vision and strategy and direct

Growth in Doctoral Nursing Programs: 2006-2016

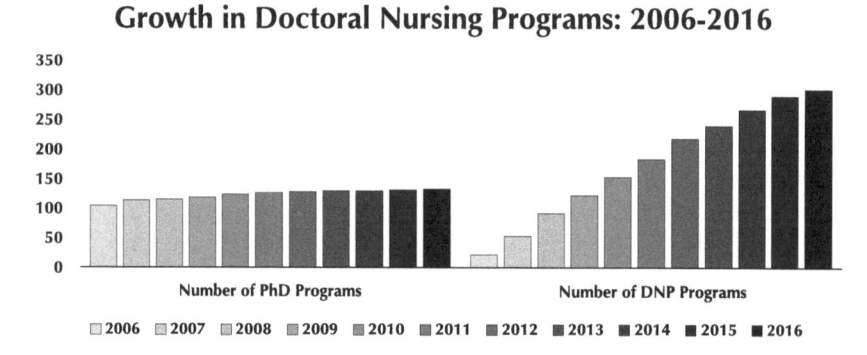

Figure 3.2. *Growth in Doctoral Nursing Programs: 2006–2016. Source: American Association of the Colleges of Nursing, June 2017.*

patient care. "The nurse manager is responsible for creating safe, healthy environments that support the work of the health care team and contribute to patient engagement. The role is influential in creating a professional environment and fostering a culture where interdisciplinary team members are able to contribute to optimal patient outcomes and grow professionally," said the AONL in 2015. The skills needed to lead at this level require both experience and continued formal education. To prepare a cadre of nurse managers who can ascend to the highest levels of nursing and hospital leadership, the nursing profession needed to set standards for degree progression in leadership positions.

Clinical leadership in nursing (the nurse manager) should not be confused with the emerging new role of the clinical nurse leader. This role was conceptualized by the AACN and a body of nursing leaders in 2003 (AACN, 2007). This new role was designed to prepare advanced generalists who would focus on transforming care at the unit level. Their role had specific aims to improve patient outcomes, reduce health care costs, and improve satisfaction of both staff and patients by focusing on eight competencies, including (1) clinician, (2) educator, (3) advocate, (4) outcomes manager, (5) information manager, (6) team manager, (7) systems analyst/risk anticipation, and (8) member of the profession (Joseph & Huber, 2015).

Dr. Carol Mest, PhD, RN, ANP-BC, Professor of Nursing and Director of Graduate Nursing Programs, has the following vision for the Executive DNP at DeSales University:

> Work on the development of the DNP Program at DeSales University commenced in 2005. The initial focus was to develop a post-Master's DNP Program in clinical leadership in order to build upon our highly successful nurse practitioner and CNS Master of Science in Nursing (MSN) programs. As the committee discussed the various position statements, definitions, white papers, and toolkits that were published by AACN and National Organization of Nurse Practitioner Faculties (NONPF), it became clear that the true vision and definition of advanced nursing practice was not restricted to direct care activities. Rather, advanced practice was defined to include 'any form of nursing intervention that influences health care outcomes for individuals or populations, including the direct care of individual patients, management of care for individuals and populations, administration of nursing and health care organizations, and the development and implementation of health policy.' (AACN, 2004).
>
> The DNP Curriculum Committee began a series of discussions regarding this expanded definition. Faculty buy-in was not immediate. The committee discussed Boyer's definition of Scholarship of Practice to further understand how an executive-focused DNP meets the vision of advanced practice nursing. In addition, we revisited the vision and outcomes of our existing MSN/Master of Business Administration (MBA) Dual Degree Program, which was launched in 1999, to ascertain how the MSN/MBA and DNP visions

and strategies might overlap and support each other. The MSN/MBA was developed in response to the demand by health care industry leaders for nurses serving in executive leadership positions to possess sophisticated skills in business administration, management, and health policy. According to our original proposal, the concurrent development of expertise in business management and in the nursing sciences affords the individual a theoretical understanding of nursing as both a scientific and practice discipline. The ultimate synthesis of these knowledge bases produces a graduate who cannot only assume an executive management role but also can impact the relationships between management and service providers. This focus and intention convinced the faculty that a DNP in Executive Leadership was not only warranted but also needed. This focus adds the dimension of administration to the research-education-clinician feedback loop.

The DNP in Executive Leadership, therefore, satisfies the intent of the DNP focus. In addition, the program allows us to continue to serve the health care industry by producing graduates who can apply administrative skills to the improvement of patient outcomes. These graduates are needed to develop the business models needed in the clinical arena to assure quality, safety, and improved outcomes for individuals and populations. Degree progression for nurse leaders that provides options for interdisciplinary knowledge and skills is critical to the continued growth of the profession. Nurse leaders who speak the language of both nursing and business have opportunities to lead organizations, to interface with all stakeholders, and to initiate change that will improve health outcomes as well as improve the environment for practicing nurses. Strategic and tactical approaches to leadership, organizational conflict, policy change, and ethical dilemmas are a significant part of the DNP in Executive Leadership curriculum.

To add an additional degree of depth to the program, an MBA option is offered as part of the DNP in Executive Leadership. Students who opt to complete the MBA take additional courses that focus on organizational and financial management, human resources, managed care, and legal and fiscal issues in health care management. Graduates of this DNP with MBA Program have gone on to achieve and successfully execute roles in health care organizations that include Chief Nursing Officer, Chief Nursing Executive, Executive Vice President of Nursing, Director of Quality and Improvement, Nurse Consultant, and director of various health care business units, to name a few. Several of these graduates are employed in top-tier academic medical centers where the impact of their DNP education can be experienced on a national level. As more nurses follow opportunities to become empowered within the profession, degrees such as this will continue to attract students who will use their education to maximize their impact on health care from a systemic, rather than solely clinical, perspective.

Building Personal Resilience

When considering the ability of an individual to positively adjust to adversity through the lens of resilience, strategies that build personal strengths include the following: (a) building positive and nurturing professional relationships; (b) maintaining positivity; (c) developing emotional insight; (d) achieving life balance and spirituality; and (e) becoming more reflective (Cross, 2015; Jackson, Firtko,& Edenborough, 2007). To survive and thrive in these environments, DNP nurse executives must role-model cogent behaviors and strengthen personal resilience in an effort to reduce their own personal vulnerability, and minimize the personal impact of adversity in the workplace. Table 3.2 offers key tactics and tools.

Additional resilience and well-being strategies acknowledge that executives must return to the "basics" in building personal strength—learning from situational experiences:

- Ongoing learning is an important element in the sustained development of a leader.
- When operating in environments where change is ever present, resilience and the capacity to learn become crucial skills.
- Leaders must role model a level of resilience and self-care in responding to crises and challenging situations. Team members seek to emulate leaders, thereby expanding their expertise in dealing with similar situational experiences.
- Daily workplace conversations should include "well-being" discussions where leaders underscore the need for all team members to practice self-compassion and finding a suitable work-life balance.

Emotional Intelligence

Goleman (1998) offer three ability clusters that characterize effective leaders. The first cluster is cognitive or intellectual ability, described as follows: (a) the content of the body of knowledge within their respective fields; (b) self-management of intrapersonal abilities as demonstrated by the speed, effectiveness, and efficiency with which they can adapt to everchanging situations and environments; and (c) interpersonal abilities, or the effectiveness and methods used to relate to others. The second and third clusters are commonly defined as emotional intelligence competencies (Goleman, 1998).

Definitions and components of EI within the literature begin with the seminal work, *Emotional Intelligence*, by Salovey and Mayer (1990), wherein they introduce the term as "a form of social intelligence that involves the ability to monitor one's own and others' feeling and emotions, to discriminate among them and to use this information to guide one's thinking and actions" (p. 189). Salovey and Mayer (1990) identified four key branches: (a) the ability to perceive emotions in oneself and others accurately; (b) the ability to use emotions to facilitate thinking; (c) the ability to understand emotions, emotional language, and the signals conveyed by emotions; and (d) the ability to manage emotions so as to attain specific

*Table 3.2 Key Tactics and Key Tools
to Build Personal Resilience in the Workplace.*

Key Tactics	Key Tools
Creating and sustaining professional relationships and networks	• Taking the time to create and maintain a network of people that can be your 'sounding board,' particularly when emotions are running high. • The more you can sustain a network of people with whom you feel secure, the more opportunities you will have to rely on the elements of this network to help you think things through, recognize your emotional triggers, and find a prudent response. • This network is a place where you know you can gather reliable feedback, whether good or bad, that will help you identify behaviors that either need to change or continue.
Maintaining a positive outlook	• Resilient people seem to be capable of consistently finding and focusing on some positive element within any situation. Whether it is a behavior, an attitude, or a frame of mind, resilience is demonstrated through the capacity to find and communicate ongoing positive elements or emotions amid any situation. • By framing things in this positive way, they seem more likely to achieve.
Identifying emotions	• An increasing number of workplaces have introduced the concepts of Emotional Intelligence (EI). • At its most basic definition, EI is the capability to enhance awareness of moment-to-moment emotions and triggers within one's own reaction to a situation, recognizing emotions and triggers within others, and managing the environment by finding ways of reducing the impact of the current stressful situation. • The use of journaling and self-reflection are oft-cited methods for developing awareness of the emotions and triggers within oneself. • A tool initially developed for teachers that can also be used is the *Meta-Moment*. At its core, the meta-moment helps to develop self-regulation in the response to triggers by allowing the individual to take a moment between the trigger and the emotional response (for more information, see RULER from the Yale Center for Emotional Intelligence (www.yale.edu/ruler).
Having an anchor of any kind (whether spiritual or religious)	• Allowing individuals to have clarity around what they define as their 'North Star' or 'True North,' which reminds them of what is truly important. When faced with a stressful situation, individuals that can reconnect with their anchor, which allows them to take a second, recognize the moment, and act accordingly.
Taking the time to reflect	• Journaling and reflective writing allow the individual to ascribe meaning to events (Jackson, 2000). • Taking a couple of minutes on a habitual basis to reflect on the day (or situation) will allow the individual to start recognizing any patterns of emotions, triggers, or behaviors, and find ways of inhabiting the knowledge within them. • Additional resources can include developing intentional attention and awareness while practicing gratitude, compassion, acceptance, forgiveness, and a higher meaning, and journaling about these events later on (Chesak *et al.*, 2015).

goals defined as: perceiving, using, understanding, and managing emotions, as illustrated in Figure 3.3.

Goleman (1995) built upon the work of Salovey and Mayer (1990) by introducing the term "EI" into leadership and development conversation throughout the world; branching out into education through programs based on social and emotional learning (SEL) and by adding to the definition "a trait not measured by IQ tests—a set of skills, including control of one's impulses, self-motivation, empathy and social competence in interpersonal relationships" (Goleman, 1995).

The five key elements as outlined by Goleman (1995) are (1) self-awareness, (2) self-regulation or discipline, (3) motivation, (4) social awareness, and (5) relationship management (otherwise known as empathy), each of these contributing to the overall composition of an individual in unique situations and relationships (see Figure 3.4).

In understanding these key elements that follow, note the overlap of ideas and techniques previously offered in discussing "resilience":

1. *Self-awareness*: The ability to know one's emotions, values, and goals and being able to recognize how they can affect those around you. One development technique includes journaling and the habitual use of reflection around any salient situations that surface during the work day. "Slowing down" also promotes self-awareness and is akin to resilience-promoting techniques. Reflecting on simple situational questions enables a clear examination of situation facts such as the following: What is really happening? What do you know for sure? What is

```
                    Emotional Intelligence
           ┌────────────┬──────────┬──────────┐
      Perceiving      Using   Understanding  Managing
                                              Emotion
```

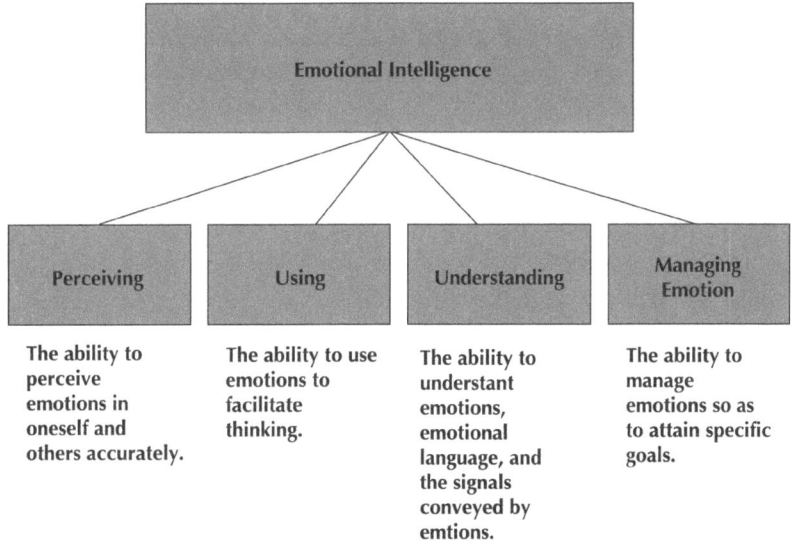

Perceiving	Using	Understanding	Managing Emotion
The ability to perceive emotions in oneself and others accurately.	The ability to use emotions to facilitate thinking.	The ability to understant emotions, emotional language, and the signals conveyed by emtions.	The ability to manage emotions so as to attain specific goals.

Figure 3.3. *Emotional Intelligence (EI); The seminal work by Salovey and Mayer (1990).*

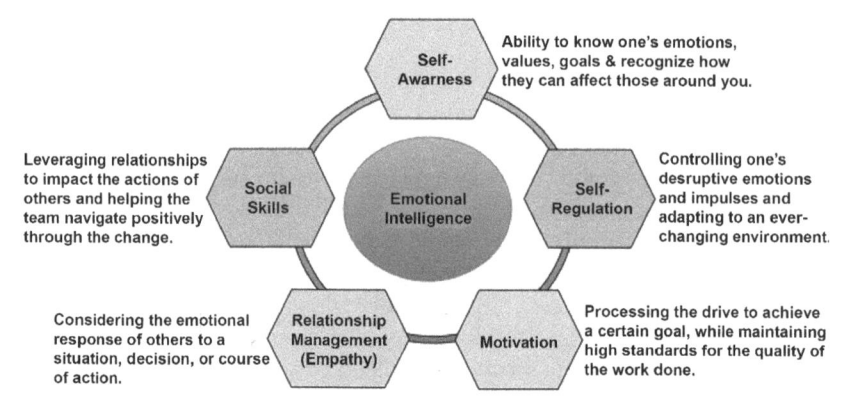

Figure 3.4. *Key Elements of Emotional Intelligence. Adapted from Goleman, 1995.*

the right response, not the emotional response? This element is resonant with the tools and ideas related to resilience.

2. *Self-regulation or discipline*: Controlling one's disruptive emotions and impulses and adapting to an ever-changing environment. An essential component to the development of self-regulation is a clear sense of direction and/or values. Clarity of values promotes decision-commitment and the development of a comfortable "accountability zone" in making difficult decisions. Since the most outward-facing behavior associated with self-regulation is the ability to maintain calm amid a storm, the leader who successfully self-regulates more easily gains the trust and support of team members.

3. *Motivation*: Possessing the drive to achieve a certain goal, while maintaining high standards for the quality of the work done. Successful leaders set a clear target, identify goals associated with a target, and finally ensure that both their actions and those of their teams are in close alignment. An effective leader knows their true motivator and easily articulates what energizes them.

4. *Social Skill*: Leveraging relationships to impact the actions of others and helping the team navigate positively through the change. Developing this skill requires listening and being fully present in the moment. Leaders successful in developing social skills reflect solid conflict management skills and the ability to effectively communicate with different audiences.

5. *Relationship Management* (Empathy): Considering the emotional response of others to a situation, decision, or course of action. Developing a sense of empathy is highly dependent on being able to 'read' the emotional reactions of others. It requires careful and curious listening, observing body language, and acknowledging feelings.

Although EI plays a role in all interactions, it is important to consider that within the realm of the DNP nurse executive, EI may play a larger role as it affects subjective well-being and a leader's work-life quality and requires a better emotional understanding of the complex situations inherent in working with the paradoxical nature of human beings.

Behavioral Styles

At the most basic level, behavioral styles are defined as a collection of observable behaviors that an individual develops over time. It is a collection of the way in which a person communicates, arranges priorities, manages time, engages with others, and organizes and communicates ideas and information. Successful DNP nurse executives exhibit the ability to develop self-awareness, identify their own areas of opportunity, and flex their style as needed. As outlined by Merrill and Reid (1981), "The modification of one's approach in order to improve an interpersonal relationship does not constitute a lack of sincerity or a Machiavellian desire to manipulate. Quite the opposite, it demonstrates respect for another person's right to be unique" (1981, p. 4).

Communication expertise plays a key role in determining the effectiveness of leaders. The Jungian Philosophy provides the foundation for instruments that measure communication styles; an understanding of this philosophy begins with a review of Carl Jung. Carl Jung, born in 1875, worked with Freud and then went on to create the school of analytic psychology; his work focused on the idea of individuation and analysis of the self-regulating psyche. Jung defined the psyche as "the totality of all psychic processes, both conscious and unconscious" (Jung, 1921). Jung was insistent on including not only the conscious mental functions (normally referred to as the mind), but also the content of both the unconscious and collective unconscious. He viewed the unconscious as "material that has been made unconscious artificially" (Campbell, 1971, p. 34) and the collective unconscious as "an absolute unconscious which has nothing to do with our personal experience (…) it goes on independently of the conscious mind and is not dependent even of the upper layers of the unconscious, untouched—and perhaps untouchable—by personal experience" (Campbell, 1971, p. 34).

The combination of both conscious and unconscious elements would become known as the *self*, defined by Jung as follows: "I have suggested calling the total personality which, though present, cannot be fully known, the *self*." (Campbell, 1971, p. 142). The *self* operates as a self-regulating system (like many living organisms or ecosystems will). As an individual develops in life, the conscious and unconscious elements of the *self* will want to develop while at the same time trying to maintain a balance between them. This desire for development is known as Individuation, a central idea in Jungian texts.

Further definitions of key elements are included in Table 3.3, as well as ideas on how each of them contributes to the development of the whole person.

Practicing components of Jung's philosophy include awareness of a preferred demonstration of being, thinking and communicating, and understanding that under conditions of stress leaders inevitably revert to an unconscious level. Behavior differences are "a result of preferences related to the basic functions our personalities perform throughout life" (Kroeger and Thuesen, 1988, p. 11).

Behavioral analysis instruments begin with the assumption that trait differences in the communication behaviors of individuals are produced by an individuals' temperament regardless of external factors such as upbringing and education. Merrill and Reid (1981) use the combination of *assertiveness* and *responsiveness* to create four distinct quadrants (and social style characteristics). In most social interactions, when people seek things from one another, they make requests and, in doing so, they may demonstrate a high level of *assertiveness* (on one end of the spectrum) or use a more passive approach (on the other end of the spectrum). The other dimension is *responsiveness*, directly related to the way in which a person responds to the requests (or demands) others make of them. On one end of the spectrum is the sociability element (a focus on relationships) on the other is a focus on tasks (see Table 3.4). When combining both axes (assertiveness and responsiveness), there are four behavioral style categories that emerge: amiable, analytical, driver, and expressive.

The first two styles (*Amiable* and *Analytical*) share low assertiveness behaviors, evidenced by a person's likelihood to ask for something, rather than demand or tell. If the person is particularly passive, he or she may not ask simply to avoid the possibility of conflict.

1. *Amiable* (High responsiveness, Low assertiveness): These individuals are people-oriented and sociable. Their higher levels of responsiveness will become evident in their higher emotional responses to others.
2. *Analytical* (Low responsiveness, Low assertiveness): These individuals are concerned with being organized, having all the facts, and being careful prior to action. They place a high value on accuracy, precision, order, and methodical approaches. They tend to be task-oriented, relying on facts and data. Lower levels of responsiveness make them less likely to have emotional content in their actions, allowing space for a higher cognitive element (they think more before responding, sometimes delaying their responses).

The second two styles (*Driver* and *Expressive*) share high assertiveness

Table 3.3 Components of Jungian Philosophy.

Component	Definition	Contributions to the Whole of the Individual
The Ego	Center of consciousness: The ego takes the most relevant information from its surrounding environment and determines how it will be used for decisions.	• This is where awareness resides and the person's sense of identity and existence manifests. • Organizes thoughts, senses, feelings, and intuition. • Determines how the person relates to the external world as either introverted or extroverted.
The Personal Unconscious	The place where irrelevant or painful information is stored and to be used at some point in the future.	• Seen as the data repository of underdeveloped and archived information that is available as needed for some future purpose.
Complexes	Diverse yet themed organization of the unconscious mind which is formed by experiences and/or reactions to experiences.	• Centered on emotions, wishes, memories and perceptions which balance the one-sided view of the ego so that development can occur.
The Collective Unconscious	The belief that people are born with a set of unique elements that either grow or languish in the environment to which they are exposed.	• These elements are influenced by various moments in the person's life (parents, relatives, major events, cultural influences, spirituality) • These elements come together and become part of the psyche and portrayed as stories and myths.
The Self	The Self is the total psyche, including the entirety of the individual's given potential.	• Drives the ability of the individual to reach their fullest potential throughout process of becoming an individual.
Persona	The element of the personality that adapts for personal convenience and is typically seen as that which brings out the person's best qualities.	• The Persona is the part that allows us to interact socially in a variety of situations with relative ease.
The Shadow	The elements of the personality which encompass personal traits that we dislike and are accessible from the conscious mind.	• The Shadow plays an important role in the balancing of the psyche, as without a well-developed shadow the individual may become preoccupied with their perception of others.
Anima and Animus	The elements of male and female in which the experiences with members of the opposite gender create individualized experiences.	• Anima and Animus are opposites, yet balance one another out in the psyche. One is not seen as better than the other.
Individuation	The quest for completeness of the human psyche.	• Individuation is the journey of a person towards attaining uniqueness that is not better or worse than another's journey.

Source: http://journalpsyche.org/jungian-model-psyche/.

behaviors evidenced by a person's tendency to tell others or demand things he or she wants, rather than asking or not saying anything. This person is more likely to address conflict head on, instead of avoiding it.

3. *Driver* (Low responsiveness, High assertiveness): Both action and goal oriented. Decisive, independent, disciplined, practical and efficient. These people will rely on facts and data, speaking and acting quickly. Their lower levels of responsiveness make them less likely to have emotional content in their actions, allowing space for a higher cognitive element (they think more before responding, sometimes delaying their responses).

4. *Expressive* (High responsiveness, High assertiveness): Primarily idea-oriented. They have little concern for routine, instead focused on the future. They tend to be sociable, stimulating, enthusiastic, and good at involving and motivating others. Their higher levels of responsiveness will become evident in their higher emotional responses to others.

These four styles can exist within an individual at any given point in time. Agile leaders are those who can adjust their style to fit both the situation and the individual. Over time, individuals will prefer one particular

Table 3.4 Communication Behavior Styles of Individuals.

	Driver	Expressive
High Assertiveness	*Both action and goal oriented.* Decisive, independent, disciplined, practical and efficient. They will rely on facts and data, speak and act quickly. Their lower levels of responsiveness make them less likely to have emotional content in their actions, allowing space for a higher cognitive element (they think more before responding, sometimes delaying their responses).	*Primarily idea-oriented.* They have little concern for routine, instead focused on the future. They tend to be sociable, stimulating, enthusiastic, and good at involving and motivating others. Their higher levels of responsiveness will become evident in their higher emotional responses to others.
	Analytical	Amiable
Low Assertiveness	These individuals are concerned with being organized, having all the facts, and being careful prior to action. They place a high value on accuracy, precision, order, and methodical approaches. They tend to be task-oriented, relying on facts and data. Their lower levels of responsiveness make them less likely to have emotional content in their actions, allowing space for a higher cognitive element (they think more before responding, sometimes delaying their responses).	These individuals are people-oriented and sociable. Their higher levels of responsiveness will become evident in their higher emotional responses to others.
	Low Responsiveness	**High Responsiveness**

style, which will start to become part of their behavioral preferences; however it is important that they receive caution about the possibility of these behaviors interfering with their true intentions (Merrill & Reid, 1981).

Change in Nursing: The Leadership Mindset of the Future

The ongoing evolution of educational standards for nurses represents a time of significant "unfreezing" (Lippitt, Watson, & Westley, 1958) for the nursing profession, a time of dramatic large-scale change in hospital leadership and clinical roles, expectations, advanced educational programs, and new professional identities. How effectively members of the profession manage the day-to-day challenges in today's health care industry while also preparing for the leadership roles in the C-Suite of the future remains uncertain. However, nursing leaders and the entire nursing profession can look for guidance to Senge and other thought leaders (1999) in large-scale change. Senge *et al.* (1999) tell us that the most successful change initiatives require large investments of time, energy, and resources; are connected to real work goals and processes that can improve performance; involve individuals who have the power to take action on the goals; balance action and reflection; and focus on increasing capacity—both individually and collectively. As a greater number of nurses aspire to top leadership roles in the health care industry, the leaders of the nursing profession must embrace their central role as capacity builders—not only for individual nurses, nurse managers, and executive colleagues, but also for the sustainability and enrichment of the nursing profession.

The nurses who become DNP leaders in hospital C-Suites—a primary audience for this textbook—and the APNs who aspire to the DNP will need to develop a new mindset and new values associated with a leadership role. According to Charan, Drotter, and Noel (2001), one of the most difficult step-by-step transitions to make in the workplace is from being an individual contributor to being a leader and then from that leader to the leadership in the C-Suite. When nurses work as individual contributors, their value depends upon their ability to achieve tasks with both efficiency and effectiveness. In contrast, as a hospital leader—whether in the C-Suite or in an advanced nursing practice—the new nurse executive must depend on a host of others to accomplish the work of the organization. As Charan *et al.* warned in 2001, leaders are obliged to embrace their organization's values as if they were their own, focus on planning the work that must be done, understand and appreciate the team's skill and knowledge, and dedicate time and energy to coaching and developing other members of the team.

In 2016, Avolio set forth a leadership development blueprint, which clearly delineates a four-level path for leaders—from self-leadership through interactive, generative, and strategic leadership. This path assumes a certain level of self-awareness and developmental readiness. As the leader moves through the blueprint, there is a complete transformation that begins, as Charan *et al.* (2001) emphasized, with an assumption of the organization's values and alignment with them. This is achieved through creating an environment in which members of the team can be engaged and fully aligned with the team's purpose within the organization. This environment is one that allows for growth, development, difficult conversations, and difficult decision-making. As leaders mature and develop, they can move away from day-to-day tasks and move into helping their team understand possibilities, developing leadership abilities in others, and serving as a role model for the ideals of the organization and the team. This balance of transactional abilities and transformational tasks is at the core of successful leaders (Avolio, 2016).

In earlier work, Avolio (2004) explained that the impact of a transformational leader extends beyond their own team: "Transformational leaders influence followers' organizational commitment by encouraging followers to think critically by using novel approaches, involving followers in decision-making processes, [and] inspiring loyalty" (p. 953). This emphasis on novelty echoes the long-standing focus from Senge *et al.* (1999) on the importance of learning and the search for "new, guiding ideas and innovations in infrastructure " within organizations (Senge *et al.*, 1999, p. 44); the belief from Swearingen (2009) that new nurse leaders are expected to learn through trial and error, like their predecessors on the team; and the recommendation from Eraut (2011) that strong DNP executive leaders create environments in which other individuals on the team are given opportunities to learn and grow through engagement with a wide variety of diverse work processes. In 2007, Eraut had identified a shift away from formally established mentors, coaches, direct supervisors, and line managers to a more informal group of "helpful others."

Thus, as Senge *et al.* (1999) suggested for those involved in change initiatives, new DNP-prepared executive leaders must work to expand their role as capacity builders. They are obliged to invest in helping their front-line clinical leaders develop a robust portfolio of skills and abilities that will positively influence staff retention. The critical importance of this leadership function for nurse leaders cannot be underestimated because, as Swearingen (2009) emphasized, "turnover in health care is higher among first-level leaders such as charge nurses, assistant nurse managers, and nurse managers" (p. 108). The continued professional development of these nurses is critical, because their work affects the management of the hospital staff, resources, and direct patient care and, ultimately, the financial health of the organization. Nursing leaders must assume responsibility for maintaining their organization's talent pipeline that requires a balance between leaders who are ready to ascend upward in the leadership ranks and the pipeline of leaders for the future (Charan et al., 2001).

Another dimension of nurses achieving higher levels of educational preparation and new leadership roles is the difficult issue of the imposter syndrome. Initially thought to exist primarily among successful women, this syndrome was first defined by Clance and Imes (1978) as ". . . an internal experience of intellectual phonies; (…) despite outstanding academic and professional accomplishments, women who experience the imposter phenomenon persist in believing that they are really not bright and have fooled anyone who think otherwise" (p.1). The syndrome has been shown to affect both genders who work in a variety of occupations.

The seminal work by Clance and Imes (1978) identified four different behaviors that were associated with the syndrome.

1. *Diligence and hard work*: Those who suffer from this syndrome are constantly afraid they will be revealed as someone who lacks the experience, knowledge, or expertise to do the job at hand. The individual falls into a continual cycle—"worry about intelligence, hard work and cover-up strategies, good grades or performance, approval and temporary good feelings"—which does not relieve "the underlying sense of phoniness [that] remains untouched" (p. 4).

2. *A sense of phoniness*: Insecurity in a new leadership role can motivate individuals to withhold their own personal opinions or to align themselves with other individuals with opinions that differed from their own.

3. *Using charm or perceptiveness to gain approval*: This behavior has a dual goal, which is to be both "liked as well as to be recognized as intellectually special" (Clance & Imes, 1978, p. 5). Unfortunately, the underlying negative self-dialogue is that if the person was indeed smart/competent, he or she would not need to use charm to gain any approval.

4. *Masking behavior*: The fourth behavior is the link between success in females and their place and acceptance in society. As defined by the authors: "as long as she maintains the notion that she is not bright, she imagines that she can avoid societal rejection" (Clance & Imes, 1978, p. 6).

The central dynamic of the impostor syndrome is an internal experience of intellectual and professional incapability despite objective evidence to the contrary (Clance & Imes, 1978). Individuals who experience this syndrome believe that their success is due to luck or error, and they live in constant fear of being unmasked as unintelligent or less capable (Clance, 1985; Harvey & Katz, 1986; Jostl, Bergsmani, Luftenegger, Schober, & Spiel, 2012).

Thus, nursing leaders who are now in transition to new heights of leadership in health care organizations—either in the C-Suite or in an advanced practice setting—must guard against self-doubt as they move forward with their professional development. As executive leaders, they will bring nursing into the center of decision-making that will guide the health care industry through the transformative times that lie ahead. This process will require them to do the following: maintain focus on developing a robust portfolio of executive leadership skills; embrace their critical roles as capacity builders, innovators, and evaluators within their health care organizations; develop and nurture an extensive network of positive and professional relationships; build bridges between patient care teams and the hospital's executive team; strengthen their resilience in the face of adversity and uncertainty; and advance their professional commitment to engaging in the relentless pursuit of new ideas and solutions that will lead to improved hospital systems and better outcomes for patients, caregivers, and hospitals.

In the new, evolving landscape of nursing leadership in 2019, the nursing profession appears to be moving forward through terrain that is new but is clearly grounded in Boyer's wise guidance from the past. Years ago, Boyer (1990) challenged professional disciplines to embrace what he envisioned as the full scope of scholarship. Such scholarship, Boyer said, involves discovery (new and unique knowledge is generated), teaching (teacher creatively builds bridges between his or her own understanding and the students' learning), application (emphasis is on the use of new knowledge in solving society's problems), and integration (new relationships among disciplines are discovered).

Chapter Takeaways

1. Large-scale change requires nurse executives to engender enthusiasm and gain support, develop detailed implementation plans, impeccably execute implementation, and then transparently monitor and evaluate.
2. Experienced nurse leaders offer competencies necessary to ensure novice nurse executive success, such as a grounded clinical subject matter expertise, an understanding of business models, and the ability to develop programs that advance safe patient outcomes while ensuring workforce stability.
3. Understanding the components of the "Imposter Syndrome" and how this phenomenon easily limits one's career may enable nurse executives to better address the syndrome's negative professional effects.
4. The continued rise in the number of DNP-prepared nurse leaders cre-

ates challenges in academia and practice as both settings struggle to define the degree components and best utilize new skills sets of program graduates.
5. Leadership skills necessary to develop high functioning teams include identifying resiliency and well-being strategies to foster growth in leaders and followers and to contribute to an engaging and rewarding work environment.

Chapter Summary

The nursing profession is in the midst of a major transition in which the preferred minimum requirement for entry into the top ranks of leadership practice is now the doctor of nursing practice. This chapter reviewed the progressive evolution of the entry level degree requirements for nurses, the parameters of the ongoing clinical research that provided the empirical evidence for the advanced standards, the large-scale change processes that are underway in health care, and the skills and perspectives that new nursing leaders must develop to succeed in their role as leaders and change agents in transforming our healthcare system into one that provides seamless, affordable, quality care. In addition, this chapter offered important discussions surrounding resilience, well-being, and emotional intelligence. A thorough discussion of behavioral styles underscored the importance of social engagement and effective communication as rooted in Jungian Philosophy.

As identified by Ketefian and Redman (2015), this transition to doctoral-level executive leadership preparation—based on the urgency for better quality, greater reliability, improved safety, patient-centeredness, efficiency, effectiveness, equity, and new leadership in health care as set forth by the IOM—will be filled with uncertainties at the individual and systems levels. What is certain, Ketefian and Redman suggest, is that in the future, there will be challenges in the graduate education of nurses. These will include, but will not be limited to, controversy about the length of DNP programs, the essential curricula that will prepare DNP nurses to assume their roles as C-Suite executives and nursing faculty, and the nature of the interaction between DNP and PhD graduate programs. Given the critical importance of the emerging decisions that lie ahead, Ketefian and Redman offered a warning for the nursing profession. As nursing moves forward, it will be essential that "careful evaluation and a deliberative progression forward" ensures that evidence is available to guide future directions. As Salmond and Echevarria (2017) reminded us, "Collecting that evidence of effectiveness and leading and participating in ongoing improvement to ensure excellence will require exquisite teamwork as excellence crosses departments, roles, and responsibilities (…)" (p. 25). Nurses must now ask themselves if they are ready.

Chapter Reflection Questions

1. As a DNP-prepared nurse leader planning to work with fellow institutional leaders to launch a massive organizational change, what critical steps must you carefully execute to achieve success?
2. Magnet-designated institutions demonstrate significantly better work environments. What factors contribute to advancing these improved work settings and how does an improved workplace environment contribute to improved patient outcomes?
3. Leaders with high EI manage their emotions in productive ways, which underpins rational decision-making, assists followers to become more effective workers and better communicators, and demonstrates sensitivity to their own and their followers' feelings and emotions. Describe a situation wherein a leader practiced a high level of EI and relate its effect on members in the workplace.
4. Overlap appears to exist between EI and resilience potentially because components of resilience (flexibility, adaptability, a positive outlook, and open and transparent communication) may be building blocks for EI. Can you identify a connection between the two? Can a leader with low or no resilience be emotionally intelligent?
5. In your role as a DNP-prepared nurse executive, consider the following cases. Can you identify the prevalent style?
   a. There is a new member on your senior leadership team, and upon meeting with this person, your intention is to break the ice and start to form a relationship. You approach in a nonthreatening way (in your mind) by telling them a joke. As soon as you do, the person stares at you blankly. You realize you have begun on the wrong foot. What happened? Which behavioral preference were you demonstrating?
   b. You are a big believer in the value of peer feedback and you approach one of your peers with the intention of providing them with fair and honest feedback by reviewing every fact in a methodical and detailed way. Halfway through the conversation, you notice things are not going well. What style were you demonstrating? How do you keep yourself from thinking your peer is not interested in your feedback?

References

Aiken, L., Clarke, S., Cheung, R., Sloane, D., & Silber, J. (2003). Education levels in hospital nurses and surgical patient mortality. *Journal of the American Medical Association, 290*(12), 1617–1623.

Altmann, T. (2011). Registered nurses returning to school for a bachelor degree in nursing: Issues emerging from a meta-analysis of the research. *Contemporary Nurse, 39*(2), 256–272.

American Association of Nurse Anesthetists. *AANA announces support of doctorate for entry into nurse anesthesia practice by 2025.* Retrieved from http://www.aana.com/newsandjournal/News/Pages/092007-AANA-Announces-Support-of-Doctorate-for-Entry-into-Nurse-Anesthesia-Practice-by-2025.aspx.

American Association of Colleges of Nursing. (2004). *AACN position statement on the practice doctorate in nursing.* Retrieved from http://www.aacnnursing.org/Portals/42/News/Position-Statements/DNP.pdf.

American Association of Colleges of Nursing. (2017). *Current DNP program statistics.* Retrieved from http://www.aacnnursing.org/News-Information/Fact-Sheets/DNP-Fact-Sheet.

American Nurses Credentialing Center. (2018). *ANCC magnet recognition program.* Retrieved from http://www.nursecredentialing.org/Magnet.

American Organization of Nurse Executives (AONE). (2015). *Nurse executive competencies.* Retrieved from http://www.aone.org/resources/nec.pdf.

Avolio, B. (2016). *The leadership development blueprint. CLST Briefing* 2016-1. Seattle, WA: Center for Leadership and Strategic Thinking.

Boyer, E. (1990). *Scholarship reconsidered: Priorities for the professoriate.* Princeton, NJ: The Carnegie Foundation for the Advancement of Teaching.

Campbell, J. (1971). *The portable Jung*, New York: Penguin.

Charan, R., Drotter, S., & Noel, J. (2001). *The leadership pipeline: How to build the leadership powered company.* San Francisco, CA: Jossey-Bass.

Chesak, S., Bhagra, A., Schroeder, D., Foy, D., Cutshall, S, Sood, A. (2015). Enhancing resilience among new nurses: Feasibility and efficacy of a pilot intervention, *The Ochsner Journal, 15*(1), 38–44.

Clance, P. R. (1985). *The impostor phenomenon: Overcoming the fear that haunts your success.* Atlanta, GA: Peachtree Publishers, Ltd.

Clance, P. R., & Imes, S. A. (1978). The imposter phenomenon in high achieving women: Dynamics and therapeutic intervention. *Psychotherapy: Theory, Research & Practice, 15*(3), 241–247.

Cross, W. (2015). Building resilience in nurses: The need for a multiple pronged approach. *Journal of Nursing Care, 4*(2).

Eraut, M. (2007). Learning from other people in the workplace. *Oxford Review of Education, 33*(4), 403–422.

Eraut, M. (2011). Informal learning in the workplace: Evidence on the real value of work-based learning (WBL). *Development and Learning in Organizations: An International Journal, 25*(5), 8–12.

Goleman, D. (1995). *Emotional Intelligence: Why It Can Matter More Than IQ.* New York: Bantam Books

Goleman, D. (1998). *Working with emotional intelligence.* New York: Bantam

Goleman, D., Boyatzis, R (2017). Emotional intelligence has 12 elements. Which do you need to work on? Harvard Business Review.

Harvey, J.C., & Katz, C. (1986). *If I'm so successful, why do I feel like a fake? The impostor phenomenon.* New York: Pocket Books.

Institute of Medicine. (2010). *The future of nursing: Leading change, advancing health.* Retrieved from http://www.nationalacademies.org/hmd/Reports/2010/The-Future-of-Nursing-Leading-Change-Advancing-Health.aspx.

Jackson, D., Firtko, A., & Edenborough, M. (2007). Personal resilience as a strategy for surviving and thriving in the face of workplace adversity: a literature review. *Journal of Advanced Nursing, 60*(1), 1–9.

Joseph, L. & Huber DL. (2015). Clinical Leadership Development and Education for Nurses: Prospects and Opportunities. *Journal of Healthcare Leadership, 7*, 55–64. Retrieved from https://doi.org/10.2147/JHL.S68071

Jostl, G., Bergsmani, E., Luftenegger, M., Schober, B., & Spiel, C., (2012). When will they blow my cover? *Zeits- chrift Fur Psychologie-Journal of Psychology. 220*(2), 109-120.

Jung, C. G. (1921). Psychological types, Collected Works, Vol. 6

Ketefian, S. & Redman, R. (2015). A critical examination of developments in nursing doctoral education in the United States. *Rev. Latino-Am. Enfermagem, 23*(3): 363–371. Retrieved from http://dx.doi.org/10.1590/0104-1169.0797.2566

Kritsonis, A. (2004-2005). Comparison of change theories. *International Journal of Scholarly Academic Intellectual Diversity, 8*(1), 1–7.

Kroeger, O., Thuesen, J. (1989). *Type Talk: The 16 Personality Types That Determine How We Live, Love and Work.* New York: Dell Publishing.

Lavizzo-Mourey, R. (2012, April 1). The nurse education imperative. *Pediatric Nursing, 38*(2), 61–62.

Lippitt, R., Watson, J., & Westley, B. (1958) *The Dynamics of Planned Change: A comparative study of principles and techniques.* New York: Harcourt, Brace & World Incorporated.

McHugh, M., Kelly, L., Smith, H., Wu, E., Vanak, J., & Aiken, L. (2013, May). Lower mortality in Magnet® hospitals. *Med Care, 51*(5), 382–388.

Merrill, D., Reid, R. (1981). *Personal Styles & Effective Performance.* New York: CRC Press.

Mitchell, G. (2013, April). Selecting the best theory to implement planned change. *Nursing Management, 20*(1), 32–37.

Salmond, S. W. & Echevarria, M. (2017). Healthcare transformation and changing roles for nursing. *Orthopedic Nursing, 36*(1), 12–25. Retrieved from http://doi.org/10.1097/NOR.0000000000000308

Salovey, P., Mayer, J. (1990). Emotional intelligence. *Imagination, Cognition, and Personality, 9*(3), 185–211.

Senge, P., Kleiner, A., Roberts, C., Ross, R., Roth, G., & Smith, B. (1999). *The dance of change: The challenge to sustaining momentum in learning organizations.* New York, NY: Doubleday.

Stichler, J. (2011, May 1). Leading change—one of a leader's most important roles. *Nursing for Women's Health, 15*(2), 166–170.

Swearingen, S. (2009). A journey to leadership: Designing a nursing leadership development program. *The Journal of Continuing Education in Nursing, 40*(3), 107–112.

Tri-Council for Nursing. (2010, May). Educational advancement of registered nurses: A consensus position. Retrieved from http://www.aacn.nche.edu/Education/pdf/TricouncilEdStatement.pdf

NANCY B. LERNER

4

The Clinical DNP Practice Environment and Leadership Transformation

Chapter Objectives

- Describe the historical antecedents of current advance practice roles.
- Discuss the transition process and barriers to transition for moving advanced practice education to the doctoral level.
- Analyze the development of DNP roles that utilize skills consistent with the essentials of DNP education.
- Discuss future possibilities for the development of new roles for DNPs, especially through the needs of the aging population.

KEY WORDS: DNP; APRN, expanded role, Long-term care

Introduction

The development of expanded roles for doctor of nursing practice (DNP) graduates, especially those who are certified advanced practice nurses (APRN), is developing. Although leadership roles for DNPs previously in leadership roles have developed, the added leadership competences for APRN DNPs still require additional explanation and demonstration. The changes in health care brought on by the Patient Care and Affordable Care Act (ACA), continually rising health care costs, and access discrepancies are changing the focus of the system and opening new opportunities. The "greying of America" and primary physician shortages have developed new roles for APRNs in long-term care and outpatient care, and these roles include the need for nurses competent in leadership, policy development, and administration providing new and exciting opportunities for DNP APRNs.

APN Role Transformation

As a practice focused doctoral degree, the DNP is tied to and a continuation of the development of multiple advanced practice nursing (APN) roles (AACN, 2006). Although the DNP was developed only 15 years ago, the evolution of APN roles has been developing for almost 50 years and, for nurse midwife and nurse anesthetist, even longer. The development of these APN roles have some of their roots in the history of the practice, especially the relationship between APNs and other health care team members. The clinical nurse specialist (CNS) role emerged as a singular specialty-focus that did not experience many of the "turf battles" of other APN groups. Midwives and nurse anesthetists developed as early specialty nurses largely due to their female gender. Physicians only adopted maternity care in the late 1800s and then only for wealthy clients (Ehrenreich & English, 1973; Wertz & Wertz, 1977). Nurses were the sole practitioners of anesthesia delivery until the advent of separate payment for the service with development of Medicare/Medicaid reimbursement which attracted large numbers of physicians (Clapesattle, 1969; Ray, 2015). Conversely, nurse practitioners (NPs) developed differently. Pediatricians began training nurses in this expanded role. The nursing profession and educational institutions were slow to embrace the new role and engage in training these "physician extenders." As the numbers and types of NPs spread, supported by physician and patient evaluation, education increasingly shifted to university-based nursing academic programs (Ford, 1979). Table 1 illustrates the timeline for the development of the APN specialties.

APN Transition to the DNP

In 2004, the American Association of Colleges of Nursing (AACN) presented its position paper on the practice doctorate as a replacement for various clinical nursing doctorates existing at that time. This document acknowledged that APNs needed additional education for the higher level of practice that society required. The paper recommended that a practice doctorate (the doctor of nursing practice) should be the basic education level for APNs, including nurse midwives, nurse anesthetists, and nurse practitioners (AACN, 2004). The move from the master's level to the DNP was recommended by 2015.

The advent of the DNP degree and designation of the degree as the preferred one for APNs has resulted in a proliferation of DNP programs in the United States (U.S.). In 2016, there were 303 existing DNP programs, with an additional 124 programs in the planning stage. There were over 25,000 students enrolled in these programs. Since the advent of DNP programs, there have been only 4,855 graduates (AACN, 2016), although the number of these graduates who are midwives, anesthetists, CNSs, and NPs could not be identified since recipients of the DNP degree include educators and nursing administration specialists. As of 2019, there exists no requirement by any state Board of Nursing to require that APNs

Table 4.1 Development of APN Specialties.

Specialty	When Developed	Formal Education Level	Accreditation	Reimbursement	Requirement for DNP for Licensure/Certification
Midwife	Biblical references	1925; Universities recommended after 1929	1955; American College of Nurse Midwives	In hospital only with MD collaboration agreement	None currently planned
Nurse Anesthetist	1860s	Late 1800s to early 1900s; Hospitals then universities 1998; 24–26-month programs	1952; American Association of Nurse Anesthetists	1986	2022 fully implemented
Clinical Nurse Specialist	Early 1900s; Referred to nurses in specialty fields especially psychiatric nursing	1974; CNS with MS as a requirement and supervised practice	1980; Specialty certification through appropriate professional society	1995; After NACCNS established	None currently planned
Nurse Practitioner	1965; Pediatric expanded role	1965; 4 months didactic and 20 months precepted clinical as a continuing education program 1970s programs moved to MS academic education	1970s; Professional organizations began certification. Certification transitioned to the AANP Certification Board who tests nationally	1997; With certification and 5 year renewal	AACN mandated DNP for NP begin in 2015 but no states have implemented yet

secure an DNP degree. The American Association of Nurse Anesthetists, however, requires that, by 2025, all candidates for certification must be educated in DNP programs.

Currently, the masters of science in nursing (MSN) is still the predominant entry level for APNs. As of 2015, 70% of schools educating APNs offered only MSN programs; of those schools offering a BSN-DNP, 65% continue to also offer MSN degree programs (Rand Corporation, 2015). Failure to require the DNP as the APN practice entry degree creates a barrier to further increasing DNP APN preparation and decreasing or fully eliminating MSN preparation. Others barriers to DNP preparation include cost, faculty resources, clinical sites and preceptors, and managing capstone projects (Rand Corporation, 2015).

DNP Role Development

The history of APN role development and corresponding practice opportunities has been a long and difficult one, of which DNPs should be cognizant. Finding locations where they can practice independently has been a struggle for nurse anesthetists, midwives, certified nurse specialists, and NPs. APNs have had to use a variety of techniques to establish their place in the health care system (Martin & Hutchinson, 1997), Because DNPs today find themselves in much the same position, the techniques used previously should be evaluated.

New DNPs describe having to explain their role and the difference between PhD and DNP practice. The lack of established mentors who are DNPs has made carving out a role, fully utilizing the DNP essentials, difficult; many APNS have found their job the same before and after their DNP education. Some APNs have even had to deal with MSN-prepared peers who do not see the need for a practice doctorate (Glaskow & Zoucha, 2011).

These DNPs also experience Chief Nursing Officer (CNO) confusion about the role in general and, specifically, the DNP/APN role. Some CNOs have a limited understanding of the clinical and population outcomes that are improved by a DNP's knowledge and skill. Without an understanding of the benefits of DNP education, the duties of DNP- and MSN-prepared NPs are treated the same (Nichols, O'Connor, & Dunn, 2014).

Understanding of APN and DNP roles

Integration of APN roles into the health care system and into cohesive interdisciplinary teams is a necessity in responding to the changing demands of the quickly evolving health care system. When developing teams for care delivery, it is imperative that administrators understand the roles and different skill sets of team members. Although APNs are accepted as valued members of outpatient teams, their role in acute care institutions is less well accepted, with ambiguity and confusion about the differing roles of CNSs and NPs (Anen & McElroy, 2017). The introduction of the role of the DNP APN has further muddied the waters, since understanding the CNS role in many places has been unclear. Clinical nurse specialist competencies include direct patient care, leadership, consultation, education, case management, and project direction (NACNS, 2017). These are similar competencies that are found in the DNP essentials and are included in NP competencies (NONPF, 2017). Hospital administrators, including nurse administrators, rely on their experience in working with APNs. Developing roles in their facilities and understanding that the use of these two different positions has been difficult for them and others in their facilities to understand. This confusion results in using APNs, especially NPs, in primarily clinical roles in direct patient care rather than utilizing the broad competencies APNs possess or using CNSs for some positions (Jokiniemi, Pietila, Kylma and Haatainen, 2016). Since 85% of hospital NPs' work time is in direct and indirect patient care, their activities are billable. These practitioners' work patterns are more easily understood by administrators than work patterns of the CNSs (Johnson, Brennan, Musil, & Fitzpatrick, 2016). One hospital-defined role for the DNP APN is leading acute care hospital NP services.

Vignette 1: The Role of the DNP in Leadership

Developing a leadership and reporting structure for NPs and physician assistants (PAs) in an academic medical center requires strategy, goal setting, and support from hospital executives. As medical directors recognized the need for advanced practice providers, integration of this role into the medical model was discussed, imagined, piloted, and revised. This required a framework for successful development of the role and integration into existing clinical teams. Recruitment, onboarding, orientation, competency-based accountability for procedures, and professional advancement required a systematic and evidence-based approach, and the doctoral education positioned this leader to develop the strategy for success. Over 10 years, the organization has developed over 230 new jobs, and the work force has grown to over 300 providers during this leader's tenure. The need for the leader to be flexible, articulate, and educated to dissect the complexity of this integration benefitted the workforce. For example, many teams practice in different ways. Surgical services had different provider gaps than unit-based teams. Surgery programs were challenged to provide more surgical experience for their trainees, requiring a skilled workforce to provide daily preoperative and postoperative management, care coordination, discharge readiness, and followup care.

Advanced practice providers actively participate in other hospital mandates, such as readmission, throughput, length of stay, discharge readiness, and hospital acquired infection rates. Key to these initiatives was the leader's inclusion at the highest organizational levels to forecast changes and to educate the workforce regarding their insight, value, and expertise in solving the challenges associated with ensuring these quality and safety initiatives.

The DNP education prepared the APN leader to understand and navigate complex health systems, evaluate the evidence, and recommend best practice guidelines at every level. There was no bias against the DNP academic degree at this organization. Instead, the degree received support and recognition. There are now 25 NPs who hold DNP credentials in this institution and participate in quality, safety, and process improvement teams as part of their roles.

Submitted by Carmel A. McComiskey, DNP, PPCNP-BC, CPNP-AC, FAANP, FAA

With regard to expanding the roles of DNP APNs, how can information on the relationship of various positions to the DNP essentials be disseminated to health care administrators? Although evidence-based information on the various roles of APNs is available in the literature and online, barriers to role dissemination exist. These include a perceived lack of time, organizational constraints and, for smaller health care facilities, lack of access to updated published material. In a Canadian survey of health care administrators including nurse administrators, almost half of survey participants wanted additional information on DNP APNs or DNP APN roles. Those administrators who requested more information wanted it disseminated through tailored strategies, such as emails, one page abstracts or briefing notes, and explanatory care plans (Carter *et al.*, 2014; Dobbins, Jack, Thomas, & Kothari, A. 2007). A potential role for DNPs who are also APNs is to work with these administrators to provide the personalized information that will help to clarify the roles of APNs in these settings, thereby facilitating the APN role expansion to use all of their competencies.

DNP APN Possibilities in an Aging and Diverse Health Care Population

In 2011, the Institute of Medicine (IOM) released its report on the future of nursing. This report emphasized that the future of health care in the U.S. required chronic disease management, increased preventive care, and increased primary care including interprofessional coordination and prevention of adverse health events. The demand to increase health services in long-term care, primary care, school health services, mental health care, and palliative care is necessary to meet future needs. The report emphasized that nurses needed to respond by assuming new roles and assuming leadership in developing a better health care system (IOM, 2010). The DNP, especially for APNs, is one important component in answering the IOM challenge.

Increase in Aging Population

The population in the U.S. is getting older and more racially diverse. In 2014, 46 million citizens in the U.S. were over 65, comprising 15% of the population. By 2030, the aging of the "baby boomers" will increase, resulting in the over 65 population increasing to 74 million, comprising 21% of the population. The racial diversity of the older population will also change. Currently whites compose 78%, with blacks at 9%, Hispanics at 8%, and Asians at 4%. By 2060, the percent of the over 65 population who identify as white will be 55%, with blacks at 12%, Asians at 9%, and Hispanics at 22% (Federal Interagency Forum on Aging-Related Statistics, 2016).

Many older Americans suffer from heart disease, cancer, stroke, diabetes, hypertension, and arthritis, and most have more than one of these conditions. Most of these conditions are costly to care for and largely preventable (CDC, 2016). It is estimated that by 2050, 16 million people over age 65 years will have dementia (Alzheimer's Association, 2016). This is important both for the long-term care population (41% to 68% of nursing home residents have dementia) and the community, in which 10% of the age 65 years and older population and up to 30% of the age 85 years and older population have dementia (Federal Interagency Forum on Aging-Related Statistics, 2016).

The increasing numbers of older adults combined with the preventable chronic diseases they have are especially important for both DNP APNS. The volume of care needs in long-term care and community care will be increasing, whereas the proportion of medical doctors (MDs) who specialize in primary care is declining. By 2025, it is estimated that an overall shortage of between 46,000 and 90,000 MDs will exist, resulting in a primary care shortage of between 12,500 and 31,100. This shortage will exacerbate since only 25% of new MDs pursue a primary care specialty (Chen *et al.*, 2013).

APNs in Long-Term Care

Medical care in nursing homes is dependent on outside contractors who have medical privileges granted by the facility. Having a medical director has been a federal requirement for nursing homes since 1974. Depending on the nursing home, these medical directors can be relatively uninvolved in the direction of the facility or very involved. Sometimes, the medical director is the physician of record for most or all of the residents, although recently they have served primarily as medical policy facilitators supervising the care others provide (Nanda, 2015). Over time, physicians have been less willing to provide care in nursing homes, perhaps because of lack of geriatric training, financial disincentives, and fears of lawsuits (Intrator *et al.*, 2015). The responsibility for resident care has largely been filled by NPs and PAs but primarily NPs, as greater practice independence has been granted to them over time. The result of this increase in the use of NPs has been increased cost-effectiveness of care, as well as decreased emergency room transfers (Lacny *et al.*, 2016). Also, NP care in nursing homes produces no difference or better overall outcomes over physician care (Lovink *et al.*, 2017). In an era in which hospital readmissions are unpaid by the Centers for Medicare and Medicaid Services (CMS) for the majority of elderly hospital patients, who have diseases known to be high for readmission, NP care in nursing homes decreased this number (Xing, Mukamel, and Temkin-Greener, 2013).

The increased aging of the population, especially those over age 85 years, should greatly increase the need for long-term care beds in future years. With the decreasing numbers of primary care physicians, combined with physician reticence to work in nursing homes, the need for highly prepared NPs in long-term care can only continue. The DNP APN can use increased skills, both in caring for the increasing acuity of nursing homes and in working with physician groups to manage large numbers of NPs working in these facilities. The skills of DNPs can also be used for development of quality control initiatives, such as decreasing emergency room and hospital transfers, improving transition of those patients who require hospitalization and reduce overall spending (Rantz, Birtley, Flesner, Crecelius, & Murray, 2016]).

Another possible new direction for DNP APNs is in the assisted living sphere. Assisted living beds, a long-term care option based on a social rather than health care model, have been increasing, whereas nursing home beds have been decreasing (Mollica, Houser, & Ujvari, 2012). Assisted living facilities are not regulated by CMS; therefore, requirements for medical care in these facilities are left to individual states. The health care needs of the residents in these facilities have been increasing, approaching the complexity of the status of NH residents (Caffrey, Harris-Kojetin, Rome, & Sengupta, 2014). The same constraints affecting the lessening number of primary care physicians and reluctance to work in long-term care can be considered a factor making assisted living facilities an increasing market for the skills of a DNP APN. Setting up APN practice involves learning about specific state regulations, identifying billing mechanisms, and negotiating with the administration. Since licensed nurses are not required for assisted living facilities in most states, the DNP APN would have to consider how to ensure appropriate nursing backup (Han, Trinkoff, Storr, Lerner, & Yang, 2016). Going even further, entrepreneurial DNP APNs could consider opening and running their own assisted living facility or group of facilities or developing a group practice of NPs who would specialize in the provision of primary care in assisted living facilities.

Vignette 2

Doctor of nursing practice education has profoundly moved me to be a consummate nursing professional. This level of education has helped me to understand myself better. It has especially helped me understand I am capable of accomplishing. It is as if I am looking through a different lens. I owned and operated an assisted living (AL) for 14 years prior to completing my DNP. I thought I had it all together. I had deficiency free surveys and felt like I knew it all. I also felt stuck because I had been doing things the same way for so many years. My work became more perfunctory and didn't require a lot of thinking. After completing the DNP, I regained my zeal for assisted living. It was a like a burst of energy and renewed strength. I began thinking of potential changes that I could make. I saw many areas that were in need of improvement, but of course I had to consider costs. I began setting up systems for tracking and documenting, creating communication tools, and developing staff education materials. With these changes, I am now able to see better workflow and improvement in resident care. I confidently share evidence-based information with my patients, staff, colleagues, and families. I have this inner drive to know more and share the knowledge. I am always reading scholarly materials and looking for conferences to attend. I've expanded my area of practice (substance abuse) and now have to establish myself in my new community. When reflecting on my participation on the MBON's Medication Technician/Delegating Nurse Committee, I feel that it is necessary to have a voice and contribute to change in an area that you are passionate about. I have prioritized participating on various committees and workgroups.

As I continue to embark upon this new journey, I have freely and openly embraced thinking out of the box. I am always looking for opportunities to discover new things and new ways of achieving change. Although acquiring DNP education was a huge sacrifice, when looking at what I have gained I have no regrets.

Submitted by Crystal Greene, DNP, AGPCNP-BC

APNs in Primary and Urgent Care

In 2001, the Institute of Medicine called for a profound change in how health care was delivered in the U.S. (IOM, 2001). Through an increase in primary and preventive care and a focus on patient-centered health care, the report proposed a fundamental shift from illness to wellness care to increase the health status of the population and reduce the costs of health care. Subsequent reports emphasized the importance of nursing in reaching these goals (IOM, 2010; AACN, 2004). The development of the DNP APN role is positioned to assist in fulfilling these goals. To focus on prevention and, at the same time, confront disparities in health care delivery, primary care in communities is key. APNs are a low cost, high quality solution to these issues. However, while ideally suited to work in primary care settings, primary care is still the purview of primary care physicians, especially in urban and suburban areas. The reduction in primary care MD specialists, combined with an increase in NPs, is poised to change that distribution (Auerbach, et al., 2013).

Nurse managed health centers, especially in states in which NPs can work independently,are assisting in the transition. DNP APNs will be needed to organize and manage the centers, provide leadership for master's-prepared NPs, and formulate policies and procedures based on evidence. These nurse leaders can also collaborate with physicians for back up and referral for more complex cases. Nurse managed clinics committed to patient-centered care and prevention can also provide a setting different from the retail centers where visits increased between 2007 and 2009, surpassing nurse managed clinics (Mehrotra and Lave, 2012). Much of the limitations to the development of nurse-managed clinics resides in the inability of NPs in certain political jurisdictions to function at the full extent of their training and experience. DNP APNs have a responsibility to work with other health care providers, policy makers, and elected officials to remove the barriers to independent practice (Cashin, Theophilos, & Green, 2017).

Table 4.2 Supply of Primary Care Practice Providers in 2010 and 2025.

Provider Type	2010 Number	2010 Percent of Total	2025 Number	2025 Percent of Total	Percent Change 2010–2025
Physicians	210,000	71	216,000	60	3
Nurse Practitioners	56,000	19	103,000	29	85
Physician Assistants	30.000	10	42,000	12	37
Total	296,000	100	361,000	100	23

Auerbach et al., 2013.

A similar opportunity for DNP APNs exists in the rapidly developing urgent care centers in the U.S., often in coordination with hospitals. These centers function as an adjunct to physician practices, which provide a limited number of office hours and rarely after-hours appointments. In addition, hospitals and consumers are anxious to eliminate non-emergent visits to crowded and expensive emergency rooms (Memmel & Spalsbury, 2017). APNs in emergency rooms often function as a "fast track" for non-critical patients, decreasing costs and wait times and freeing physicians for patients with severe threats to health. Using APNs in urgent care centers allows these centers this same benefit (Memmel & Spalsbury, 2017). APNs in urgent care have been found to deliver care that is similar in quality to MD care (University of California, 2013).

Vignette 3

I have been the Manager of Quality & Education of a large health care system's ambulatory clinics since October 2013. Armed with my MSN with a focus on education, I felt qualified, capable, and successful in creating, teaching, and facilitating multiple projects and seminars. I approached each project as it was handed to me with little thought of a framework or structure. My methods changed dramatically in the fall of 2016 when I began my DNP journey.

I was recently notified of a break in my organization's system around the influenza vaccine administration plan. I was tasked with "fixing" the break. Previously I would have developed an education plan and rolled it out. My current approach is different in that I think in complex adaptive systems and mind maps. System problems are not linear but complex in nature, with a chaotic pattern similar to atoms in a closed beaker. The ability to look at the problem from "30,000 feet" gives new insight on dissection of the problem and the solution. The project began with identification of the problem within a framework. Extensive research was done through CINAHL, PubMed, and Medline]. Implementation of the Six Sigma quality improvement method of reducing defects through the phases of define, measure, analyze, improve, and control (DMAIC) guided progression of the project. In the measure and analyze phases, data points were collected to determine influenza vaccine rates from the previous 2 years and medication errors with a root-cause analysis to determine gaps in care and processes. For the implementation phase, a mind map was designed with influenza vaccine administration in the center and multiple arcs extending from the nucleus. Each arc led to a multidisciplinary subtopic that consisted of senior leadership, IT, nursing education, infection prevention, and pharmacy. Based on the research, a multidisciplinary approach has been shown to be more effective in implementation of influenza vaccine programs than a single-armed approach for implementation and sustainability. The project was rolled out to all of the primary care and pediatric offices within the organization through educational modules completed via WebEx, then recorded for purposes of review, remediation, and new employee education. The control phase for sustainability will consist of weekly measures of metrics and patient safety events as data points, chart audits, and weekly communication with clinic managers.

Management of ambulatory clinics, whether for a system or for individual centers, is a good role for DNPs to consider. The role combines both leadership and management skills and the need for advanced clinical knowledge.

Joyce Falkenhan, MSN, RN; DNP anticipated 5/2019

Emerging Roles

Through the increased learning experiences in a variety of patient settings and greater refinement in assessment, practice, and application of doctoral competency as described in Essential VIII, many practice locations both old and new are available to the DNP APN (AACN, 2006). These possible practice areas include wound care, pain management, and other subspecialties (Kaasalainen, *et al.*, 2016; Looman, *et al.*, 2013). Another interesting venue for practice that has the potential to expand is home visits for chronic disease management. Residential visits are a small component of all Medicare visits but ones in which APNs have a significant percentage. For example, large numbers of severely disabled adults reside in a community. It is estimated that three to four million adults in the community have three or more activity of daily living deficiencies and one million are bedbound (Ornstein *et al.*, 2015). Medical specialization and technology advancement decreased what formerly a frequently used techniques to see patients, but NPs are a natural group to manage these patients, decreasing at least the cost of ambulance transportation and often expensive hospital readmission (Yao *et al.*, 2017). DNP APNs, in addition to doing home visits themselves, could collaborate with MD groups to expand their practices through supervision and marketing of a NP home care division. Entrepreneurial DNPs can consider creating and marketing their own teams in this new and open field.

Another interesting possibility for DNP APN practice is the expanding area of care coordination. As hospitals and CMS work to reduce readmission, the importance of providing and coordinating care for patients with multiple co-morbidities becomes crucial. Although APNs have not focused in this area, their skills in assessment, diagnosis, and treatment can contribute to developing a coordinated approach and bring together multiple specialists and facilities. DNPs with experience in Essential V, interprofessional collaboration, have the skills to successfully do this coordination and help institutions to decrease readmission through timely care coordination. These DNP APNs can intervene at the first sign of exacerbation of an illness to obtain necessary intervention and prevent a problem.

Care coordination, long-term care, outpatient and urgent care, and home care are especially important considering the possible profound changes in payment mechanisms that have occurred recently and will continue to occur. Some of the recent changes in payment mechanisms involve hospital readmissions which, CMS, followed quickly by other insurers, failure to reimburse. The readmissions reduction program developed in 2012 as an outgrowth of the ACA (CMS, 2012) has reduced the readmission rate by 7.9% for Medicare patients, 5.8% for privately insured patients, and 4.0% for uninsured patients. CMS has also created a four model Bundled Care Initiatives, which use pilot projects involving the four models. The first model is the traditional Medicare payment system, but models 2 to 4 test retrospective payments and prospective payments, which include all locations, including medication for an episode of illness. Awardees can be acute care hospitals, skilled nursing facilities, physician group practices, home health agencies, inpatient rehabilitation facilities, and long-term care hospitals that trigger an episode of care (CMS, 2017a). To profit financially from bundled payments requires strict care coordination as well as the utilization of less expensive providers. Working in this new potential payment mechanism, both clinically and intraprofessionally, and in a policy perspective, is an opportunity for DNP APNs with experience in Essentials I, II, IV, and V (AACN, 2006).

Also, in line with CMS cost reduction strategies is the Medicare Waiver, which has been in effect since 1982. Maryland, the only state to retain the waiver, has agreed to initiate the Care Redesign Program (CRP). This program, which allows CMS to pay for hospitals for uninsured care in Maryland, will have hospitals reimbursed for the total cost of care on a per capita basis (population in surrounding communities) not per admission basis (CMS, 2017b). This project, like the bundled payment project, addresses the health care system payment method in the U.S. to decrease the rising cost of medical care and to increase its quality.

Chapter Takeaways

1. APN specialties including the nurse midwife, nurse anesthetist, clinical nurse specialist, and nurse practitioner originated at different times in nursing history, with the nurse midwife and nurse anesthetist beginning with nurses as the only practitioner.

2. Assisted living, a social model, provides a prime market for DNP APN entrepreneurs to own and manage a facility.
3. Emerging roles for APNs include managing urgent care centers, supervising home care of disabled individuals, and directing care coordination. Each role fills a vital need in the expanding care networks of patient centered medical home and accountable care organizations.

Chapter Summary

Over the last 50 years, the development of the multiple roles of advanced practice nurses (APNs) and the environments in which they practice have been dramatic. APNs now work in and are an integral part of the health care system. Unfortunately, there are still many barriers to full practice, including misunderstandings about the differing roles and impediments to APN self-governance. The development of the DNP APN role, educated in evidenced-based practice and inter-professional collaboration, is an advancement of the role designed to enable APNs to lead in improving the health care system and the health of served populations.

Chapter Reflection Questions

1. How do you envision DNP education influencing how you perform your current role?
2. What can the DNP community do to influence the acceptance of the DNP entry into APN practice?
3. What role do you envision for yourself following the granting of your DNP degree?

References

Alzheimer's Association. (2016). *Alzheimer's disease facts and figures*. Retrieved from https://www.alz.org/documents_custom/2016-facts-and-figures.pdf.

American Association of College of Nursing (2004). AACN *Position statement on the practice doctorate in nursing*. Retrieved from http://www.aacnnursing.org/DNP/Position-Statement.

American Association of Colleges of Nursing (2006). *The essentials of doctoral education for advanced nursing practice*. Retrieved from http://www.aacnnursing.org/DNP/DNP-Essentials.

American Association of Colleges of Nursing (2015). *The Doctor of Nursing Practice: Current Issues and Clarifying Recommendations Report from the Task Force on the American Association of Colleges of Nursing (2015). The Doctor of Nursing Prac-*

tice: Current Issues and Clarifying Recommendations Report from the Task Force on the Implementation of the DNP. August 2015

American Association of College of Nursing (2016). DNP fact sheet. Retrieved from http://www.aacnnursing.org/News-Information/Fact-Sheets/DNP-Fact-Sheet

American Association of Nurse Anesthetists (2018). Retrieved from https://www.aana.com/search?keyword=mandated%20DNP.

Anen, T., & McElroy, D. (2017). The evolution of the new provider team: Driving cultural change through data. *Nursing Administration Quarterly 41*(1), 4–10.

Auerbach, D. I., Chen, P. G., Friedberg, M. W., Reid, R., Lau, C., Buerhaus, P. I., & Mehrotra, A. (2013). *Nurse-managed health centers and patient-centered medical homes could mitigate expected primary care physician shortage.* Retrieved from http://survey.hshsl.umaryland.edu/?url=http://search.ebscohost.com/login.aspx?direct=true&db=edswss&AN=000326841400012&site=eds-live.

Caffrey, C., Harris-Kojetin, L., Rome, V., & Sengupta, M. (2014). Characteristics of residents living in residential care communities, by community bed size: United States, 2012. *NCHS data brief*, 171, 1–8.

Carter, N., Dobbins, M., Peachey, G., Hoxby, H., Ireland, S., Akhtar-Danesh, N., & DiCenso, A. (2014). Knowledge transfer and dissemination of advanced practice nursing information and research to acute-care administrators. *CJNR: Canadian Journal of Nursing Research, 46*(2), 10–27. Retrieved from http://survey.hshsl.umaryland.edu/?url=http://search.ebscohost.com/login.aspx?direct=true&db=psyh&AN=2015-05754-002&site=eds-live.

Cashin, A., Theophilos, T., & Green, R. (2017). The internationally present perpetual policy themes inhibiting development of the nurse practitioner role in the primary care context: An Australian–USA comparison. *Collegian, 24*, 303–312. doi:10.1016/j.colegn.2016.05.001.

Centers for Disease Control and Prevention (2016). Chronic disease overview. Retrieved from https://www.cdc.gov/chronicdisease/overview/index.htm.

Centers for Medicare and Medicaid Services (CMS) (2012). *Readmissions Reduction Program (HRRP).* Retrieved from https://www.cms.gov/medicare/medicare-fee-for-service-payment/acuteinpatientpps/readmissions-reduction-program.html.

Centers for Medicare and Medicaid Services (CMS) (2017a). *Bundled Payments for Care Improvement (BPCI) Initiative: General Information.* Retrieved from https://innovation.cms.gov/initiatives/bundled-payments/.

Centers for Medicare and Medicaid Services (CMS) (2017b). *The Maryland all-payers model care redesign program.* Retrieved from https://innovation.cms.gov/Files/x/md-allpayer-crdfaq.pdf.

Chen, C., Petterson, S., Phillips, R. L., Mullan, F., Bazemore, A., & O'Donnell, S. D. (2013). Toward graduate medical education (GME) accountability: Measuring the outcomes of GME institutions. *Academic Medicine: Journal of the Association of American Medical Colleges, 88*(9), 1267–1280. doi:10.1097/ACM.0b013e31829a3ce9.

Clapesattle, H. (1969). *The doctors Mayo.* Minneapolis, Minnesota: University of Minnesota Press.

Dobbins, M., Jack, S., Thomas, H., & Kothari, A. (2007). Public health decisionmakers' informational needs and preferences for receiving research evidence. *Worldviews on*

Evidence-Based Nursing, 4(3), 156–163. Dobbins, M., Rosenbaum, R., Plews, N., Law, M., & Fysh, A. (2007)

Ehrenreich, B., English, D. (1973) Witches, midwives and nurses: A history of women healers. Old Westbury, N.Y.: The Feminist Press.

Federal Interagency Forum on Aging-Related Statistics (2016). *Older americans 2016: Key indicators of well-being*. Retrieved from https://agingstats.gov/docs/LatestReport/Older-Americans-2016-Key-Indicators-of-WellBeing.pdf.

Ford, L. C. (1979). A nurse for all settings: The nurse practitioner. *Nursing Outlook, 27*(8), 516521. Retrieved from http://survey.hshsl.umaryland.edu/?url=http://search.ebscohost.com/login.aspx?direct=true&db=cmedm&AN=257381&site=eds-live.

Glasgow, M. E. S., & Zoucha, R. (2011). Role strain in the doctorally prepared advanced practice nurse: The experiences of doctor of nursing practice graduates in their current professional positions. In H. M. Dreher, M. E. Smith Glasgow, H. M. Dreher (Ed) & M. E. Smith Glasgow (Ed) (Eds.), (pp. 213-226). New York, NY: Springer Publishing Co. Retrieved from http://survey.hshsl.umaryland.edu/?url=http://search.ebscohost.com/login.aspx?direct=true&db=psyh&AN=2012-04605-022&site=eds-live .

Han, K, Trinkoff, A. M., Storr, C. L., Lerner, N. B., Yang, B. (2016). Variation across U.S. assisted living facilities: Admissions, resident care needs, and staffing. *Journal of Nursing Scholarship*. Epub ahead of print (00:0) 1-9, doi 10.1111/jnu.12262.

Institute of Medicine (2001). *Crossing the Quality Chasm*. Retrieved from http://www.nationalacademies.org/hmd/~/media/Files/Report%20Files/2001/Crossing-the-Quality-Chasm/Quality%20Chasm%202001%20%20report%20brief.pdf.

Institute of Medicine (2010). *The future of nursing: Leading change, advancing health*. Retrieved from http://nationalacademies.org/hmd/reports/2010/the-future-of-nursing-leading-change-advancing-health.aspx.

Intrator, O., Miller, E. A., Gadbois, E., Kofi Acquah, J., Makineni, R., Tyler, D., & Acquah, J. K. (2015). Trends in nurse practitioner and physician assistant practice in nursing homes, 2000–2010. *Health Services Research, 50*(6), 1772. Retrieved from http://survey.hshsl.umaryland.edu/?url=http://search.ebscohost.com/login.aspx?direct=true&db=edb&AN=111343157&site=eds-live.

Johnson, J., Brennan, M., Musil, C. M., & Fitzpatrick, J. J. (2016). Practice patterns and organizational commitment of inpatient nurse practitioners. *Journal of the American Association of Nurse Practitioners, 28*(7), 370–378. doi:10.1002/2327-6924.12318.

Jokiniemi, K., Pietila, A. M., Kylma, J., & Haatainen, K. (2016). Advanced nursing roles: A systematic review. *Nursing and Health Sciences, 14*(3) 290–307.

Kaasalainen, S., Wickson-Griffiths, A., Akhtar-Danesh, N., Brazil, K., Donald, F., Martin-Misener, R., . . . Dolovich, L. (2016). The effectiveness of a nurse practitioner-led pain management team in long-term care: A mixed methods study. *International Journal of Nursing Studies, 62*, 156-167. doi:10.1016/j.ijnurstu.2016.07.022.

Lacny, S., Zarrabi, M., Martin-Misener, R., Donald, F., Sketris, I., Murphy, A. L., . . . Marshall, D. A. (2016). Cost-effectiveness of a nurse practitioner-family physician model of care in a nursing home: Controlled before and after study. *Journal of Advanced Nursing, 72*(9), 2138. Retrieved from http://survey.hshsl.umaryland.edu/?url=http://search.ebscohost.com/login.aspx?direct=true&db=edb&AN=116935196&site=eds-live

Looman, W. S., Presler, E., Erickson, M. M., Garwick, A. W., Cady, R. G., Kelly, A. M., & Finkelstein, S. M. (2013). Article: Care coordination for children with complex special health care needs: The value of the advanced practice nurse's enhanced scope of knowledge and practice. *Journal of Pediatric Health Care, 27*, 293–303. doi:10.1016/j.pedhc.2012.03.002

Lovink, M. H., Persoon, A., Koopmans, R. T. C. M., Van Vught, A. J. A. H., Schoonhoven, L., & Laurant, M. G. H. (2017). Effects of substituting nurse practitioners, physician assistants or nurses for physicians concerning healthcare for the ageing population: A systematic literature review. *Journal of Advanced Nursing, 73*(9), 2084-2102. doi:10.1111/jan.13299

Martin, P. D., & Hutchinson, S. A. (1997). Negotiating symbolic space: Strategies to increase NP status and value. *The Nurse Practitioner, 22*(1), 89. Retrieved from http://survey.hshsl.umaryland.edu/?url=http://search.ebscohost.com/login.aspx?direct=true&db=cmedm&AN=9004312&site=eds-live

Mehrotra, A. & Lave, J.R. (2012). Visits to retail clinics grew fourfold from 2007 to 2009, although their share of overall outpatient visits remains low. *Health Affairs 31*(9) 2123–2129.

Memmel, J., & Spalsbury, M. (2017). Urgent care medicine and the role of the APP within this specialty. *Disease-a-Month, 63*, 105–114. doi:10.1016/j.disamonth.2017.03.001

Mollica, R. L., Houser, A. N., & Ujvari, K. (2012). Assisted living and residential care in the states in 2010. *AARP Public Policy Institute*, 58. Retrieved from http://www.aarp.org/content/dam/aarp/research/public_policy_institute/ltc/2012/residential-care-insight-on-the-issues-july-2012-AARP-ppi-ltc.pdf

Nanda, A. (2015) The roles and functions of medical directors in nursing homes. *Rhode Island Medical Journal*. Retrieved from http://www.rimed.org/rimedicaljournal/2015/03/2015-20-ltc-nanda.pdf

National Association of Clinical Nurse Specialists (NACNS). (2017) *Policy Affecting CNSs*. Retrieved from http://nacns.org/advocacy-policy/policies-affecting-cnss/scope-of-practice/

National Organization of Nurse Practitioner Faculties (2017). *Competencies for nurse Practitioners*. Retrieved from https://www.nonpf.org/page/14?.

Nichols, C., O'Connor, N., & Dunn, D. (2014). Exploring early and future use of DNP prepared nurses within healthcare organizations. *Journal of Nursing Administration, 44*(2), 74–78. doi:10.1097/NNA.0000000000000029

Ornstein, K. A., Kelley, A. S., Siu, A. L., Federman, A. D., Leff, B., Roberts, L., . . . Ritchie, C. S. (2015). *Epidemiology of the homebound population in the united states*. Retrieved from http://survey.hshsl.umaryland.edu/?url=http://search.ebscohost.com/login.aspx?direct=true&db=edswss&AN=000357604400028&site=eds-live .

Rand Corporation (2015). Rand Health Quarterly. Retrieved from https://www.ncbi.nlm.nih.gov/pmc/articles/PMC5158236/

Rantz, M.J.,Birtley, N.M., Flesner,M., Crecelius, C. & Murray, C. (2017) Call to action: APRNs in U.S. nursing homes to improve care and reduce costs. Nursing *Outlook 65*(6), 689–696.

Ray, W.T. & Desai, S.P. (2016). Original contribution: The history of the nurse anesthesia profession. *Journal of Clinical Anesthesia 30*: 51–58.

University of California. Berkeley forum: a new vision for California's healthcare system; 2013. Retrieved from http://berkeleyhealthcareforum.berkeley.edu/wp-content/uploads/Appendix-IX.-Nurse-Practitioners-and-Physician-Assistants-Initiative-Memorandum.pdf

Wertz, R.W., Wertz, D. C. (1977). *Lying-In: A history of childbirth in America.* New York: The Free Press

Xing, J., Mukamel, D. B., & Temkin-Greener, H. (2013). Hospitalizations of nursing home residents in the last year of life: Nursing home characteristics and variation in potentially avoidable hospitalizations. *Journal of the American Geriatrics Society, 61*(11), 1900–1908. Retrieved from http://survey.hshsl.umaryland.edu/?url=http://search.ebscohost.com/login.aspx?direct=true&db=gnh&AN=EP91929553&site=eds-live

Yao, N., Rose, K., LeBaron, V., Camacho, F., & Boling, P. (2017). Increasing role of nurse practitioners in house call programs. *Journal of the American Geriatrics Society, 65*(4), 847–852. Retrieved from http://survey.hshsl.umaryland.edu/?url=http://search.ebscohost.com/login.aspx?direct=true&db=gnh&AN=EP122576428&site=eds-live

KARI A. MASTRO
JOAN GLEASON-SCOTT
CHRISTA PREUSTER

5

Healthcare System Transformation, Quadruple Aim, and Quality Improvement

Chapter Objectives

- Identify the key external drivers that guide quality improvement initiatives.
- Describe the concept of the "quadruple aim" and its application to the current practices in the delivery of care within a health care system.
- Describe the role of the DNP nurse executive in driving the AHRQ quadruple aims objectives.
- Evaluate current research and evidence-based practices in quality and safety.
- Describe patient and family-centered care and the role of the patient and family in both quality and safety.

KEY WORDS: Healthcare Transformation, Quadruple Aim, Quality Improvement, Healthcare Quality; Healthcare Safety; Workforce Burnout; Evidence-Based Practice

Introduction

Donabedian theory—the theory that examines relationships among structure, process, and outcomes (SPO)—is recognized as a leading platform for quality and safety improvement in health care (Donabedian, 1980). Donabedian's SPO model suggested that structures influence processes, which in turn influence outcomes. In relation to health care transformation and improvements in both quality and safety, Donabedian's model suggested that structures (interprofessional respect/dignity, information and knowledge sharing, participation and shared decisionmaking, collaboration and engagement) support processes (such as full engagement of the interprofessional team) and result in positive outcomes, such as excellent patient and staff satisfaction, high quality and safety outcomes, the ability of the patient to provide self-care, and reduced health care costs.

Donabedian's theory provides a guide to the transformation of health care through the development of structures that support processes of care that in turn lead to excellence in safety and quality of care. The ability to create the type of structures needed for process improvement and to lead teams through process improvement and the measurement of outcomes is an essential competency in the doctor of nursing practice (DNP) nurse executive's practice.

The Delivery of Safe, Reliable, and Effective Care

It is essential for the DNP nurse executive to develop a solid foundation in the leadership competencies associated with leading the modern health care system. As the health care system evolves, DNP nurse executives must be nimble in their approach to ensuring that the clinical teams are supported, that the culture within the health care system maintains a strong focus on safety, and that quality patient-centered care across a continuum can be provided at the lowest cost possible.

Doctorally prepared C-Suite nurse executives must understand the challenges to transformation of the American health care system and must be involved in creating approaches to navigate those challenges that ensure high performance in quality, safety, and satisfaction with patient care. Many national organizations have been working to provide health care system executives with structural guidance on transformational strategies. These transformational strategies—grounded in evidence-based practice and research—have been identified by health care organizations that innovate, develop, test, and measure the outcomes of novel practices within their organizations. One example is the Institute for Healthcare Improvement (IHI), which provides resources and research findings that have been developed by experts with significant experience in quality and safety improvement. Another is the American Organization for Nursing Leadership (AONL) (formerly the American Organization of Nurse Executives), whose Nurse Executive Competencies (AONE, 2015) underscore some of the key proficiencies nurse leaders must develop and exhibit to advance safety and quality improvements.

The Institute for Health Care Improvement

The primary focus of the IHI is providing health care organizations with support that enables the provision of safe and reliable care and the building of highly reliable systems that provide that care. In 2017, the IHI published a white paper, *A Framework for Safe Reliable, and Effective Care* (Frankel, Haraden, Federico, & Lenoci-Edwards, 2017) that focused on creating systems of safety. The report provided a framework (see Figure 5.1) that helps health care organizations constantly and methodically learn to improve pa-

Healthcare System Transformation, Quadruple Aim, and Quality Improvement 95

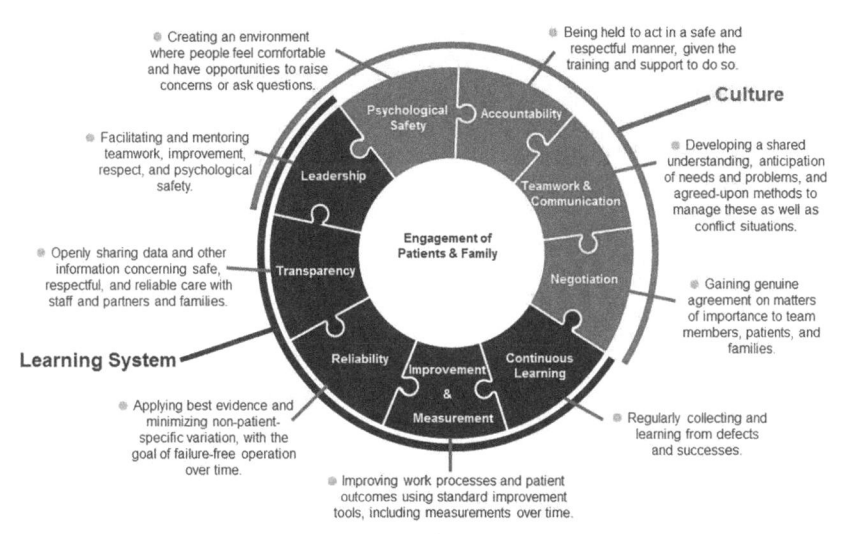

Figure 5.1. *Framework for Safe, Reliable, and Effective Care. Source: Frankel, Haraden, Federico, & Lenoci-Edwards, 2017.*

tient safety by developing the appropriate culture and learning systems that ensure patient safety.

The two domains within this framework—culture and learning systems—work synergistically. When all components are fully operational, the organization has the ability to provide safe, reliable, and effective quality care to patients.

Leadership

Each domain has four components with *Leadership* as the common component. In this construct, *Leadership* is not defined by title but by the role the individual plays in creating a culture of safety and reliability. The role of the "leader," whether formal or informal, is important in both domains, because the leader works to create a safe environment in which reliable care can be delivered and excellence in clinical outcomes can be achieved. The primary responsibilities for *leadership* include the following:

- *Guarding the learning system*: Fully engaging in the work of self-reflection that leads to transparency; understanding and applying improvement science, reliability science, and continuous learning; and inspiring such work throughout the organization.
- *Creating psychological safety*: Making sure that anyone in an organization, including patients and their families, can comfortably voice concerns, suggestions, and ideas for change.
- *Fostering trust*: Creating an environment of non-negotiable respect, en-

suring that individuals feel their opinions are valued, and any negative or abusive behavior is addressed swiftly and satisfactorily.
- *Ensuring value alignment*: Applying organizational values to every decision, whether in service of safety, effectiveness, patient-centeredness, timeliness, efficiency, or equity (Frankel *et al.*, 2017, p. 10).

Culture

The *culture* domain includes four components: psychological safety, accountability, teamwork and communication, and negotiation. *Psychological safety* allows for welcomed feedback and input. In a psychologically safe environment, anyone can raise a concern without the fear of seeming incompetent or being judged. The environment is one of respect, innovation, and safety from criticism and judgment. *Accountability* is defined as "the importance of holding people to account for their actions, but not for flaws in processes or systems" (Frankel *et al.*, 2017, p. 12). *Teamwork and communication* occur when "effective groups develop norms of conduct that lead to shared understanding, that anticipate needs and problems, and that use agreed-upon methods to manage situations—including those that involve conflict" (Frankel *et al.*, p. 14). *Collaborative negotiation* is an approach "that yields workable solutions that manage resources, provide the best options for patients, and preserve the relationships between parties" (Frankel *et al.*, p. 16).

Learning System

The learning system domain also has four distinct components: transparency, reliability, improvement and measurement, and continuous learning (and leadership). *Transparency* is the act of ensuring that staff, patients, families, and the community know how decisions are made and how performance is achieved. Transparency among clinicians, patients, between organizations, and the community is defined differently for each of these groups:

- *Transparency among clinicians* exists when there is no fear of giving suggestions, pointing out problems, or providing feedback.
- *Transparency with patients*, specifically after an adverse event, involves clearly describing what happened and what is being done to prevent it from happening again.
- *Transparency between organizations* includes sharing best practices and applying lessons learned.
- *Transparency with the community* requires robust information sharing so that patients can make informed decisions and easily access the care they need." (Frankel *et al.*, 2017, p. 17).

Organizations that achieve high levels of *reliability* have strong structures and processes in place that are evidence-based, tested, and measured consistently. The foundational principles for ensuring a reliable, safe system include the following:

- *Standardization*: This involves designing processes so that individuals do the same thing the same way every time. Standardization makes it easier to train others on the processes, and it becomes more apparent if the processes fail and where they fail, enabling the organization to better target improvements.
- *Simplification*: Greater complexity reduces the possibility of success, because there are more opportunities for mistakes, and the staff may avoid processes that are too difficult or time consuming. Simplified processes, however, make it easy for people to do the right thing.
- *Reduction of autonomy*: Health care professionals have historically functioned autonomously by making decisions based on personal preference, experience, and individual beliefs. However, this can result in variations in care and less consistent outcomes. To achieve greater reliability, organizations must set the expectation that care delivery follows evidence-based best practices, unless contraindicated for specific patients.
- *Highlight deviation from practice*: Clinicians sometimes have good reasons for departing from standardized processes. Smart health care organizations create environments in which clinicians can apply their expertise intelligently and deviate from protocols when necessary, but also relentlessly capture these deviations for analysis. After analysis, the new insights can lead to educating clinicians or altering the protocol, both of which result in greater reliability. (Frankel *et al.*, 2017. p. 18).

Improvement and measurement use a systematic improvement approach to understand a defect and systematically improve it while measuring both process and outcomes of the improvement plan. There are many different models for improvement methodologies such as LEAN, Six, Sigma, Value Stream Mapping, PDSA (Plan, Do, Study Adjust), and DMAIC (Define, Measure, Analyze, Improve, Control).

The final learning system concept is *continuous learning*, which is defined as a "proactive and real-time identification and prevention of defects and harm" (Frankel *et al.*, 2017, p. 24). The essence of continuous learning is grounded in the notion that a journey to excellence never ends, because processes must be consistently reviewed, measured, and refined.

It is essential for all hospital leaders, including the DNP nurse executive, to effectively ensure that all members of the health care team understand the evidence-based practices of these domains. Most importantly, DNP nurse executives must work to create an organizational culture with a learning system composed of transparency, reliability, continuous improvement with measurement, and continual learning. In this type of culture, individuals working within the system will feel safe to raise concerns and ask questions, and teamwork with effective communication will flourish. Ultimately, this environment leads to safer, more reliable, and effective care for patients.

The IHI is an important resource for the DNP nurse executive who will be responsible for effectively designing improvement projects that improve quality of care across the health care organization. Over 38 white papers have been developed, and this number continues to grow as the health care system evolves. These IHI resources are grounded in the latest evidence-based practice and align with two key essentials for doctoral education for advanced practice nurses: (1) organizational and systems leadership for quality improvement and systems thinking and (2) interprofessional collaboration for improving patient and population health outcomes.

The Evolution of the Quadruple Aim

The Agency for Healthcare Research and Quality (AHRQ) quadruple aim guides the work of health care organizations in the improvement of patient and organizational outcomes. The quadruple aim focuses on ensuring the highest patient satisfaction and best experience, reducing health care costs, and improving quality and safety while also addressing workforce burnout. The ultimate goal is the optimization of health system performance and high quality patient care.

It is essential for all DNP nurse executives to have the knowledge and capability to execute nursing strategies that improve the safety and quality of patient care. The primacy of quality care is patient and staff safety. Nurse executives in DNP programs study the science of safety, methods for ensuring safety, and application of safety principles and regulations. DNP nurse executives must maintain current knowledge of existing regulatory and accreditation standards, such as the Centers for Medicare and Medicaid Services (CMS) Pay for Performance program and the Hospital Accreditation Standards from The Joint Commission. In addition, understanding the science of quality methods, data-driven decision support, and the science of patient safety are essential competencies for DNP nurse executives.

The Triple Aim

In 2008, Berwick, Nolan, and Whittington first described the Triple Aim as simultaneously improving population health, improving the patient experience of care, and reducing per capita cost (Berwick, Nolan, & Whit-

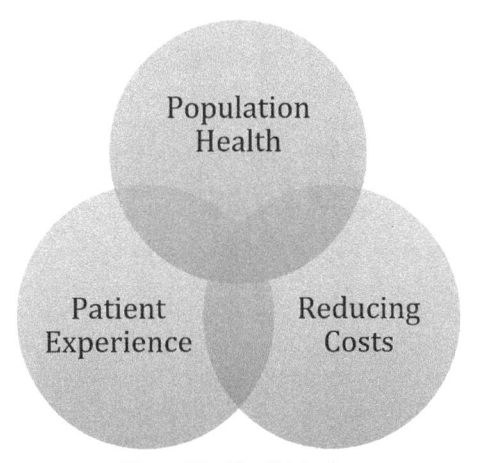

Figure 5.2. *The Triple Aim.*

tington, 2008). In 2012, the IHI's Innovation Series included a white paper, "A Guide to Measuring the Triple Aim: Population Health, Experience of Care, and Per Capita Cost" (Stiefel & Nolan, 2012).

As the Triple Aim became integrated in the health care community, the three aims became the foundation from which health care organizations identified priorities in improvement initiatives. The IHI outlined the essential principles of the Triple Aim and identified metrics, measurement principles, and strategies for improvement, which health care system leaders could use to effectively assess the operational performance within their organizations while they prioritized quality improvement initiatives.

The primary goal of the Triple Aim was to improve the health of the population. Two secondary goals include (1) improving the patient experience and (2) reducing costs while contributing to the achievement of the primary goal (Berwick *et al.*, 2008). Ultimately, the three goals were defined as improving the patient care experience, improving the health of populations, and reducing the per capita cost of health care,

These three aims have provided the guidance and the foundation for identifying priority projects, including quality and patient safety initiatives. External driving forces continue to establish priorities which, in turn, support the delivery of quality care in a safe and costeffective way. These external influences include The CMS Pay for Performance programs, which include, but are not limited to, Value-based Purchasing, Hospital Acquired Conditions, and the Readmissions Reduction Program; The Joint Commission Hospital Accreditation Standards in Leadership, Performance Improvement and Patient Safety; and population health programs selected for reimbursement payments withheld for Medicaid, uninsured patients, and patients who have signed up for governmental exchange programs (Stiefel & Nolan, 2008).

The Triple Aim provided essential principles for the identification of metrics, measurement principles, and strategies for improvement, which enabled health care system leaders to effectively assess the operational performance within their organizations while prioritizing quality improvement initiatives. There are many available data sources for each of the three dimensions: (1) patient care experience, (2) outcomes of care, and (3) cost of care.

Figure 5.3 is an example of how a health care system can use the Triple Aim as a platform for identifying priority focus areas within the annual strategic quality and safety plan. The illustration includes metrics that the organization in the example endorsed to evaluate (1) performance in the delivery of quality care, (2) the patient experience of care, and (3) the cost of care. Each source of measurement includes metrics that have been standardized by regulatory and/or accreditation bodies. Although the selection of metrics may change over time, the definitions are established and standardized by the external agencies.

Legislative and regulatory changes in the Patient Protection and Affordable Care Act (ACA) of 2010 called for an increased focus on access to high quality, affordable health care for all Americans. The National Strategy for Quality Improvement (NQS) supports the incorporation of evidence-based standards that support the development of quality and patient safety programs. An understanding of this content is essential for the DNP

The IHI Triple Aim

Population Health

Inpatient/Outpatient Services
AHRQ Patient Safety Indicators
Leapfrog Safety Practices
CMS Hospital Acquired Conditions
Value Based Purchasing Metrics

AMI, HE, PNE Mortality Rates
Patient Centered Medial Home

Experience of Care
Overall Rating of Hospital
Communication with MDs
Hospital Environment
Responsiveness of Staff
Discharge Information

Per Capita Cost

Efficiency/Hospital Level Cost of Care
CMS VBP: Medicare Spending per Beneficiary
CMS Readmissions Reduction Program
Cost of Care/DRG

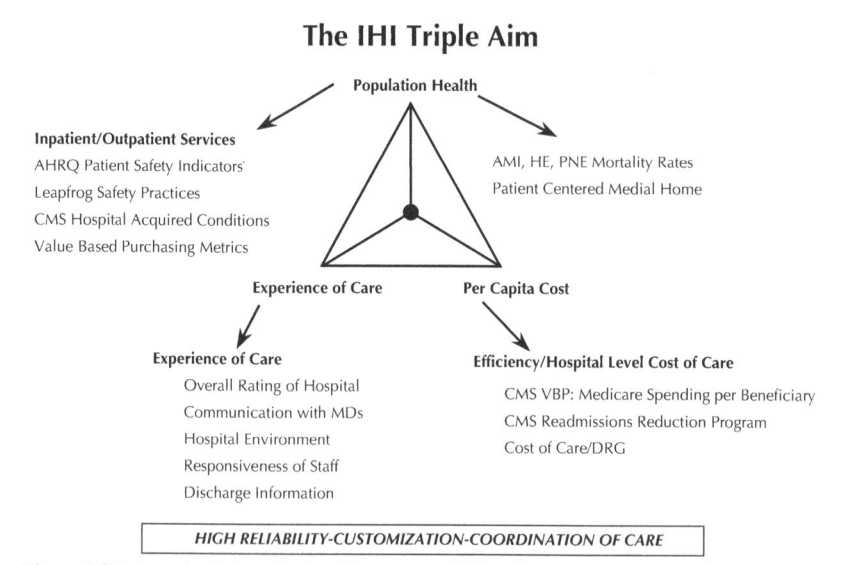

HIGH RELIABILITY-CUSTOMIZATION-COORDINATION OF CARE

Figure 5.3. *Example of Organization Priorities to Address Components of the Triple Aim. Adapted from: Stiefel, M. and Nolan, K. (2012). A Guide to measuring the triple aim: Population health, experience of care, and per capita cost. IHI Innovation Series white paper. Cambridge, Massachusetts: Institute for Healthcare Improvement; 2012. (Available on www.IHI.org).*

VBP Domains

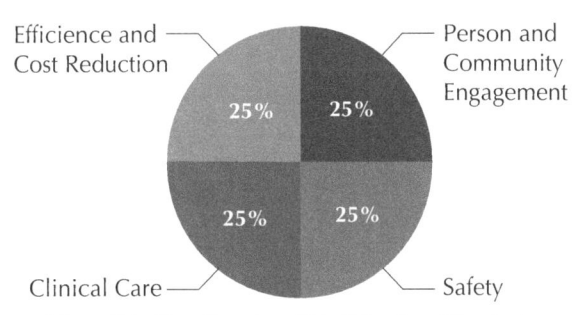

Figure 5.4. *Four Domains within Value Based Purchasing.*

nurse executive who is working with health care systems executives to drive and sustain quality of care. To advance these aims, the NQS suggests focuses on six priorities: (1) Making care safer by reducing harm caused in the delivery of care; (2) Ensuring that each person and family is engaged as partners in their care; (3) Promoting effective communication and coordination of care; (4) Promoting the most effective prevention and treatment practices for the leading causes of mortality, starting with cardiovascular disease; (5) Working with communities to promote wide use of best practices to enable healthy living; and (6) Making quality care more affordable for individuals, families, employers, and governments by developing and spreading new health care delivery models (Agency for Healthcare Research and Quality, 2018).

Value Based Purchasing

Value based purchasing (VBP), the nation's first pay-for-performance program for acute care, was set forth in Section 1886(o) of the Social Security Act. VBP changed the focus in healthcare from quantity to quality. The DNP nurse executive and all hospital executives are accountable for providing the strategic direction and operations that maximize Medicare's fee-for service reimbursement, which can be affected by fee-for-service. As shown in Figure 5.4, there are four domains within VBP.

The data used for fiscal year reporting is retrospective, with different reporting periods for each of the four domains. The VBP payments are based on a point system that recognizes each hospital's achievements on metrics since the last reporting period. If the hospital exceeds the national measures, points are awarded, whereas points are deducted if the hospital does not exceed the national expectations. The points determine the amount of reimbursement.

Achievement points, calculated for each metric from the baseline period, are based upon a comparison of individual hospitals with the national benchmark. *Improvement points* are awarded to hospitals based upon their individual improvement for each metric, as compared to the baseline performance period. Table 5.1 summarizes the retrospective dates for each metric of the VBP, along with domains, measures, and baseline period and performance periods for 2019.

Since the data for each performance period are evaluated retrospectively, the DNP nurse executive must focus on ensuring that the performance measures are met and exceed projected outcomes. In addition, the approach must be multidisciplinary with a keen focus on developing the type of organizational structures and processes that support exemplary outcomes in each domain. Although quality and patient safety are paramount to any hospital, contextual knowledge of the financial implications of key quality drivers is essential for all hospital executives, including the DNP nurse executive. Shared accountability—across the entire organization—is essential because frontline leaders can identify strategies and solutions for quality and safety for every patient, family, and colleague.

The Hospital Acquired Conditions Reduction Program

The Hospital Acquired Conditions (HAC) Reduction Program is a Medicare pay-for-performance program that supports CMS's long-standing effort to link Medicare payments to health care quality in the inpatient hospital setting. Section 3008 of the ACA established the HAC Reduction Program, which was designed to encourage hospitals to reduce conditions that were acquired during hospital stays.

Table 5.1 Value Based Purchasing Domains, Measures, and Performance Periods for Calendar Year 2019.

Domain/Measure	Baseline Period	Performance Period
Clinical Care: 30-Day Mortality Measures	July 1, 2009–June 30, 2012	July 1, 2014–June 30, 2017
Clinical Care: Total Hip Arthroplasty (THA)/Total Knee Arthroplasty (TKA) Complication Measure	July, 1 2010–June 30, 2013	January 1, 2015–June 30, 2017
Person and Community Engagement: Hospital Consumer Assessment of Healthcare Providers and Systems (HCAHPS) Dimensions	July 1, 2010–June 30, 2013	January 1–December 31, 2017
Safety: Elective Delivery Prior to 39 Completed Weeks Gestation (PC-01)	January 1–December 31, 2015	January 1–December 31, 2017
Safety: Healthcare-Associated Infection (HAI) Measures	January 1–December 31, 2015	January 1–December 31, 2017
Efficiency and Cost Reduction: Medicare Spending Per Beneficiary (MSPB)	January 1–December 31, 2015	January 1–December 31, 2017

Beginning with fiscal year 2015 discharges (effective October 1, 2014), the HAC Reduction Program requires the Secretary of Health and Human Services (HHS) to adjust payments to hospitals that rank in the worst-performing 25% of all subsection (d) hospitals on HAC quality measures. Hospitals with a total HAC score greater than the 75th percentile of all total HAC scores (the worst-performing quartile) are subject to a 1% payment reduction. For example, for fiscal year 2018, the payment adjustment applies to all Medicare discharges between October 1, 2017, and September 30, 2018. The payment reduction, realized when CMS pays hospital claims, occur in two domains.

Domain 1—Safety

Fifteen percent of the HAC score is calculated by the composite Patient Safety 90 score, which includes the following individual measures:

- PSI 03—Pressure Ulcer Rate
- PSI 06—Iatrogenic Pneumothorax Rate
- PSI 08—In-Hospital Fall with Hip Fracture Rate
- PSI 09—Perioperative Hemorrhage or Hematoma Rate
- PSI 10—Postoperative Acute Kidney Injury Requiring Dialysis Rate
- PSI 11—Postoperative Respiratory Failure Rate
- PSI 12—Perioperative Pulmonary Embolism or Deep Vein Thrombosis Rate
- PSI 13—Postoperative Sepsis Rate
- PSI 14—Postoperative Wound Dehiscence Rate
- PSI 15—Unrecognized Abdomino-pelvic Accidental Puncture/Laceration Rate

Domain 2—Infections

The HAC reduction program is also based upon hospital acquired infections (HAIs), which account for 85% of the total score. These infections include catheter-associated urinary tract infections (CAUTIs), surgical site infections (SSI), methicillin resistant *Staphylococcus aureus* (MRSA), catheter-associated bloodstream infections (CLABSIs), and *Clostridium difficile* (CDI) infection.

The CAUTI and SSI measures use National Health Safety Network (NHSN) chart abstracted surveillance data. The MRSA and CDI measures use NHSN laboratory surveillance data, which hospitals report annually to NHSN for infections. Figure 5.5 represents the methodology for calculating scores for the HAC data. With retrospective data, the DNP nurse executive and other members of the C-Suite team identify the domains that are at risk for quality and financial penalties.

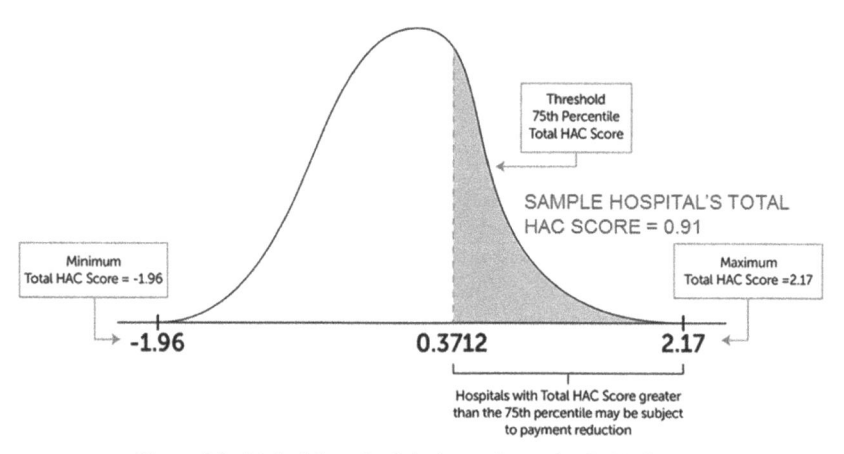

Figure 5.5. *Methodology for Calculating Scores for the HAC Data.*

Here is an example of a quality and safety plan developed by a C-Suite team that included the DNP Chief Nursing Officer, the hospital's Chief Quality Officer, and the Chief Medical Officer. In this scenario, the role of the DNP nurse executive is to be a transparent and present leader who provides real-time performance solutions that improve quality and reduce Medicare penalties. The ultimate goal is reducing HACs by using targeted aims based on the organization's performance. A gap analysis and prioritization matrix, generated by the Quality Department, was aligned with the underperforming areas. The executive team identified the following steps for reducing HACs: Charters established for improvement activities for CAUTI and CLABSI reduction and implemented by the frontline clinical staff and managers. Changes in departmental quality and safety reporting aligned with clinical and financial areas for focus at the Performance Improvement Committee and at front-line clinical staff and manager meetings.

Increased partnership with external groups, such as state hospital associations, share and learn best practices. Daily focus of clinical priorities occurs with concurrent collaboration with front-line clinical staff, quality staff, case management, and clinical documentation staff. Development of communication "maps," such as intranet communication on quality and safety successes, educational reviews, quality counsels achievements for frontline clinical staff ensure active engagement.

Hospital Readmission Reduction Program

The Hospital Readmission Reduction Program began in 2012, as CMS began a reduction in payments for the Inpatient Prospective Payment System (IPPS). Readmissions within 30 days of discharge from the hospital for acute myocardial infarction (AMI), heart failure (HF), pneumonia, chronic obstructive pulmonary disease (COPD), hip/knee replacement (THA/TKA), and coronary artery bypass graft surgery (CABG) are the diagnoses that qualify under the program. Excessive readmissions are based on a statistical method that utilizes an observed vs. expected ratio.

This program has been an influential factor in shifting a major focus in health care from providing care in acute care hospitals to outpatient and home-based services. Theoretically, population interventions and the effective management of the transitions of care can help to avoid excessive readmission. Thus, every DNP nurse executive who practices in an acute care hospital must provide the vision and leadership needed to keep patients recovering at home with the necessary knowledge, treatment, and support services.

Transition to the Quadruple Aim

The evolution of the Triple Aim to the Quadruple Aim added a key component in ensuring that patients receive the best care possible: that from health care providers. The increasing demands on health care professionals have resulted in increased stress, increased anxiety, decreased job satisfaction, a low sense of self-accomplishment, and ultimately burnout (Waterman, Garbutt, & Hazel, *et al.*, 2007). The evolution of the Triple Aim to the Quadruple Aim addresses this critical missing component. The focus of this fourth aim is to improve work life balance and decrease burnout in health care providers.

Achieving the goals of the Triple Aim in health care organizations has come with challenges. The increased demands on health care professionals have produced increased anxiety and stress, decreased job satisfaction, and a low sense of self-accomplishment, which ultimately caused burnout (Waterman, *et al.*, 2007). Symptoms of burnout have been noted across specialties and across disciplines and are related to the increased demands of care delivery.

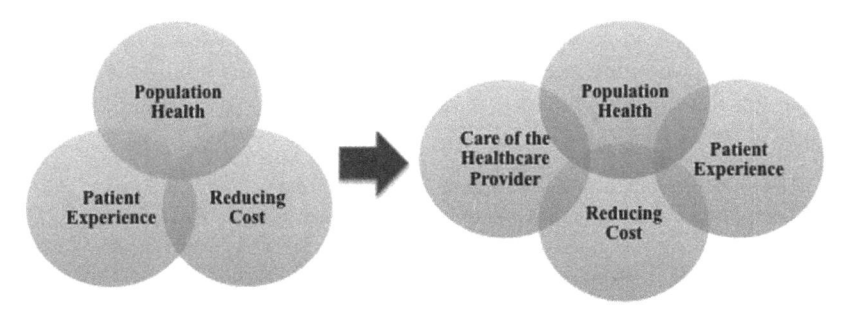

Figure 5.6. *Triple Aim to Quadruple Aim.*

Table 5.2 Signs of Burnout.

• Feelings of exhaustion
• Loss of passion
• Frequent absences from work
• Changes in mood
• Easily frustrated
• Social isolation
• Feelings of hopelessness
• Loss of appetite
• Anxiety and depression
• Apathy towards patients
• Weakened immune system
• Consumed with thoughts of work
• Disconnected from work
• Inability to manage schedule
• Decreased efficacy

Chockinov & Breitbart, 2009.

Many nurses have reported working conditions that are not conducive to providing high quality, patient-centered care (McHugh, Kutney-Lee, Cimiotti, Sloane, & Aiken, 2011). Burnout within the health care workforce threatens the health care industry's ability to achieve the original goals of Triple Aim. For example, it has been shown that dissatisfaction among care providers is associated with lower rates of patient satisfaction (McHugh, *et al.*, 2011), and that burnout among nurses and other caregivers leads to an increases in errors and in health care costs.

Normalization of Deviance. Simply acknowledging the signs of burnout among health care providers is not enough to ensure that quality and safety standards are met in today's hospitals. The Lucian Leape Institute's report, *Through the Eyes of the Workforce: Creating Joy, Meaning, and Safer Health Care* (Lucian Leape Institute, 2013), identified the connection between workplace safety and patient safety and emphasized that recognizing and correcting harmful behaviors in clinical practices is the responsibility of all health care leaders. Respect, protection, and support are essential behaviors needed to ensure workplace safety and safe quality care. The following case scenario described in Leape Institute's report illustrates how some behaviors and practices can cause psychological and physical harm.

> "'Jane Doe' is an experienced surgical technician. She was exposed to a large volume of body fluid while assisting in a surgical case. Rather than scrub out, disinfect, and exchange her scrubs and gown, she proceeded in the case while the saturated gown and scrub shirt served as a vehicle to infect a small lesion on her arm associated with a rash. No one on the surgical team challenged her decision, offered to call a relief scrub tech,

or stopped the line. The pace of the case and the schedule for the day were protected. She developed a severe infection that required months of treatment." (Lucian Leape Institute, 2018)

This case illustrates a work culture in which the staff fails to address the immediate needs of a team member, while they continue to focus on the usual work procedure. The continual pressure to remain on schedule limits the staff's ability to change practices, which in turn has negative consequences. This case illustrates the "normalization of deviance," which is defined as "The gradual process through which unacceptable practice or standards become acceptable. As the deviant behavior is repeated without catastrophic results, it becomes the social norm for the organization." (Boe, 2018). In the above case, normalization of deviance occurred in response to the constant pressure of meeting time goals. When normalization of deviance is imbedded within an organization, the team's perception of the *wrong* processes is changed and defended. Over time, the deviant practices become the norm.

Advancing the Fourth Aim: The Role of the DNP Nurse Executive

As a C-Suite leader, the DNP nurse executive is obligated to identify deviant nursing practices that have become the norm, determine the root cause(s) of the practice, and develop counter measures that can change the behavior. After the counter measures are implemented, the DNP nurse executive, along with his or her quality leader colleagues, must assign accountability metrics to the process improvement that ensure that monitoring occurs and sustainability is achieved. Involvement of the front-line clinical nurse is essential in this process.

The Future of Nursing: Leading Change, Advancing Health (2010) asserts that "nursing has a critical contribution in healthcare reform and the demands for a safe, quality, patientcentered, accessible, and affordable healthcare system" (IOM, 2010). Nursing is the largest segment of the health care workforce, and nurses who serve in leadership positions exert influence in practice environments, the patient experience, health care quality, and cost per capita.

In 2017, sixteen experts from around the United States (U.S.) met to discuss the role of the nurse leader in the Quadruple Aim. Nursing leaders from the American Academy of Nursing Expert Panel on Building Health System Excellence convened the invitational meeting, entitled *Nursing Leadership and the Quadruple Aim: Framing Contribution and Influencing the Future*, to advance the role of nursing leaders as the architects of health care. One of the major themes that emerged included the desired qualities and competencies needed by nurse leaders to successfully support the Quadruple Aim (Figure 5.7).

Most importantly, the prevailing theme of the meeting moved from the traditional definition of a "nurse leader" to that in which *all nurses, regardless of their official title,* are leaders who must drive the outcomes associated with the Quadruple Aim (Bowels, *et al.*, 2018). As leaders, nurses are change agents and conveners, who are responsible for bringing others together to address issues, problems, and opportunities. As shown in Figure 5.7 and defined by the expert panel, the essential competencies of DNP nurse executives who serve as change agents and conveners include the following (Bowles, *et al.*, 2018):

- *Influence*: the ability to persuade others based on authority, communication traits, knowledge-based competencies, status, and timing
- *Advocate*: an examination of options using unbiased interpretation of scientific evidence to promote a policy option most desirable for society
- *Innovate*: the nurse as leader improves or develops a new idea, practice, or object for adoption that results in a beneficial outcome

According to Bowles *et al.* (2018), these core competencies are prerequisites for all nurse leaders, and they must be purposefully addressed at each stage of nurses' careers and across all care delivery practices, education, research, and policies.

Core Competencies for All Nurse Leaders to be Change Agents and Conveners

Influence — *Advocate* — *Innovate*

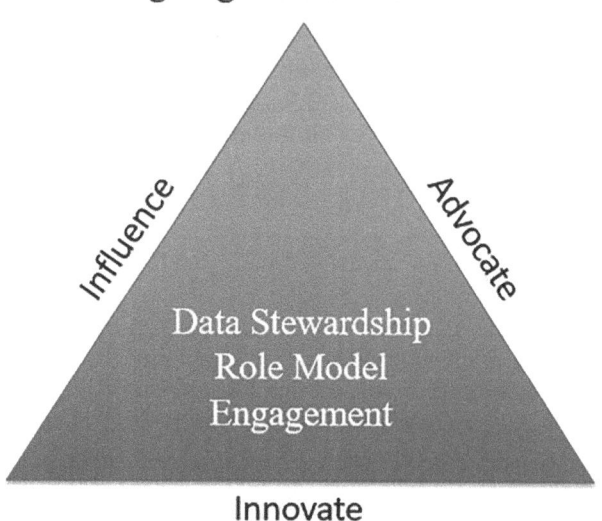

Data Stewardship
Role Model
Engagement

Figure 5.7. *Nurse Leader as Convener and Change Agent to Support Quadruple Aim. Source: Adapted from Bowels, J. et al (2018). The Role of the Nurse Leader in Advancing the Quadruple Aim. Nurse Leader, 16 (4), p. 245.*

Evidence-Based Practice Programs and The DNP Nurse Executive

The DNP nurse executive is charged with developing solutions that improve quality and safety within the healthcare organization. The process of evaluating nursing care and patient outcomes began with Florence Nightingale's use of a systematic approach to patient care and statistical analysis of data and has been evolving since that time. Current quality care outcomes linked to the practice of nursing have evolved from this process. These nursing practice quality indicators as defined by the American Nurses Association (ANA) capture the patient outcomes of nursing care (American Nurses Association, 2013). These indicators—classified as structural, process, or outcome—identify structures of care and care processes that are unique to nursing and that influence the care outcomes of patients.

Evidence-based practice. In 2003, The (IOM established a goal that by 2020, the majority of health care practices and decisions would be evidence-based, which is defined as the use of the most current published evidence in making decisions and developing standards for patient care. The goal demonstrated the IOM belief in the value and patientfocused benefits of evidence-based practice (EBP). Evidence-based practice is essential, given the increasing demands by the public and all health professionals for improvement in the safety and quality in health care. The use of the latest research and evidence in defining best practice, rather than supporting existing practices, demands that DNP nurse executives, in collaboration with the frontline clinical nurses, participate in conducting and interpreting research, and applying new knowledge.

The National Database of Nursing Quality Indicators (NDNQI), established in 1998 by the ANA, is the single national nursing database that provides quarterly and annual reporting of structure, process, and outcome indicators which evaluate the contribution of nursing to patient care outcomes. The ANA created the NDNQI as part of the Safety and Quality Initiative (NDNQI, 2011), with goals of providing participant hospitals with national comparative unit level data for use in quality improvement activities and with developing national data on the relationships between nurse staffing and patient outcomes.

This database captures the outcome data of patient care that are a direct result of the practice of nursing. These data are compared at the unit or department level to national benchmarks to provide the baseline for continued quality and safety improvement initiatives. It is the role of the DNP nurse executive to interpret the data and to develop structures that support improvement strategies and the processes needed to achieve the outcomes specific to the nurse practice quality indicators. Some examples of the nursing practice quality indicators are the prevention of central line bloodstream infections (CLBSIs), CAUTIs, patient falls with injury, and hospital acquired pressure ulcers.

Described below is an example of a comprehensive approach to reducing central line blood stream infections in a hospital system led by a DNP nurse executive. The project was designed to ensure zero harm to patients by achieving and sustaining zero CLBSI. The nurse executive began with the development of a project charter, which is shown in Figure 5.8.

The nurse executive then formed a multidisciplinary professional team to review potential evidence-based strategies that could achieve zero CLABSI. The interventions and accomplishments of the team are described below:

Interventions to Date

2013 Accomplishments

- Established unit-level champion teams in each ICU
- Created a CLABSI Case Review tool to drill-down on the factors that may have contributed to the CLABSI and to learn how to prevent future events
- Implemented a CLABSI Case Review huddle process, in which Infection Prevention & Control (IP&C) sends the Case Review tool to the ICU champion teams and an interdisciplinary team reviews the event
- Developed a central line monitoring tool to be used during weekly rounds on patients who currently have a central line
- Initiated weekly workgroup calls, including leadership from IP&C, Nursing, Nursing Education, Vascular Access, and Quality and Patient Safety
- Developed and launched CLABSI e-learning modules for nursing
- American Association of Critical-Care Nurses (AACN) Clinical Scene Investigator (CSI) Academy grant awardees implemented unit-based teams to improve quality of patient care, including CLABSI-related projects

2014 Accomplishments

- Developed a process to summarize data from the CLABSI case reviews and reported trends at various hospital committees/groups (e.g., Inter-ICU Committee, IP&C monthly meetings)
- Implemented new infection prevention products and processes: Curos antiseptic port protectors
- OneLink needless endcaps
- Regular alcohol pads to "scrub the hub"
- Considering new hemodialysis endcaps and port protectors
- Considering use of midline catheters
- Produced a video on central line maintenance techniques
- Monitored Chlorhexidine (CHG) bathing compliance and, where applicable, identified barriers and implement improvements
- Added defaulted CHG bathing parameter to all flowsheets in Allscripts
- Drafted automated report of CHG bathing documentation compliance

Project Title: CLABSI Prevention	Start date: Q3 2013	Est. completion date: Q4 2015

PROBLEM STATEMENT
As of July 2014, the ICU CLABSI standardized infection ratio (SIR) was 0.42 (95% CI 0.291-0.591), which is significantly worse than the top performing U.S. hospitals (the national SIR at the 25% percentile was 0.20, FY 2015 Hospital Performance).

Patients with a central venous catheter (CVC) are at risk for CLABSI, but this risk can be mitigated through adherence to evidence-based practices during insertion, maintenance, and removal of the CVC.

The hospital has been monitoring CLABSI since 2009 in admitted patients in both ICUs and non-ICUs, and although the SIR has recently decreased (from 0.58 in 2013), several units have CLABSI rates that are higher than national benchmarks.

PURPOSE/BUSINESS CASE
CLABSIs are preventable hospital-acquired infections that lead to patient harm. In addition, patients with a CLABSI often have increased LOS, as well as increased costs of care ($3,700-$39,000 per episode).

The CLABSI SIR is publicly reported and is included as a value based purchasing measure.

GOAL STATEMENT
To be within the top 25% of U.S. Hospitals by achieving a CLABSI SIR of 0.20 or less by June 2015.

KEY OUTCOMES AND TARGETS

Metrics	Current	Target	By When
CLABSI SIR (ICU)	0.42 (Jan-Jun 2014)	< 0.20	Jun 2015
% of ICUs below NHSN pooled mean CLABSI Rate	53% (Aug-TD 2014)	> 80%	Mar 2015
CHG Bathing Compliance	84% (Oct 2014)	> 95%	Dec 2014

PROJECT SCOPE
Process Start: CVC Insertion (including choice of CVC type and insertion site)

Process Stop: CVC Removal

Sub-processes: CVC Maintenance, including daily assessment of necessity, compliance to cleaning CVC hubs and injection ports, use of antiseptic-containing port protectors, compliance to daily CHG baths, and dressing assessment and changes

Suppliers/customers:
Inpatients in ICUs and non-ICUs where CVCs are used
Frontline clinicians: MDs, PAs, NPs, RNs

TEAM	Name	Title	Department
Project Sponsor		VP Nursing,	Nursing
Process Owner(s)		Director of Nursing	Nursing
QPSI Facilitator		QPSI Manager	QPS
Team Members *Ensure all stakeholders/ departments (suppliers/customers are represented)*		Program Dir. Nursing Ed. Program Dir. Nursing Ed. Instructor Coordinator Nursing Ed. Clinical Nurse	Nursing Education
		Dir. Oper. Bus. Admin. DON, Epidemiology	IP&C
		Patient Care Director	Vascular Access
Additional Support/ Resources Required	Physician Leadership, Strategic Sourcing, Information Technology, Patient/Family Advisor		

Figure 5.8. *CLBSI Prevention Project Charter.*

Future Strategies to Reach ZERO

- Identify roles and responsibilities of CLABSI Project Team members:
  — Implement accountability structure for CLABSI events (including plan to proactively monitor performance on a less frequent basis for high-performing units)
- Enhance the CLABSI Case Review Process:
  — Decrease the expected turn-around time on the reviews from one week to 72 hours
  — Include unit medical directors and directors of nursing on the notification emails
  — Automate CLABSI case reviews, including the data collection and reporting
- Ensure consistent practice on major CLABSI prevention strategies through monitoring and continuous improvement:
  — CHG bathing (consider trialing CHG wipes for areas with high SIR)
  — Use of antiseptic containing port protectors
  — Daily assessment of continued use of CVC (including more quickly converting patients from IV to PO medications)
  — Rates of types of CVC and insertion sites used (including decision process for choosing these)
  — Reduce the number of IV connections/filters used
  — Convert patients from IV to PO medications in timely manner
  — Engage patients and family in CLABSI prevention through focused education and awareness
  — Identify roles and responsibilities of CLABSI Project Team members

A critical part of this process was defining how success was going to be measured. Although the ultimate outcome measure was sustained achievement of zero CLABSI, the team identified process measures that would ensure compliance with the reduction initiative, as shown in Table 5.3.

The next step in the process was developing and implementing an accountability plan that would confirm that decisions made by the interdisciplinary team were applied in practice and monitored for compliance.

A process also needed to be identified for CLABSI reoccurrences. The nurse executive and the team developed a case review instrument that was to be completed for all patients identified with a CLABSI as shown in Table 5.10. The data were analyzed for trends, which then guided additional improvement strategies were implemented, monitored and measured as shown in Figure 5.11..

Table 5.3 Example of Process Measures Identified for CLABSI Reduction.

Metric Name	Brief Definition	Target
CLABSI SIR (ICU)	The combined CLABSI standardized infection ratio for all ICUs, as determined by the NHSH guidelines.	≤ 0.2
CLABSI SIR (non ICU)	The combined CLABSI standardized infection ratio for all non-ICUs, as determined by the NHSH guidelines.	≤ 0.5
Percent of ICUs Below NHSN Pooled Mean CLABSI Rate	The percentage of ICUs that are performing better than the pooled mean national CLABSI rate, per the latest NHSN data.	≥ 80%
CHG Bathing Compliance	The percentage of ICU patients with documentation of a CHG bath within the past 36 hours. (Excludes neonatal ICU, patients < 2 months of age, patients allergic to CHG, patients with an ICU LOS < 2 days.)	≥ 95%
Antiseptic-Containing Port Protector Compliance	The percentage of central line end caps with antiseptic-containing port protectors in place	≥ 95%
Documentation of Daily Assessment Compliance	The percentage of patients with a central line who have documentation of daily assessment of necessity for the line.	≥ 95%
Hand Hygiene Compliance	The percentage of compliance to correct hand hygiene protocols.	≥ 98%

The Role of Patients and Families in Quality and Safety Outcomes

The Institute for Patient and Family-Centered Care (IPFCC) defined the partnership with patients as an "approach to the planning, delivery, and evaluation of health care that is grounded in mutually beneficial partnerships among health care providers, patients, and families. It redefines the relationships in health care by placing an emphasis on collaborating with people of all ages, at all levels of care, and in all health care settings." (IPFCC, 2018). As shown below in Figure 5.12, Mastro, Flynn, & Preuster (2014) synthesized the existing literature and developed a parsimonious theoretical model of patient and family-centered care (PFCC). The model outlines sequenced phases of partnership development in PFCC, as well as propositional statements about the associations between PFCC and outcomes.

The PFCC theoretical model is well supported in the literature. The 2014 published review by Mastro *et al.* (2014) demonstrated that the defining attributes of PFCC include the development of a caring and trusting relationship; the leveling of power, information and knowledge sharing; participation and shared decision-making; and dignity and respect (Coyne, 2006; Curtis-Tyler, 2010; D'Amour, Ferranda-Videla, Rodriguez, & Beaulieu, 2005; Eldh, Ehnfors, & Ekman, 2004; Hobbs, 2009; Hook, 2006; Kin-

Instructions	
(1) IP&C RN: Upon confirming a CLABSI, notify Nurse Manager and champion team with background information (2) Nurse Manager: Schedule an immediate huddle with champion team members & IP&C RN. If possible, include members of the patient's care team. (3) Champion team (incl. IP&C RN): Huddle to review this worksheet. (4) Nurse Manager: Send completed Case Review Worksheet to QPSI Manager within 1 week (5) Nurse Manager & Director of Nursing: Within 1 week of confirmed CLABSI and team huddle, meet with VP of Nursing to review team's analysis & improvement plans. (6) Nurse Manager: Report out about overall insights from the review huddle during the monthly IP&C meeting.	
Unit of CLABSI acquisition	Reviewer(s)
Patient Name / MRN	Patient Age / Gender
Primary diagnosis	Organism
IP&C REVIEW	
(1) Date of first positive blood culture	[Complete b & c if more than one central line]
(2) Central line insertion location (unit/dept) (a) (b) (c)	
(3) Insertion date/time (a) (b) (c)	
(4) Insertion site (a) (b) (c)	
(5) Type of central line (a) (b) (c)	
(6) Is there documentation that the central line insertion checklist was used? (a) (b) (c)	
CHAMPION TEAM REVIEW	[refer to CL described in a / b / c above]
(7) Indication for central line (a) (b) (c)	
Complete # 8-11 only if blood stream infection occurred fewer than 7 days after insertion date (#3)	
(8) Name/level/supervision of practitioner who inserted line (a) (b) (c)	
(9) If the insertion site is internal jugular or femoral (#4), what was the reason for choosing this site instead of subclavian? (a) (b) (c)	
(10) Does documentation support that insertion was performed emergently? (a) (b) (c)	
(11) If patient is from ED, does ED physician note contain details of the insertion? (a) (b) (c)	
(12) Was line inserted with ultrasound and/or fluroroscope guidance? (a) (b) (c)	
(13) Was the central line antibiotic impregnated (write "N/A" for a PICC)? (a) (b) (c)	

(continued)

Figure 5.10. *Example of the Case Review Instrument Used Post CLABSI Identification.*

CHAMPION TEAM REVIEW, CONT.			
(14) Was the central line used for blood draws?	(a)	(b)	(c)
(15) Was TPN/IL infused in the days preceding the CLABSI?	(a)	(b)	(c)
(16) Were IV fluids administered via CL?	(a)	(b)	(c)
(17) Was the catheter declotted with TPA within 2–3 days of CLABSI?	(a)	(b)	(c)
IN THE DAYS PRIOR TO THE INFECTION:			
(18) Were there any procedures during which a catheter was accessed?	(18)	(19) If yes, what type of procedure(s)?	(19)
(20) Were there other notable incidents? (cardiac arrest, emergent reintubation, etc)	(20)		
(21) Were there any issues with appropriate backflow from line or other flushing issues?	(21)		
(22) Date of last documented dressing change?	(22)	(23) Was dressing intact and labeled appropriately?	(23)
(24) Was CL tubing changed and dated per policy (every 4 days, except for TPN/IL and blood tubing which is daily)?	(24)	(25) What kind of dressing covered the line (circle all that apply)?	(a) CHG Tegaderm (b) Non-CHG Tegaderm only (c) Non-CHG Tegaderm w/gauze (d) Island Dressing (e) IV 3000 Dressing (f) Other:
(26) Describe the appearance of the insertion site:	(26)	(27) Did patient have daily CHG bath 3 days prior to CLABSI?	(27)
(28) Do all end ports of the CL have a Curos port protector in place, when the CL is not in use? (mark "N/A" if CL has been discontinued)	(28)	(29) If the CL tubing has a 3-way stop-cock, do all ports on the stop-cock have needleless valves (OneLink)? (mark "N/A" if CL has been discontinued)	(29)

Figure 5.10 (continued). *Example of the Case Review Instrument Used Post CLABSI Identification.*

CLABSI by Central Line Type

[Pareto chart showing frequency by central line type: PICC, Non-tunneled TL, Non-tunneled DL, Introducer-PA, Tunneled DL, Introducer, Atrial Catheter, with cumulative percent line reaching 100%]

54% of the central lines associated with a CLABSI were a PICC or non-tunneled TLC

(a)

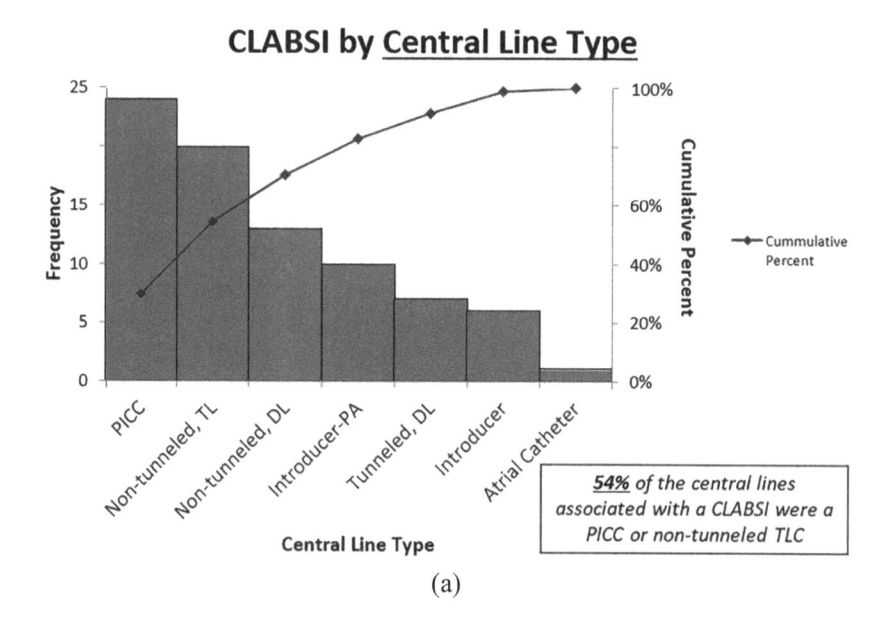

Variation in number of days between insertion and CLABSI event

[Histogram showing frequency of lines associated with a CLABSI by number of days between insertion and event, ranging from 3-4 days through 56-166 days]

59% of CLABSI occurred at least **one week after insertion** of the central line.
Average = 14.8 days (exc. Outlier); Median = 9 days

(b)

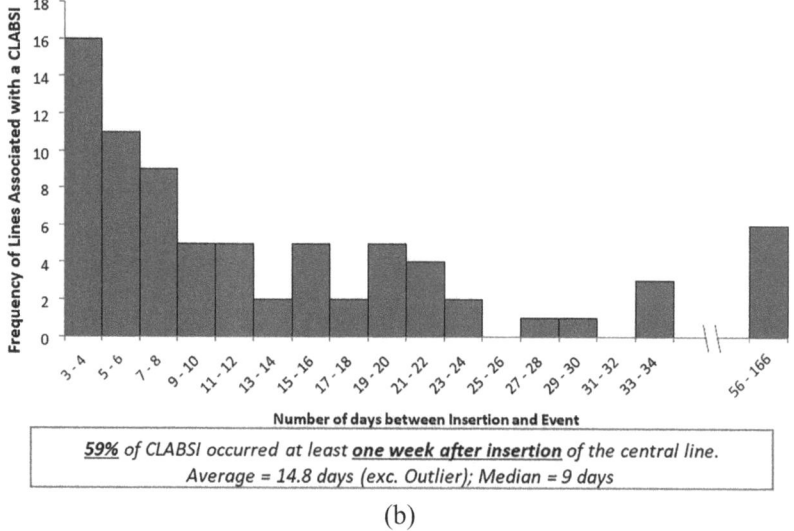

Figure 5.11. *Example of Data That Were Collected and Analyzed from the CLABSI Case Review Instrument.*

CLABSI by Insertion Site

(c)

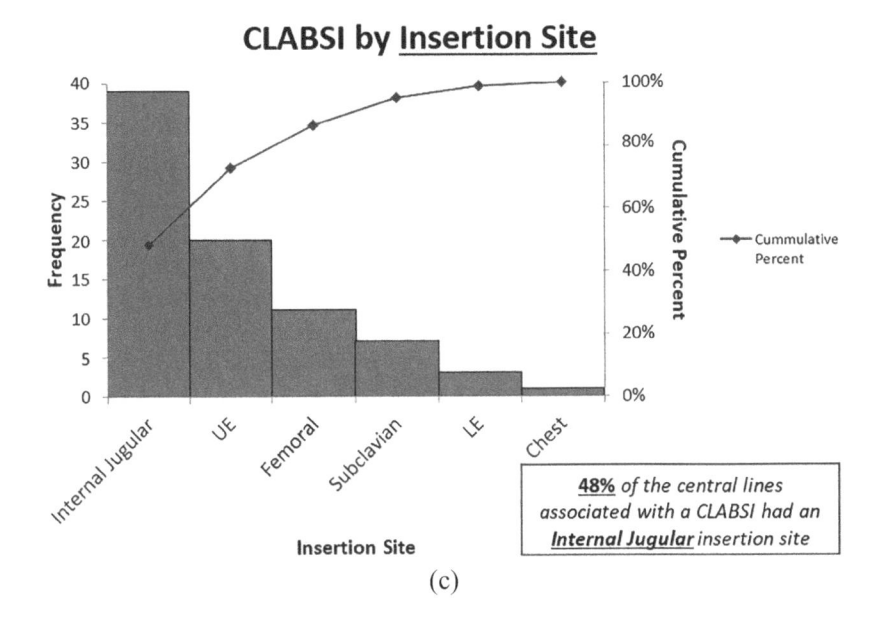

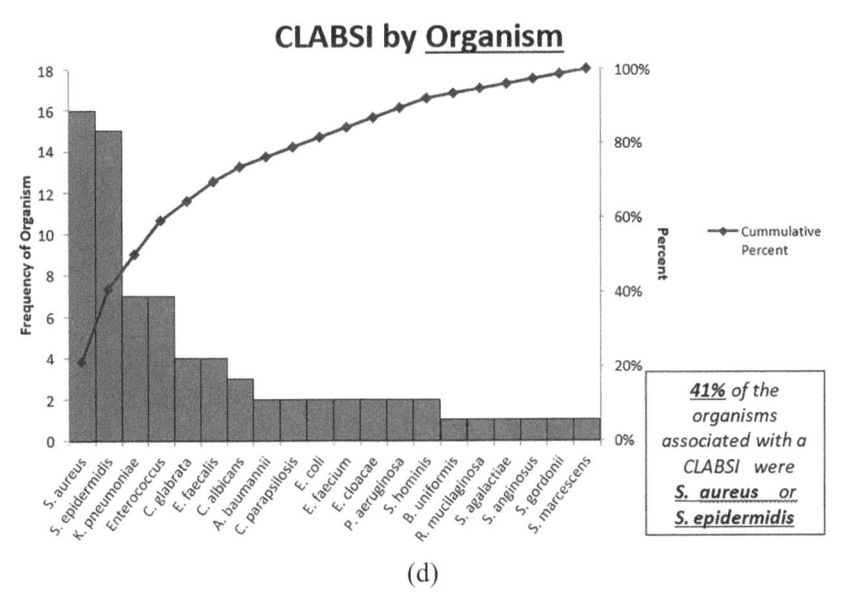

48% of the central lines associated with a CLABSI had an **Internal Jugular** insertion site

CLABSI by Organism

(d)

41% of the organisms associated with a CLABSI were **S. aureus** or **S. epidermidis**

Figure 5.11 (continued). *Example of Data That Were Collected and Analyzed from the CLABSI Case Review Instrument.*

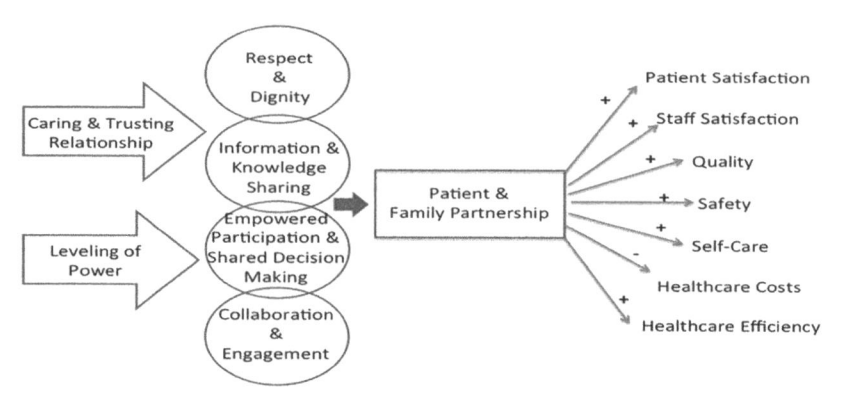

Figure 5.12. *Theoretical Model of Patient and Family-Centered Care. Source: Mastro, Flynn, & Preuster, 2014.*

naman & Bleich, 2004; Klein, *et al.*, 2011]; Sahlsten, Larsson, Sjostrom, & Kaety, 2008). The development of a caring and trusting relationship and the leveling of power are critical for PFCC and the patient to fully engage in her/his care. Once actualized, this leads to the empowerment of the patient to participate as a full partner in care and care decisions (Coyne, 2006; Curtis-Tyler *et al.*, 2010; D'Amour *et al.*, 2005; Eldh *et al.*, 2004; Gallant, Leaulieu, & Carnevale, 2002; Harbaugh, Tomlinson, & Kirschbaum, 2004; Hobbs, 2009; Hook, 2006; Kettunen, Poskiparta, & Karhila, 2003; Klein *et al.*, 2011; Sahlsten *et al.*, 2008).

From a health care provider perspective, information and knowledge sharing is enhanced when the provider shares knowledge of health and illness and the patient/family shares personal experiences of the illness, social and family support, values, beliefs, and culture. This creates a stronger partnership (Hook, 2006; Latta, Dick, Parry, & Tamura, 2008; Klein *et al.*, 2011; Macdonald, Liben, Carnevale, & Cohen, 2012). Shared decision making is achieved through empowered participation, in which the provider and the patient/family share in the decisions of care through the development of mutually agreeable goals (Eldh *et al.*, 2004; Hobbs, 2009; Hook, 2006). This relationship between the provider and the patient/family is critical to the success of a strong partnership (Mastro *et al.*, 2014). The leveling of power, in which the provider surrenders power and control to become an equal partner with the patient/family, is critical because, without it, partnership cannot be realized (Coyne, 2006; Curtis-Tyler, 2010; Eldh *et al.*, 2004; Hobbs, 2009; Hook, 2006). The final attribute is that of respect and dignity. In partnership with patients and families, the provider must have respect for the patient and family and "openly listen to and honor the patient and family's perspectives and choices" (Piper, 2011. p. 127). When the patient's/family's views are seen as the most valuable contributions to the planning of their care and together, a full partnership is realized (Johnston et al., 2006; Hook, 2006; Hutchenfield, 1999; Stahlsten et al., 2008).

In review of the existing empirical literature, Mastro et al. (2014) developed propositional statements about the associations between patient/family partnership and outcomes. They proposed that after full patient/family partnership is achieved, outcomes such as improvements in patient satisfaction, staff satisfaction, quality, safety, self-care, and health care efficiency could be achieved, along with reductions in health care costs. After the health care provider fully engages patients and families as partners in care, Mastro et al. (2014) propose and the literature supports the improvement of quality and safety outcomes of care.

The Role of the Patient and Family in Care Trajectory

The patient and family have a role in ensuring the highest quality and best safety, because they are full partners in the type of care in which the voice of the patient and/or family is active and valued as care decisions are made and as quality and safety are ensured. Mastro et al. (2014) describe this partnership as a unique relationship that develops from a foundation of care and trust and a leveling of power between the health care provider and the patient/family. Dignity and mutual respect, information and knowledge sharing, empowered patient/family participation with shared decision-making, and collaboration and engagement are the key components that the DNP nurse executive must ensure are present at the patient's bedside.

The patient and family as full partners in care aligns with all eight DNP essentials as defined by the American Association of the Colleges of Nursing. Patient and Family Centered Care is the latest cutting-edge scientific underpinning for evidence-based practice in nursing. This is grounded in interprofessional collaboration that drives quality and safety outcomes, transforms health care within acute care, and ensures the improvement of health outcomes of the population.

As the DNP nurse executive advances the practice of nursing and creates a culture focused on patients and their families as full partners in every aspect of care, initiatives that improve the nation's health and the health of populations will be successful. With patient and families as partners in care, the DNP nurse executive will advance the practice of nursing and the outcomes for patients through advocacy and the type of health care policy advancement that ensures that the patient/family remain at the center of health care decisions.

Future Projections

The future of health care will continue to evolve as payers continue to push health care systems to perform with the highest possible quality, safety, and patient satisfaction with care. Health care systems will increasingly be held accountable for ensuring healthy work environments that have excellent patient outcomes with the highest safety at the lowest costs. Health care systems will need to continue on the journey of becoming high reliable organizations that function beyond the walls of the acute care hospitals and throughout the entire continuum of care.

Chapter Takeaways

1. The classic framework and tools for ensuring quality and safety standards through evidence-based practice are in place in health care organizations.
2. A comprehensive review of the Quadruple Aim and methodologies for ensuring all four components are met with success.
3. Advancing to the Quadruple Aim and caring for those who are caring for patients is a key element of the DNP nurse executive's role. Without a clear focus on balancing the increased demands on health care professionals, these is risk of increased anxiety and stress, decreased job satisfaction, and a low sense of self-accomplishment, which ultimately results in burnout.
4. An example of a comprehensive approach to ensuring zero harm to patients while assuring that patients and families are actively engaged and partnered in care.

Chapter Summary

The content of this chapter supports the DNP nurse executive's success in leading the strategies needed for the transformation of health care. From the development of a solid foundation in the competencies needed for leading the changing modern health care system, approaches that ensure that the clinical teams are supported and the culture within and throughout the health care system has a strong focus on high reliability, driving quality outcomes, and engaging and partnering with patient/families to drive sustained change at the lowest cost possible, this chapter has described a framework for safe, reliable, and effective care. This chapter is intended to advance the knowledge of the nurse executive as they drive not only clinical change but also serve as change agents and conveners engaged in advocacy, influence, and innovation.

Chapter Reflection Questions

1. In the delivery of safe, reliable, and effective care, what how do external drivers affect the outcomes of care?

2. What are the four objectives of the Quadruple Aim? How have these objectives changed health care delivery?
3. What are the domains and components of safe, reliable, and effective care? How does the DNP nurse executive effectively ensure that all members of the health care team understand the evidenced-based practices of these domains?
4. What are the domains of value-based purchasing and what is the role of the DNP nurse executive in the achievement of outcomes in these domains?
5. In the development of solutions to improve quality and safety within the health care organization, how does the practice of nursing affect patient outcomes? What is the role of the DNP nurse executive in ensuring quality patient care outcomes?
6. What is the role of the patient/family in quality and safety? How does enabling that role affect health outcomes of a population? In partnering with patients/families, which DNP essential competencies are fulfilled?

References

Agency for Healthcare Research and Quality (2018). About the national quality strategy. Content last reviewed March 2017. *Agency for Healthcare Research and Quality*, Rockville, MD. Retrieved from http://www.ahrq.gov/workingforquality/about/index.html.

American Nurses Association (ANA) (2013). *Framework for measuring nurses contribution to care coordination*. Retrieved from https://www.nursingworld.org/~4afbd6/globalassets/practiceandpolicy/health-policy/framework-for-measuring-nurses-contributions-to-care-coordination.pdf.

American Organization of Nurse Executives (AONE) (2015). *Nurse executive competencies*. Retrieved from http://www.aone.org/resources/nec.pdf.

Balik, B., Conway, J., Zipperer, L., Watson, J. (2011). *Achieving an Exceptional Patient and Family Experience of Inpatient Hospital Care*. IHI Innovation Series white paper. Cambridge, Massachusetts: Institute for Healthcare Improvement. Retrieved from www.IHI.org

Berwick, D. M., Nolan, T. W., Whittington, J. (2008). The triple aim: Care, health, and cost. *Health Affairs, 27*(3), 759–769.

Boe, R. (2018). Retrieved from http://lmcontheline.blogspot.com/2013/01/the-normalization-of-deviance-if-it-can.html.

Bowels, J., Adams, J., Batcheller, J., Zimmermann, D., & Pappas, S. (2018). The role of the nurse leader in advancing the quadruple aim. *Nurse Leader, 16*(4), 244–248.

Chockinov, H., & Breitbart, W. (2009). Handbook of psychiatry in palliative medicine (2nd ed.). Oxford, England: Oxford Press (pp. 236–240).

Coyne, I. (2006). Consultation with Children in Hospital: Children, Parents', and Nurses' perspectives. *Journal of Clinical Nursing, 15*, 61–71.

Curtis-Tyler, K. (2010). Levers and Barriers to Patient-Centered Care with Children:

Findings from a Synthesis of Studies of the Experiences of Children Living with Type 1 Diabetes or Asthma. *Child: Care, Health and Development, 37*(4), 540–550.

D'Amour, D., Ferranda-Videla, M., Rodriguez, L.M., *et al.* (2005). The Conceptual Basis for Interprofessional Collaboration: Core Concepts and Theoretical Frameworks. *Journal of Interprofessional Care*, Supplement 1, 116–131.

Donabedian, A. (1980). *The definition of quality and approaches to its assessment.* Ann Arbor, MI: Health Administration Press.

Eldh, A.C., Ehnfors, M., Ekman, I. (2004). The Phenomena of participation and no-participation in Health Care-Experiences of Patients Attending a Nurse-Led Clinic for Chronic Healthcare. *European Society of Cardiology, 3*(3), 239-246.

Frankel, A., Haraden, C., Federico, F., Lenoci-Edwards, J. (2017). A Framework for Safe, Reliable, and Effective Care. White Paper. Cambridge, MA: *Institute for Healthcare Improvement and Safe & Reliable Healthcare.*

Gallant, M., Leaulieu, M., Carnevale. F. (2002) Partnership: An Analysis of the Concept within the Nurse-Client Relationship. *Journal of Advanced Nursing, 40*(2), 149–157.

Harbaugh, B., Tomlinson, P., Kirschbaum, M. (2004). Parents' Perceptions of Nurses' Caregiving Behaviors in the Pediatric Intensive Care Unit. *Issues in Comprehensive Pediatric Nursing, 27*, 163–179.

Hobbs, J. (2009). A Dimentional Analysis of Patient-Centered Care. *Nursing Research, 58*(1), 52–62.

Hook, M. (2006). Partnering with Patients-A Concept Ready for Action. *The Author. Journal compilation*, 133–143.

Institute for Healthcare Improvement, (2018). Retrieved from http://www.ihi.org/resources/pages/ViewAll.aspx?FilterField1=IHI_x0020_Content_x0020_Type&FilterValue1=94ee13e7-06de-453a-b053-979131880fc5&Filter1ChainingOperator=And&TargetWebPath=/resources&orb=Created

Institute for Patient and Family Centered Care. (2018). Retrieved from http://www.ipfcc.org/about/pfcc.html.

Institute of Medicine. (2010). The future of nursing: Leading change, advancing health. Retrieved from http://books.nap.edu/openbook.php?record_id=12956&page=R1

Johnston, A., Bullock, C., Graham, J., *et al.* (2006). Implementation of Case-Study Results of Potentially Better Practices for Family-Centered Care: The Family-Centered Care Map. *Pediatrics, 118*(2),108–114.

Kettunen, T., Poskiparta, M., Karhila, P. (2003). Speech Practices that Facilitate Patient Participation in Health Counseling-A Way to Empowerment. *Health Education Journal, 62*, 326–340.

Kinnaman, M., Bleich, M. (2004). Collaboration: Aligning Relationships to Create and Sustain Partnerships. *Journal of Professional Nursing, 20*(50), 310–322.

Klein, S., Wynn, K., Ray, L., *et al.* (2011). Information Sharing during Diagnostic Assessments: What is Relevant for Parents?. *Physical and Occupational Therapy in Pediatrics, 31*(2), 120–132.

Latta, L., Dick, R., Parry, C., *et al.* (2008). Parental Responses to Involvement in Rounds on a Pediatric Inpatient Unit at a Teaching Hospital: A Qualitative Study. *Academic Medicine, 83*(3), 292–297.

Lucian Leape Institute. (2013). Through the Eyes of the Workforce: Creating Joy, Meaning, and Safer Health Care. Boston, MA: National Patient Safety Foundation. Retrieved from https://c.ymcdn.com/sites/npsf.site-ym.com/resource/resmgr/LLI/Through-Eyes-of-the-Workforc.pdf

Macdonald, M., Liben, S., Carnevale, F., et al. (2012). An Office or a Bedroom? Challenges for Family-Centered Care in the Pediatric Intensive Care Unit. *Journal of Child Health Care, 16*(3), 237–249.

Mastro, K.A., Flynn, L., Preuster, C. (2014). Patient- and Family-Centered Care: A National Call to Action for New Knowledge and Innovation. *The Journal of Nursing Administration, 44*(9), 446–451.

McHugh, M.D., Kutney-Lee, A., Cimiotti, J.P., Sloane, D.M., Aiken, L.H., (2011). Nurses' widespread job dissatisfaction, burnout, and frustration with health benefits signal problems for patient care. *Health Affairs, 30*(2), 202–210.

National Database of Nursing Quality Indicators (NDNQI). (2011). National database of nursing quality indicators-NDNQI: Taking your quality improvement data to the national level [PowerPoint slides]. Retrieved from https://www.nursingquality.org/documents/public/NDNQI%20Info.pps

Piper, L. (2001). The Ethical Leadership Challenge: Creating a Culture of Patient- and Family-Centered Care in the Hospital Setting. *The Health Care Manager, 30*(2), 125-132.

Pronovost, P. J., et al. (2013). Demonstrating high reliability on accountability measures at the Johns Hopkins Hospital. *The Joint Commission Journal on Quality and Patient Safety, 39*(12), 531–544.

Sahlsten, J.M., Larsson, I., Sjostrom, B., et al. (2008). An Analysis of the Concept of Patient Participation. *Nursing Forum, 43*(1), 2–11.

Stiefel, M., Nolan, K. (2012). A Guide to Measuring the Triple Aim: Population Health, Experience of Care, and Per Capita Cost. IHI Innovation Series white paper. Cambridge, Massachusetts: Institute for Healthcare Improvement; Retrieved from www.IHI.org

Waterman, A.D., Garbutt, J., Hazel, E., Dunagen, W. C., Levinson, W., Fraser, V. J., & Gallagher, T. H. (2007). The emotional impact of medical errors on practicing physicians in the United States and Canada. *Joint Commission Journal on Quality and Patient Safety, 33*(8), 467–476.

PETRA GOODMAN

6

Clinical Research, Quality Improvement, and the DNP Nurse Executive

Chapter Objectives

- Identify the research process knowledge and skills that DNP nurses should acquire.
- Detail the essential components of a collaborative approach to maximize research capacity.
- Discuss the DNP nurse role and accountability in quality improvements.
- Describe and delineate the quality metrics collected for multiple organizations.
- Present various methods for identification, development, and analysis of quality improvement initiatives.

KEY WORDS: Research, research process, collaborative research, quality improvement, quality metrics, quality improvement methods, dashboards

Introduction

Health care organizations must integrate research and quality improvement into the delivery of care to create innovative, effective, safe, timely, and fiscally responsive processes; to validate practice; and to demonstrate compliance with state and national directives. The DNP nurse, as a C-Suite executive, not only develops and implements evidence-based nursing care, but also must also actively engage in research and quality improvement. The DNP nurse executive must attain competence in research to address clinical problems, demonstrate the value of nursing practice, generate new evidence, sustain evidence-based nursing, and appraise current practice, systems of care, and health care organization processes and population outcomes. Similarly, the DNP nurse executive must be proficient in quality improvement strategies to facilitate safe practice, prevent harmful events, and improve care processes and patient outcomes. In terms of research, this chapter reviews the significance of the research process to the DNP nurse executive, delineates research competencies needed by DNP nurse executives, and presents a collaborative approach to maximize research capacity. In reference to quality improvement, the chapter discusses the role of the DNP in quality improvement, describes multiple quality metrics that health care organizations measure, and presents various methods for identification, development, implementation, and analysis of quality improvement initiatives.

The DNP Nurse and Clinical Research

Today, professional health organizations and policy-making bodies are emphasizing the importance of research for the development of and validation of nursing practice. In 2001, the Institute of Medicine (IOM), in a report, *Crossing the Quality Chasm: A New Health System for the 21st Century*, recommended that health care systems bridge the gap between practice and research, in which practice is based on research evidence and research priorities are based on problems identified in practice (IOM, 2001a). Then in 2010, *The Future of Nursing: Leading Change, Advancing Health*, reinforced research priorities for transforming nursing practice. Priorities addressed scope of practice, nursing residencies, teamwork, technology, and the value of nursing practice (IOM, 2010).

The American Nurses Credentialing Center (ANCC) represents an influential organization within nursing. A component of the ANCC, the Magnet® Recognition Program, awards Magnet® status to health care organizations that demonstrate nursing excellence in nursing practice, management, and leadership and exemplary nursing participation in organizational structure and systems (ANCC, 2014). Magnet® status equates to nursing excellence and is recognized as distinguishing outstanding health care organizations. Due to the high honor affiliated with achievement of Magnet® status, health care organizations seek to achieve such recognition. One of the five components in the Magnet® model, "new knowledge, innovations, and improvements," focuses on "new models of care, application of existing evidence, new evidence, and contributions to the science of nursing," (https://www.nursingworld.org/organizational-programs/magnet/magnet-model/). To acquire Magnet® status, organizations must demonstrate system-wide implementation of nursing research to include evidence of systems that integrate nursing research into operations and processes. Moreover, nurses must validate contribution of nursing research to patient care, the organization, and the profession. Clearly, the Magnet® requirements indicate the significance of research for recognition of an organization as a Magnet® facility. As advanced practice nurses (APNs) with knowledge and skills representative of components of the research process, DNP nurses will be instrumental to organizations in the development, implementation, and integration of nursing research within their organization, whether for the achievement or sustainment of Magnet® status.

In 2006, the American Association of Colleges of Nursing (AACN) defined core competencies for the DNP academic program accreditation in *The Essentials of Doctoral Education for Advanced Nursing Practice* (AACN, 2006). The core competencies acknowledge that research validates nursing practice and provides processes for evaluation of nursing practice, health outcomes, and systems of care. Based on this recognition, the competencies indicate that DNP nurses "should be able to . . . use science-based theories and concepts to determine the nature and significance of health and health care delivery phenomena (AACN, 2006, p. 9)

> . . . use analytic methods to critically appraise existing literature and other evidence to determine and implement the best evidence for practice; design and implement processes to evaluate outcomes of practice, practice patterns, and systems of care within a practice setting, health care organization or community against national benchmarks to determine variances in practice outcomes and population trends . . . use information technology and research methods to collect appropriate and accurate data to generate evidence for nursing practice, inform and guide the design of databases that generate meaningful evidence for nursing practice, analyze data from practice, . . . predict and analyze outcomes, and examine patterns of behavior and outcomes." (AACN, 2006, p. 12).

The competencies identify that DNP nurses will need research process skills to not only translate evidence into practice, but also to appraise current practice, systems of care, health care organization processes and population outcomes, generate evidence, and inform, guide, and develop improved processes.

To respond to professional organizations' mandates, achieve the highest standards of nursing excellence, and bridge the gap between science and practice, health care organizations expect DNP nurses to critically analyze practice with rigorous research evaluation processes. Although the primary role of the DNP is to translate evidence into practice and conduct practice inquiry to inform practice, practice improvement requires a command of research methods. Knowledge of concept analysis facilitates determination and evaluation of the conceptualizations, attributional characteristics, and operational measures of health terms and procedures. Understanding of theory promotes query and evaluation of the conceptual frameworks that support practice and systems within the facility. Appropriate framing of researchable questions generated from observations and discussions identifies innovative practices and systems and those requiring validation. Understanding of research design and methods, data management, and statistical analyses promotes the DNP's competence in critical appraisal of the literature to identify the best evidence for practice. Fundamental

Table 6.1 Application of Research Process Knowledge and Skills.

- Develop and evaluate models and methods of disseminating and sustaining evidence-based clinical guidelines in clinical practice and program development
- Evaluate evidence-based clinical guidelines' impact on quality of care, access, and cost
- Critique and evaluate how organizational, structural, financial, and policy decisions impact cost, quality, and accessibility of health care
- Complete analyses to identify health disparities and variables and processes that account for variation in therapeutic effects
- Evaluate outcomes of practice and systems of care against national benchmarks to determine effectiveness and variances in practice outcomes and population trends
- Design, direct, and evaluate quality improvement methodologies to promote safe, timely, effective, efficient, equitable, and patient-centered care and compliance with benchmarks
- Evaluate integration of nursing processes and outcomes into health information technology (HIT) systems
- Identify and evaluate the impact of health information technologies on effectiveness, efficacy, and quality of nursing care delivery
- Implement trend analyses on innovative and current practices, programs, models of care, and systems to identify improvements and problems for which early corrective actions can be executed and the impact on human capital, logistical and operational requirements, efficacy, cost, access, quality, policy impact, and sustainability
- Analyze attributes of translation research that improve integration and sustainability for populations, organization, staff, providers, financiers, and policymakers

Lauver & Phalen, 2017; Magyary, Whitney, & Brown, 2006

knowledge and skills of statistics inclusive of descriptive statistics, t-test, analysis of variance, chi-square, correlation, non-parametric tests, repeated measures, and linear, multiple, and logistic regression provides ability to conduct descriptive and inferential analyses of processes and outcomes (Lauver & Phalen, 2017; Polancich, James, Miltner, Smith, & Moneyham, 2018). Armed with knowledge and skills related to the research process, the DNP nurse applies her competence in multiple ways, as outlined in Table 6.1.

Equally important, the DNP must possess knowledge and skills related to qualitative research. Knowledge of qualitative research methods such as interviews, observations, and focus groups allows the DNP to explore the experience of patients, families, staff, and care providers to gain input from multiple perspectives. Access to such rich narrative data enhances understanding about clinical phenomena and can provide a unique perspective related to the value of practice (Magyary *et al.*, 2006). Qualitative approaches enrich the depth of understanding to inform practice and systems.

Collaboration to Increase Research Capacity

Even with the DNP's research process knowledge and skills, converging research with practice is challenging and requires merging of expertise across fields, such as practice and academia, and across disciplines to coalesce divergent perspectives, maximize knowledge of methods and systems, and create innovative approaches (Magyary et al., 2006). To contribute to nursing care through the development and integration of nursing knowledge as charged by the IOM's (2010) report, *The Future of Nursing: Leading Change, Advancing Health*, DNP nurses need to collaborate with PhD nurses, whether in clinical settings or academia. Moreover, the *Essentials of Doctoral Education for Advanced Nursing Practice* (AACN, 2006) indicates that "both research- and practice-focused doctoral programs in nursing . . . share a commitment to the advancement of the profession" (p. 3). Essential VI addresses "interprofessional collaboration for improving patient and population health outcomes (AACN, 2006, p. 14). Because of the divergent perspective and frameworks yet complementary skills and expertise between DNP and PhD nurses, they can collaborate to advance clinical and translational research validating the research as contributing to the advancement of nursing care. Collaborative relationships between research and practice focused nurses generates research ideas and projects, which contribute to the advancement of nursing knowledge, improve access, and promote quality of nursing care (Zinn et al., 2011).

Prior to initiation of collaborative efforts, DNP nurses must obtain support from executive leadership, departmental directors and other administrators, nursing managers, clinicians, and other decision-makers and stakeholders, whose advocacy, processes, approvals, and resources impact the success of the collaboration. Such support facilitates integration of research into the complexities and realities of clinical practice and service system models. To acquire support, the DNP nurses must articulate to organizational stakeholder how the academic institution's strategic plan will contribute to the mission of the organization and to the delivery and quality of care.

To establish a mutually beneficial partnership, the DNP nurses along with nursing leadership and administrative and clinical nurses must establish with academic faculty common ground which facilitates sharing of resources (Hendrix, Matters, West, Stewart, & McConnell, 2011). Likewise, the collaboration must support individual organizational goals as well as the goals of the academic institution and faculty (Soltani et al., 2017). The more the goals and objectives between the clinical and academic setting align, the better the continuity and lower likelihood of conflicts (Soltani et al., 2017). Moreover, inclusion of academic partners in organizational activities and committees, such as practice, research, EBP, QI, and professional development councils, facilitates sustainment of the relationship beyond the organizational affiliation agreements or memorandums of understandings.

To foster collegiality and trust, the DNP and clinical nurses must establish shared governance with the academic faculty. To ensure shared governance, the partners must develop a formalized research agreement annotating formal expectations and deliverable and tangible results. The agreement must identify the collaboration's mission and vision so that alignment of these goals in comparison to the health care organization's and academic institution's mission and vision can be assessed. The agreement outlines each organization's and academic institution's roles and responsibilities, including the purpose, research goals, and objectives, with identification of each partner's contributions to the objectives, planning and implementation of the study, meeting participation, tracking of performance, availability of any funding, key dates, and hosting of networking opportunities (Boland, Kamikawa, Inouye, Latimer, & Marshall, 2010; Soltani et al., 2017). To ensure that each partner supports the collaborative agreement, evaluation parameters are developed to measure adherence to responsibilities, tasks, and timelines. Evaluation metrics include task assignment and execution; achievement of proposed outcomes, time required to achieve tasks and proposed outcomes, and investment of resources and expected return on investment (Kirschling & Erickson, 2010). In summary, the agreement specifies the strategic and operational plan in support of the collaborative relationship, and metrics evaluate adherence to the plan. Each partner is actively involved in the drafting and revision of the agreement to create a sustainable collaboration.

Implementation requires that respect be extended to individuals' areas of expertise. Each individual works from his or her strengths and educational preparation. Table 6.2 identifies the responsibilities for the academic and clinical staff.

Although DNP nurses and other clinical nurses, as well as academic faculty, execute their respective responsibilities based on their strengths, multiple tasks require the joint efforts of both partners. For example, both clinical and academic team members collaborate on the use or development of data collection tools, data management, and analysis. Clinical staff and faculty are both identified as investigators on the research proposal. Finally, based on their collaborative contributions, both clinical nurses and academic faculty need to publish and present. They need to collaborative disseminate their efforts and innovations to advance nursing knowledge and science.

The collaborative research team must be receptive to feedback from all members and maintain consistent and effective communication. An atmosphere of openness demonstrating acknowledgement of controversial issues facilitates collaborative efforts. (Hendrix et al., 2011). Due to intervening factors that may impact timelines or alteration of invested resources, the research team members must accede to such realities. However, such issues warrant further explication for both the clinical nurses' and the academic faculty's need to fully understand the other entities' time horizons and expectations regarding return on the investment (Hendrix et al., 2011). The research team must maintain a consistent dialogue about

Table 6.2 Faculty and Clinical Staff Responsibilities.

DNP and Clinical Staff Responsibilities	Faculty Responsibilities
Provide clinical expertise and practice focus	Provide research expertise to ensure reliable and valid results
Direct how the study should be implemented within the setting and assist researchers with understanding the clinical context in which the research will be conducted	Lead the development of the design and methodology
Identify effective changes when unintended barriers surface	Develop plan for participant compensation
Facilitate access to patients and insights into unique clinical issues	Develop human subject protection plan
Inform the faculty and research team members of workflow and staffing levels to facilitate recruitment, participant selection, and participant participation	Develop informed consent
Actively engage the clinic staff to facilitate study progression	Provide letters for the nurses' annual performance reviews
Provide updates on data collection to the staff	Develop budget
Ensure consistent appreciation is extended to staff	

Gettrust, Hagle, Boaz, & Bull, 2016; Hendrix et al., 2011; Zinn et al., 2011.

the research project, benefits, accomplishments, barriers, and ways to overcome barriers (Soltani et al., 2017). Regular meetings and e-mail correspondence facilitate decisionmaking and discussions to maintain progress toward study completion and review research processes. Development of a website can facilitate discussion forums and document sharing, notifications, and project calendar.

To promote engagement of clinic staff in research, the research team must actively engage clinical staff. Clinical nurses should be informed of research projects and allowed to participate as needed. The nurses can assist the research team with understanding the clinical unit from which patients may be recruited, identify potential barriers and facilitators, and assist with recruitment and participant selection. In addition, such nurses function as unit champions for research projects. Research team members can implement educational programs that teach the research process to clinical staff. Following completion of the research project, clinical staff personnel are acknowledged for their contributions. The staff members participate in presentation of study findings, particularly within the clinical organization, such as during Nursing Grand Rounds, and participate in preparation of oral and poster presentations at local and national conferences (Gettrust et al., 2016). Inclusion of and recognition of clinical staff in research promotes nursing staff's knowledge of and interest in research and future participation in research endeavors, which contributes to expansion of research and building of research capacity within the organization.

The benefits reaped from collaborative research efforts are multiple. Table 6.3 outlines the benefits for both clinical nursing and academic faculty.

To facilitate nurses' participation in addressing emerging health care needs, the DNP nurse is the key individual for bridging the gap between practice and academia. The DNP nurse cultivates a climate of clinical inquiry across the health care organization by explaining the research process and engaging stakeholders and staff. Active and equal involvement in the study design and research development proposal, implementation, analysis, and follow-on discussion of findings demonstrates the value of research to not only nursing practice, but also to health outcomes, models of delivery of care, systems, and organizational processes. Such efforts validate that nursing can "make a difference" at the individual, system, and organizational levels. The next section highlights that it is incumbent upon DNP nurses to also acquire competency in quality improvement to further optimize health care delivery.

Table 6.3 Benefits of Collaborative Research Between Clinical Nurses and Academic Faculty.

- Strengthened partnerships
- Improvement in patient care and outcomes
- More rigorous evaluation of outcomes
- Expanded publication of results from shared projects and their outcomes
- Direct insight into current clinical issues that require research to inform practice
- Enculturation of nursing science within clinical settings
- Evidence of a comprehensive plan of care that ensures exemplary professional practice and high-quality patient outcomes
- Information sharing and networking
- Access to a larger variety of skill sets with differing strengths, expertise, and organizational and material resources
- Growth of research trajectories
- Faculty who aspire to keep their program of research grounded in practice and relevant to the bedside have the ability to participate in addressing clinical questions
- Clinical staff exposure to research
- Clinical staff receipt of assistance with developing and implementing research projects
- Increase in the skill set of both clinical nurses and nursing faculty
- Each organization's own growth in research capacity
- Reciprocal interactive processes whereby the bi-directional exchange of perspectives, values, expertise, and resources culminate in a commitment toward improving health care
- Sustainment of evidence-based innovative practices that address the daily realities of service systems and, thereby, bridge the gap between science and service

Boland et al., 2010; Hatfield et al., 2016; Hendrix et al., 2011; Magyary et al., 2006; Soltani et al., 2017.

The DNP Nurse and Quality of Care

In response to a report, *To Err is Human: Building a Safer Health System*, which disclosed that between 44,000 to 98,000 people die from medical errors each year (IOM, 1999), the IOM (2001) issued another report calling for improvements in the quality and safety of care. The six aims for improving health care included safety, effectiveness, patient-centered care, timeliness, efficiency, and equitability. Likewise, in 2001, the *Envisioning the National Healthcare Quality Report* developed a design and robust content for an annual National Healthcare Quality Report (NHQR) (Committee on the National Quality Report on Health Care Delivery; IOM, 2001). The Agency for Healthcare Research and Quality (AHRQ), an agency in the Department of Health and Human Services (HHS), assumes responsibility for the annual NHQR. The report defines the quality measures, characteristics of measures, and data sources for collection of data related to measures and provides criteria for designing and producing the quality report. Then in 2010, *The Future of Nursing: Leading Change, Advancing Health*, reinforced the accountability for contributing to the six aims and evaluation of quality outcomes for practice, care delivery models, and information technology initiatives.

The DNP nurse, as a C-Suite executive, maintains a practice-focus to not only develop and implement evidence-based nursing care, but also to sustain evidence-based nursing to improve quality practice and care. The DNP C-Suite nurse leader maintains accountability for contributing to AHRQ's six aims designed to improve health care quality. This key role for the DNP nurse is supported in *The Essentials of Doctoral Education for Advanced Nursing Practice* (AACN, 2006), which indicates that DNP nurses should have the "needed advanced competencies for increasingly complex practice, faculty, and leadership roles, enhanced knowledge to improve nursing practice and patient outcomes, and enhanced leadership skills to strengthen practice and health care delivery" (p. 5). In addition, *Essential II: Organizational and Systems Leadership for Quality Improvement and Systems Thinking*, states that "DNPs must be proficient in quality improvement strategies" (p. 10). Moreover, the Essentials highlight that the DNP must acquire competencies in system processes, business, finance, economics, and health policy to integrate with their expert knowledge of populations and clinical practice to facilitate continuous quality improvement (AACN, 2006). The Quality and Safety Education for Nurses (QSEN) Institute prepares nurses with the knowledge, skills, and attitudes to continuously improve the quality of the health care systems (Cronenwett *et al.*, 2007). The competencies are: patient-centered care, teamwork and collaboration, evidence-based practice, quality improvement, safety, and informatics. Within each competency, reference to the required skills, knowledge, and attitudes provides detailed expertise necessary for successful doctoral-level practice. For example, nurses need to be competent in the utilization of informatics to measure quality, lead teams, solicit team members, and establish effective collaboration of teamwork. Their knowledge base must enable them to complete root cause analyses and to demonstrate familiarity with the responsibilities of other departments and services to highlight cause-effect diagrams that explicitly delineate processes of care. Furthermore, they must understand measurement and variation to evaluate quality and, in the process, develop effective strategies to improve care (Cronenwett *et al.*, 2007).

Quality care is defined as "the degree to which health care services for individuals and populations increase the likelihood of desired health outcomes and are consistent with current professional knowledge," (IOM, 1990, p. 21). Systems and processes determine outcomes of care. This definition supports Donabedien's (1980) description of quality care as consisting of three elements: structure, process, and outcomes. The administrative, informational, therapeutic, diagnostic, and support services; governance; and systems represent the structure of the organization. Material and human resources and the organizational schematic serve as structure, which ranks as a critical factor for the successful development and implementation of quality improvement projects (Donabedian, 1980). Process refers to all required actions of a QI project. Actions may include technical, clinical, administrative, and interpersonal processes. Process oriented indicators may include adherence to regulatory requirements, integration of resources, and number of patients served. Finally, outcomes refer to the effect of the project on patients, populations, delivery of care, hospital costs, and other factors. Outcome measures include financial viability of clinical services, improved clinical outcomes, new models of care and education, satisfaction of staff and clients, reduced costs, and improved patient safety indicators. In practice, it is important to measure both process and outcome measures to evaluate the effectiveness of the processes intended to improve care. Measuring one without the other may result in conclusions that may not support the improvement of quality of care. The elements of structure, process, and outcomes are apparent in the definition of continuous quality improvement (CQI), which is defined as "a structural organizational process for involving personnel in planning and executing a continuous flow of improvements to provide quality healthcare that meets or exceeds expectations and usually involves a common set of characteristics," (Sollecito & Johnson, 2013, pp 4–5).

The IOM reports resulted in major changes not only directly in health care facilities, but also in the development of new legislation and regulations in multiple government departments and agencies, such as the Centers for Medicare and Medicaid Services (CMS), U.S. Food and Drug Administration (FDA), Centers for Disease Control and Prevention (CDC), Occupational Safety and Health Administration (OSHA), The Joint Com-

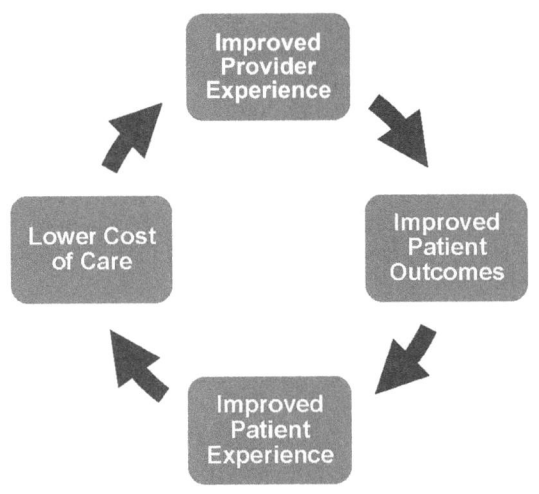

Figure 6.1. *Quadruple Aims. Adapted from Summit Strategic Solutions (2018). Courtesy of Diane B. Stoy.*

mission (TJC), and AHRQ (Finkelman, 2017). Furthermore, the reports led to the development of the Institute for Healthcare Improvement, which in turn, created the "Triple Aims" to optimize health for individuals and populations (Berwick, Nolan, & Whittington, 2008). The three aims were as follows: (1) Improving the patient experience of care, (2) Improving the health of populations, and (3) Reducing the per capita cost of health care (Berwick *et al.*, 2008). In 2008, Berwick, Nolan, and Whittington established these three dimensions to identify broader goals that were linked to facilitate achievement of health care improvement initiatives. Since its origins, a fourth dimension, improving the life of health care providers, clinicians, and staff, has been added and today the aims are referred to as the "Quadruple Aims" (Figure 6.1) (Bodenheimer & Sinsky, 2014). The IOM reports also influenced the development of the 2010 Patient Protection and Affordable Care Act (ACA) and resulted in the establishment of the National Quality Strategy.

Quality Improvement Initiative: The National Quality Strategy (NQS)

The ACA established the National Quality Strategy (NQS), which addressed the need for a national quality improvement framework (Burstin, Leatherman, & Goldmann, 2016; HHS, AHRQ, 2017). The Quadruple Aims provide the basis for the NQS (HHS, AHRQ, 2017). The six priorities include (1) Making care safer by reducing harm caused in the delivery of care; (2) Ensuring that each person and family is as partners in their care; (3) Promoting effective communication and coordination of care; (4) Promoting the most effective prevention and treatment practices for leading causes of mortality; (5) Working with communities to promote wide use of best practices to enable healthy living; and (6) Making quality care more affordable for individuals, families, employers, and government by developing and distributing new healthcare delivery models (HHS, AHRQ, 2017). Nine levers, which represent "a core business function, resource, and/or action that stakeholders can use to align to the strategy," facilitate meeting the aims (Figure 6.2) (HHS, AHRQ, 2017).

Federal health care programs apply the NQS, and the AHRQ (HHS, AHRQ, 2017) recommends that private and public health care programs adopt the NQS, although it is not required. However, multiple private and public health care organizations provide data for the NQS report. Figure 6.3 presents an overview of the NQS highlighting the linkage between levers, priorities, and aims. The implementation of the NQS considers factors such as health care trends, state and national health care policies and legislation, professional standards, state and federal requirements, and reporting of quality measures for reporting systems and third-party payers (HHS, AHRQ, 2017). The NQS has been key in stimulating development of national metrics and aggregate reports focusing on the measurement of quality indicators in health care organizations. The next section highlights some of the various organizations and the quality care metrics they mandate or recommend for measurement of quality improvement.

Organizations Measuring Health Care Quality

The Centers for Medicare and Medicaid Services

The Centers for Medicare and Medicaid Services (CMS) bases its quality improvement goals on four principles: (1) Eliminate racial and ethnic disparities, (2) Strengthen infrastructure and data systems, (3) Enable local innovations, and (4) Foster learning organizations (CMS, 2016). The overall vision for the CMS Quality Strategy is to optimize health outcomes by improving quality and transforming the healthcare system (CMS, 2016). Its quality goals are as follows:

1. Make care safer by reducing harm caused in the delivery of care
2. Strengthen patient and family engagement as partners in care
3. Promote effective communication and coordination of care
4. Promote effective prevention and treatment of chronic disease
5. Work with communities to promote best practices of healthy living
6. Make care affordable

Lever	Icon	Design	Example
Payment		Reward and incentivize providers to deliver high-quality, patient-centered care.	Join a regional coalition of purchasers that are pursuing value-based purchasing.
Public Reporting		Compare treatment results, costs, and patient experience for consumers.	A regional collaborative may ask member hospitals and medical practices to align public reports to the National Quality Strategy aims or priorities.
Learning and Technical Assistance		Foster learning environments that offer training, resources, tools, and guidance to help organizations achieve quality improvement goals.	A Quality Improvement Organization may disseminate evidence-based best practices in quality improvement with physicians, hospitals, nursing homes, and home health agencies.
Certification, Accreditation, and Regulation		Adopt or adhere to approaches to meet safety and quality standards.	The National Quality Strategy aims and priorities may be incorporated into continuing education requirements or certification maintenance.
Consumer Incentives and Benefit Designs		Help consumers adopt healthy behaviors and make informed decisions.	Employers may implement workforce wellness programs that promote prevention and provide incentives for employees to improve their health.
Measurement and Feedback		Provide performance feedback to plans and providers to improve care.	A long-term care provider may implement a strategy that includes the use of Quality Assurance and Performance Improvement data to populate measurement dashboards for purposes of identifying and addressing areas requiring quality improvement.
Health Information Technology		Improve communication, transparency, and efficiency for better coordinated health and health care.	A hospital or medical practice may adopt an electronic health record system to improve communication and care coordination.
Workforce Development		Investing in people to prepare the next generation of health care professionals and support lifelong learning for providers.	A medical leadership institution may incorporate quality improvement principles in their training.
Innovation and Diffusion		Foster innovation in health care quality improvement, and facilitate rapid adoption within and across organizations and communities.	Center for Medicare & Medicaid Innovation tests various payment and service delivery models and shares successful models across the Nation.

Figure 6.2. *National Quality Strategy Levers. Reproduced from U.S. Department of Health and Human Services (2017). National quality strategy: Using levers to achieve improved health and health care. Retrieved from https://www.ahrq.gov/workingforquality/about/nqs-fact-sheets/index.html.*

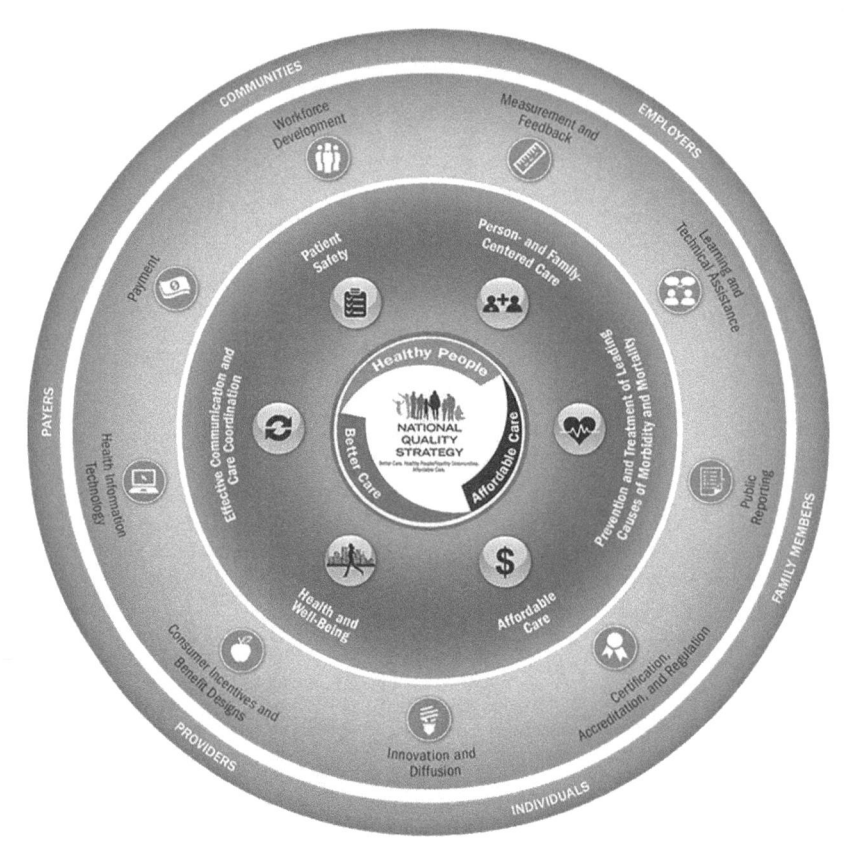

Figure 6.3. *National Quality Strategy: How It Works. Source: Reproduced from U.S. Department of Health and Human Services (2017). National quality strategy: Overview [PowerPoint presentation]. Retrieved from https://www.ahrq.gov/workingforquality/nqs-tools/briefing-slides.html.*

The CMS uses a variety of measures to assess quality. The measures focus on highly prevalent conditions in the Medicare beneficiary populations, such as heart disease, pneumonia/influenza, diabetes, joint disease/arthritis, cancer, renal disease, and chronic obstructive pulmonary disease, and on other topics such as health information technology, patient safety, patient experience, health disparities, end-of-life and palliative care, and preventive care (CMS, 2018). The CMS collects data on quality measures for multiple reporting systems, such as hospital inpatient and outpatient quality reporting, hospital readmission reduction reporting, hospital value-based purchasing, Medicaid, Medicare Advantage, Healthcare Effectiveness Data and Information Set (HEDIS) quality measure rating system, ambulatory surgical center quality reporting, inpatient psychiatric facility quality reporting, and many others (CMS, 2018).

The CMS also developed and maintains *The Consumer Assessment of*

Healthcare Providers and Systems (CAHPS), which collects patient satisfaction data (CMS, 2018). The surveys focus on the patient's, and sometimes family's, experience with and ratings of health care providers, health plans, and health care settings. The patient experience surveys differ from patient satisfaction surveys. The CAHPS survey asks how the patient or family experienced or perceived their care. Numerous CAHPS surveys exist specific to hospitals, home health, fee-for-service facilities, the Medicare Advantage and the Prescription Drug Plan, in-center hemodialysis, adult Medicaid recipients, hospice, accountable care organizations, outpatient and ambulatory surgery, the Merit-Based Incentive Payment System, and home and community-based services (CMS, 2018).

As of October 2012, Medicare implemented a system of value-based purchasing for hospitals. Hospital Value-Based Purchasing (VBP) rewards hospitals based primarily on quality measures, and not quantity, of care provided to Medicare patients (CMS, 2011). Medicare provides payment based on how well hospital perform on each VBP measure compared with other hospitals' performances and how much the hospital improves their performances on each measure compared with their baseline period. Therefore, performance assesses achievement and improvement. If a hospital rates at or above the benchmark (average [mean] performance of the top 10% of hospitals during the baseline period), it receives 10 achievement points. However, if the hospital rates below the achievement threshold (performance at the 50th percentile [median] of hospitals during the baseline period), it receives 0 achievement points. For improvement, if the hospital rates at or above the benchmark, it receives 9 points. If the hospital rates below the baseline period score, it receives 0 improvement points. The CMS pays based on the hospitals' summated points for achievement and improvement.

The *Hospital Consumer Assessment of Healthcare Providers and Systems* (HCAHPS) survey measures patient satisfaction with rendered hospital services. Consistency points are awarded by comparing an individual hospital's HCAHPS survey dimension rates during the performance period to all hospitals' HCAHPS survey rates from a baseline period (CMS, 2011). To calculate the total performance score, the greater of either the hospital's achievement or improvement points for each measure are combined to determine a score for each domain; each domain score is multiplied by a specified weight (percentage), and the weighted domain scores are summed. The CMS provide the measures grouped by domains. Table 6.4 provides the fiscal year 2019 CMS Hospital Value-Based Performance Program measures.

The CMS, as well as numerous organizations such as The National Quality Forum, the Joint Commission, the Agency for Healthcare Research and Quality, and third-party payers, collect data on hospital-acquired condition (HAC) measures. CMS classifies HACs as follows (CMS, 2005):

1. High cost, high volume, or both
2. Identified through the International Classification of Diseases as complicating or major complicating condition that when present and included in secondary diagnoses may result in a higher-paying diagnosis-related group (DRG), the diagnosis classification system developed by CMS
3. Conditions that are reasonably preventable through use of evidence-based guidelines

Although the types of HACs may change from year to year, the CMS provides no payment for HACs nor can Medicaid or Medicare patients be personally charged for the additional care needs. The conditions for 2018 are as follows (CMS, 2018):

1. Foreign object retained after surgery
2. Air embolism
3. Blood incompatibility
4. Stage III and IV pressure ulcers
5. Falls and trauma: Fractures, dislocations, intracranial injuries, crushing injuries, burns, other injuries
6. Manifestations of poor gylcemic control: Diabetic ketoacidosis, non-ketotic hyperosmolar coma, hypoglycemic coma, secondary diabetes with ketoacidosis, secondary diabetes with hyperosmolarity
7. Catheter-associated urinary tract infections (CAUTI)
8. Vascular catheter-associated infection such as central line associated blood stream infections (CLABSI)
9. Surgical site infection, mediastinitis, following coronary artery bypass graft
10. Surgical site infection following bariatric surgery for obesity: Laparoscopic gastric bypass, gastroenterostomy, laparoscopic gastric restrictive surgery
11. Surgical site infection following certain orthopedic procedures: Spine, neck, shoulder, elbows
12. Surgical site infection following cardiac implantable electronic device
13. Deep vein thrombosis pulmonary embolism following certain orthopedic procedures: Total knee replacement, hip replacement
14. Iatrogenic pneumothorax with venous catheterization

National Committee for Quality Assurance

The National Committee for Quality Assurance collects data for the

Table 6.4 FY2019 CMS Hospital Value-Based Performance Program Measures.

Measure ID	Measure Description	Domain
CAUTI	Catheter-Associated Urinary Tract Infection	Safety
CLABSI	Central Line-Associated Blood Stream Infection	Safety
CDI	Clostridium difficile Infection (C. difficile)	Safety
MRSA	Methicillin-Resistant Staphylococcus aureus Bacteremia	Safety
PC-01	Elective Delivery Prior to 39 Completed Weeks Gestation	Safety
SSI	Surgical Site Infection: Colon, Abdominal Hysterectomy	Safety
MORT-30-AMI	Acute Myocardial Infarction (AMI) 30-Day Mortality Rate	Clinical Care
MORT-30-HF	Heart Failure (HF) 30-Day Mortality Rate	Clinical Care
MORT-30-PN	Pneumonia (PN) 30-Day Mortality Rate	Clinical Care
THA/TKA	Total Hip Arthroplasty (THA) and/or total Knee Arthroplasty (TKA)	Clinical Care
MSPB	Medicare Spending per Beneficiary (MSPB)	Efficiency and Cost Reduction
HCAHPS Survey	Communication with Nurses Communication with Doctors Responsiveness of Hospital Staff Communication about Medicines Hospital Cleanliness and Quietness Discharge Information 3-Item Care Transition Overall Rating of Hospital	Person and Community Engagement

Reproduced from Centers for Medicare and Medicaid Services (2017). Hospital value-based purchasing. Medicare Learning network booklet. Retrieved from https://www.cms.gov/Outreach-and-Education/Medicare-Learning-Network-MLN/MLNProducts/downloads/Hospital_VBPurchasing_Fact_Sheet_ICN907664.pdf.

Healthcare Effectiveness Data and Information Set (HEDIS), which includes 90 measures across six domains: effectiveness of care, access/availability of care, experience of care, utilization and risk adjusted utilization, health plan descriptive information, and measures collected using electronic clinical data systems (NCQA, 2018). Examples of focus for measures include BMI, weight counseling, immunizations lead screening, breast and cervical cancer screening, care for older adults, medication management, diabetes care, follow-up after Emergency Department visits, well-child visits, and many others (NCQA, 2018). The NCQA collects data directly from health plans and preferred provider organizations (PPO) through the Healthcare Organization Questionnaire and collects non-survey data from the Interactive Data Submission System (NQAS, 2018). The HEDIS data facilitates establishment of national performance statistics and benchmarks.

The Agency for Healthcare Research and Quality

The AHRQ provides free software to health care organizations to collect and submit data to AHRQ based on designated indicators. This allows health care organizations to compare their data to national benchmarks. AHRQ provides a variety of programs to health care organizations and providers for the collection of data related to specific indicators.

The AHRQ quality indicators measure health care quality that exists in real time in hospital inpatient administrative data (HHS, AHRQ, 2018). These indicators are specific for acute care hospitals and, as such, cannot apply to other settings, including long-term care, outpatient services, emergency department, or hospice. Applicability excludes other populations, such as mental health, substance abuse, readmission, surgery, or rehabilitation. The AHRQ indicators are categorized into five modules: prevention quality indicators, inpatient quality indicators, patient safety indicators, pediatric quality indicators, and home and community-based indicators (HHS, AHRQ, 2018). The inpatient quality indicators include 28 provider-level indicators for which data is collected from the hospital inpatient discharge data (HHS, AHRQ, 2018). The indicators are grouped into four categories:

1. *Volume indicators* are indirect measures of quality based on counts of admissions during which certain intensive, high-technology, or highly complex procedures were performed. They are based on evidence suggesting that hospitals performing more of these procedures may have better outcomes.
2. *Mortality indicators* for inpatient procedures include procedures for which mortality has been shown to vary across institutions and for which evidence suggests that high mortality may be associated with poorer quality of care.
3. *Mortality indicators for inpatient conditions* include conditions for which mortality has been shown to vary substantially across institutions and for which evidence suggests that high mortality may be associated with deficiencies in the quality of care.
4. *Utilization indicators* examine procedures for which use varies significantly across hospitals and for which questions have been raised about overuse, underuse, and misuse.

Prevention quality indicators focus on preventing additional hospitalizations or are used to indicate the need for early intervention to avoid complications or negative health outcomes. The data are collected from inpatient discharge data. Pediatric quality indicators examine care for pediatric patients in hospitals. Home and community-based services indicators focus on Medicaid beneficiaries who are receiving home and community-based services. Patient safety indicators examine hospital complications and adverse events, particularly following surgery, procedures, and childbirth.

The National Healthcare Quality and Disparities Report

The AHRQ reports on the status of healthcare quality and disparities in the National Healthcare Quality and Disparities Report (HHS, AHRQ, 2018). The report is mandated by Congress to provide a comprehensive overview of the quality of health care and disparities in care experienced by different racial and socioeconomic groups. The report addresses over 250 indicators across various areas, such as access to care, care coordination, patient- and family-centered care, effective treatment, women's health, and health care for Hispanics and Blacks.

The National Quality Measures Clearinghouse

The National Quality Measures Clearinghouse (NQMC) provides evidence-based quality measures and measure sets (HHS, AHRQ, NQMC, 2015). The goal is to provide more consistent measures of quality and provide a resource that organizes measures so that health care organizations and providers have a more accessible source of multiple measures. The measures focus on two categories, health care delivery measures and population health measures. Health care delivery measures focus on care delivered to individuals and populations defined by their relationships to clinicians, clinician delivery teams, delivery organizations, or health insurance plans. Population health measures address individual or population health issues defined by residence in a geographic area or a relationship to an organization that is not designated as to provide health care services (e.g., schools and prisons) (HHS, AHRQ, NQMC, 2015). Figure 6.4 describes the NQMC domain framework

National Quality Forum

The National Quality Forum (NQF) requires reporting on a listing of identified serious events (Table 6.5). The NFQ considers a serious reportable event to be "unambiguous, largely, if not entirely, preventable, serious, and any of the following: (1) Adverse; (2) Indicative of a problem in a healthcare setting's safety systems; and (3) Important for public creditability or public accountability" (NQF, 2011). The serious reportable events comprise those that are of concern to both the public and health care providers, identifiable and measurable, feasible to include in a reporting system, and of a nature such that the risk of occurrence is significantly influenced by the policies and procedures of the health care facility (NQF, 2011). The reporting facilitates, on a national level, identification of the magnitude of the event, evaluation of the events, and development of preventive measures.

NQMC Domain Framework

Measures Related to Health

- **Health Care Delivery Measures**: Measures of care delivered to individuals and populations defined by their relationship to clinicians, clinical delivery teams, delivery organizations, or health insurance plans. Denominators for these measures are defined by some form of affiliation with a clinical care delivery organization, e.g. recipients of health care, health plan enrollees, clinical episodes, clinicians, or clinical delivery organizations.
  - Clinical Quality Measures
    - Process
    - Access
    - Outcome
    - Structure
    - Patient Experience
  - Related Health Care Delivery Measures
    - User-Enrollee Health State
    - Management
    - Use of Services
    - Cost
  - Clinical Efficiency Measures
    - Efficiency

- **Population Health Measures**: Measures that address health issues of individuals or populations defined by residence in a geographic area or a relationship to organizations that are not primarily organized to deliver or pay for health care services (such as schools or prisons). The responsibility for "performance" typically falls to public officials, public health agencies, or organizations that are not primarily deliverers of care.
  - Population Health Quality Measures
    - Population Process
    - Population Access
    - Population Outcome
    - Population Structure
    - Population Experience
  - Related Population Health Measures
    - Population Health State
    - Population Management
    - Population Use of Services
    - Population Cost
    - Population Health Knowledge
    - Social Determinants of Health
    - Environment
  - Population Efficiency Measures
    - Population Efficiency

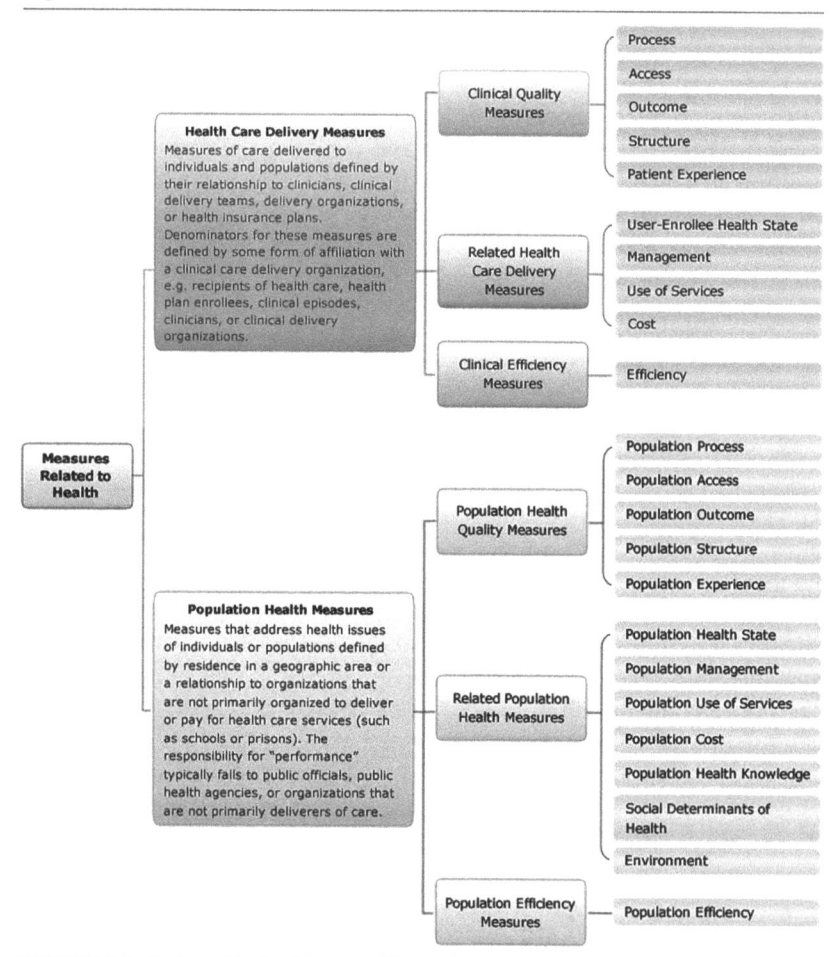

FIGURE 6.4. *National Quality Measures Clearinghouse Domain Framework. Reproduced from Agency for Healthcare Research and Quality (September 10, 2018). Retrieved from https://www.ahrq.gov/gam/summaries/domain-framework/index.html.*

The Joint Commission

The Joint Commission (TJC), an independent, not-for-profit organization, accredits and certifies health care organizations and health care programs (TJC, 2018). In 1999, TJC introduced the ORYX initiative for hospital quality measurement to integrate quality improvement into accreditation (TJC, 2018). This initiative required hospitals to collect and transmit data to TJC for a minimum of four core measures sets: acute myocardial infarction (AMI), heart failure (HF), pneumonia (PN), and preg-

Table 6.5 National Quality Forum Serious Reportable Events.

Surgical or Invasive Procedure Events

- Surgery/invasive procedure performed on the wrong site or wrong patient
- Wrong surgical/invasive procedure performed on a patient
- Unintended retention of a foreign object in a patient after surgery or invasive procedure
- Intraoperative or immediately post-operative post-procedure death in a normal, healthy patient

Product or Device Events

- Patient death/serious injury associated with the use of contaminated drugs, devices, or biologics, the use or function of a devise for other than intended use or function, or with intravascular air embolism

Patient Protection Events

- Discharge/release of a patient, who is unable to make decisions, to other than an authorized person
- Patient death/serious injury associated with patient elopement (disappearance)
- Patient suicide, attempted suicide, or self-harm that results in serious injury

Care Management Events

- Patient death/serious injury associated with a medication error, unsafe administration of blood products, resulting from the irretrievable loss of an irreplaceable biologic specimen or from failure to follow-up or communicate laboratory, pathology, or radiology test results; or a fall while being cared for in a healthcare setting
- Maternal death/serious injury associated with labor or delivery in a low-risk pregnancy
- Death/serious injury of a neonate associated with labor or delivery in a low-risk pregnancy
- Any Stage 3, Stage 4, or unstageable pressure ulcers acquired after admission/presentation to a healthcare setting
- Artificial insemination with the wrong donor sperm/egg

Environmental Events

- Patient/staff death or serious injury associated with an electric shock
- Any incident in which systems designated for oxygen or other gas to be delivered to a patient contains no gas, the wrong gas, or are contaminated by toxic substance
- Patient/staff death or serious injury associated with a burn incurred from any source in the course of a patient care process
- Patient death/serious injury associated with the use of physical restraints or bedrails

Radiologic Events

- Death/serious injury of a patient or staff associated with the introduction of a metallic object into the MRI area

Potential Criminal Events

- Any instance of care ordered by or provided by someone impersonating a licensed healthcare provider (e.g., physician, nurse, or pharmacist)
- Abduction of a patient/resident
- Sexual abuse/assault on a patient or staff member
- Death/serious injury of a patient or staff member resulting from a physical assault

Reproduced from the National Quality Forum, List of Serious Reportable Events. Retrieved from http://www.qualityforum.org/Topics/SREs/List_of_SREs.aspx.

nancy and related conditions (PR). Since the introduction of the initiative, the measures have been subsumed under other measures or replaced, and multiple additional measure sets have been added. The current measures include AMI, perinatal care, the emergency department, children's asthma care, hospital outpatient, early hearing detection and intervention, immunization, stroke, venous thromboembolism, substance use, tobacco treatment, and hospital-based inpatient psychiatric services (TJC, 2017a). TJC categorizes the core measures into accountability and nonaccountability measures and incorporates standards-based expectations for minimum performance on accountability measures against which health care organizations are surveyed and requirements for improvement (RFIs) can be made (TJC, 2018). TJC performance measures are closely aligned with CMS quality reporting measures. Today, TJC has shifted from ORYX to electronic clinical quality measures (e-CQM) requiring electronic reporting by all health care facilities.

TJC also identifies key safety goals (TJC, 2018). These goals are established based on the information TJC receives from its health care organizations and are specified in accordance with the type of health care organization (e.g., ambulatory care, acute care hospital). The 2018 goals focus on patient identification, staff communication, medication safety, safe use of false alarms, prevention of infection, identification of patient safety risks (suicide focus), and prevention of mistakes in surgery (TJC, 2018). Health care organizations accredited by TJC must use the National Patient Safety Goals as one of their critical continuous quality improvement guides. Data about the goals are collected by individual health care organizations and submitted to TJC, who describes the data in aggregate form to assess progress in meeting the annual goals and then shares the aggregate data with health care organizations and others.

In 1996, TJC implemented a Sentinel Event Policy to identify major unexpected events that happen to patients resulting in major negative outcomes, such as unexpected death or a critical physical or psychological complication that can lead to major alterations in the patient's health, and to assist hospitals with prevention of such events. A sentinel event is a patient event that "results in death, permanent harm, or severe temporary harm and intervention required to sustain life," (TJC, 2017b, no page). The types of sentinel events are determined by the type of health care organization (eg, ambulatory care, nursing care center, or hospital). Table 6 lists events considered sentinel events in a hospital setting. Accredited hospitals are expected to identify and respond to all sentinel events.

Press Ganey—The National Database of Nursing Indicators

The National Database of Nursing Indicators (NDNQI) is the only nursing database that tracks specific nursing-sensitive indicators related to nursing structure, process, and patient outcomes. The original database was developed with American Nurses Association (ANA) support and administered through several university nursing programs, but is now administered through Press Ganey (Finkelman, 2018). Health care organizations voluntarily participate in the database. Currently, 2,000 health care organizations and 98% of Magnet-recognized health care organizations participate (Press Ganey, 2016). The database provides a monitor for relationships between its specific indicators and outcomes. The list of indicators includes nursing hours per patient day; nursing turnover rate; nosocomial infections; patient falls; patient falls with injury; pressure ulcer rate; pediatric pain assessment, intervention, and reassessment; pediatric peripheral intravenous infiltration; psychiatric physical/sexual assault; restraints; staff mix; job satisfaction; practice environment; and education/certification (Montalvo, 2007).

Table 6.6 Hospital-Related Sentinel Events.

- Suicide of any patient receiving care, treatment, and services in a staffed around-the-clock care setting or within 72 hours of discharge, including from the hospital's emergency department
- Unanticipated death of a full-term infant
- Discharge of an infant to the wrong family
- Abduction of any patient receiving care, treatment, and services
- Any elopement (unauthorized departure) of a patient from a staffed around-the-clock care setting (including the Emergency Department), leading to death, permanent harm, or severe temporary harm to the patient
- Hemolytic transfusion reaction involving administration of blood or blood products having major blood group incompatibilities (ABO, Rh, other blood groups)
- Rape, assault (leading to death, permanent harm, or severe temporary harm), or homicide of a staff member, licensed independent practitioner, visitor, or vendor while on-site at the hospital
- Invasive procedure, including surgery, on the wrong patient, at the wrong site, or that is the wrong (unintended) procedure
- Unintended retention of a foreign object in a patient after an invasive procedure, including surgery,
- Severe neonatal hyperbilirubinemia (bilirubin > 30 milligrams/deciliter)
- Prolonged fluoroscopy with cumulative dose > 1,500 rads to a single field or any delivery of radiotherapy to the wrong body region or > 25% above the planned radiotherapy dose
- Fire, flame, or unanticipated smoke, heat, or flashes occurring during an episode of patient care
- Any intrapartum (related to the birth process) maternal death
- Severe maternal morbidity (not primarily related to the natural course of the patient's illness or underlying condition) when it reaches a patient and results in permanent harm or severe temporary harm

Reproduced from The Joint Commission Comprehensive Accreditation Manual for Hospitals (CAMH), July 1, 2017. Retrieved from https://www.jointcommission.org/assets/1/6/CAMH_SE_0717.pdf.

Dashboards

To track these metrics, health care industry C-Suite executives, including chief nurse officers, create dashboards, a performance scorecard, that rates the progress of quality improvements projects and compliance with required metrics (Figure 6.5). The dashboards report progress in a concise and clear manner using statistical charts and figures to illustrate the status of measures. Most U.S. hospitals, greater than 80%, have dashboards (Kroch et al., 2006). The measures relate to clinical quality, safety, patient satisfaction, financial indicator, employee factors, daily operations management, and strategic objectives (Kroch et al., 2006). Required and incentivized reporting metrics requested by CMS and TJC are reflected in the dashboards. In a study examining hospital dashboards (Kroch et al., 2006), findings indicated that hospitals that use dashboards for monitoring QI projects are more likely to be high-quality performers. A factor contributing to this relationship is that the dashboard communicates progress on QI projects to executive leadership who, in turn, hold lower level managers accountable for failure to meet expected outcomes on QI projects. Findings also highlighted that improved QI performance is linked to engagement of QI committees, clinicians including nurses, and other QI experts in development and monitoring of QI metrics included in dashboards (Kroch et al., 2006).

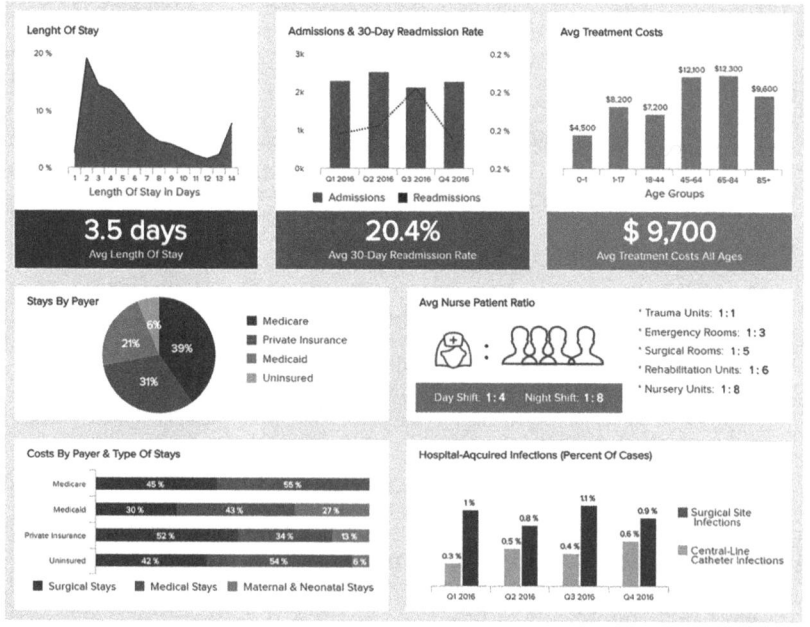

FIGURE 6.5. *Hospital Dashboard. Reproduced from https://www.datapine.com/images/hospital-performance-dashboard.png. Reprinted with permission from Datapine © 2018.*

Quality Improvement Methods

Each health care organization selects the methods it will use for identification, development, implementation, and analysis of its quality improvement initiatives. DNP-prepared nurse executives must understand these methods and their application to successfully participate in QI initiatives. With the increasing emphasis on quality improvement since the publication of the Quality Chasm report in 1999, the health care industry has witnessed an expansion in the development of measures. The following presents an overview of the most common methods used for quality improvement projects.

Root Cause Analysis

Root cause analysis (RCA) assumes that most errors are caused by systems and not individual staff. The RCA process "allows the analyst or analyzing team to identify the exact issue, identify the reason for the occurrence of the problem, and develop means to prevent the issue from recurring or reduce the probability that it will happen again," (HHS, AHRQ, 2013). The RCA process includes the following steps (HHS, AHRQ, 2013):

1. Select the team to complete the RCA. The team should include experts related to the event as well as management staff.
2. Create a flowchart
3. Examine the flowchart for areas of failure
4. Use team methods to assist the team in discussing and identifying underlying causes
5. Use CQI tools to compare collected data to possible root causes
6. Redesign the process for improvement based on the analysis results
7. Initially through a pilot project, implement the changes. Readjust the process based on analysis and again implement the revised process on a larger scale. Continue until the desired outcomes are achieved.

The RCA should provide a clear and comprehensive identification of the problem and options for preventing further occurrences of the problem. Evidence or best practice should be used to support the new process. TJC requires its accredited health care organizations to use an RCA for analysis of sentinel events. The corrective action plan identifies the strategies that the hospital intends to implement to prevent future occurrences of the sentinel event.

Failure Mode and Effects Analysis

Failure mode and effects analysis (FMEA) is a prospective method to prevent errors or harm by attempting to identify ways a process could fail, estimate the probability and consequences of each failure, and then act to prevent the potential failures from occurring (Institute for Healthcare Improvement [IHI], 2017). FMEA requires identification of all steps in the process and a description of potential problems with each step, impact, and probability. FMEA includes review of the process and identification of the failure mode, cause, and effect. The team also evaluates the likelihood that a failure mode would occur and the likelihood that a failure mode would not be detected. Severity of the failure mode is also determined. Multiplication of the likelihood of occurrence, the likelihood of detection, and the severity calculates a risk profile number, which is used to develop actions to reduce the occurrence of failure (IHI, 2017). Because it is a prospective process, it represents a preventive approach to reduce risk of harm to the patients and staff. FMEA is suited for evaluation of a new process prior to implementation to assess the effect of the new process on existing systems, patients, and staff. The IHI provides an on-line quality improvement essentials toolkit for a failure modes and effects analysis.

Plan-Do-Study-Act

The plan-do-study-act (PDSA) (Figure 6.6) is a rapid cycle change method (IHI, 2012; Langley *et al.* 2009). In Step 1, Plan, the team describes a plan for a change. The team establishes objectives and predictions of the outcome and plans for the test of change. The planning phase is where the objective and specific changes to be tested are identified. Planning considers who, what, when, where, and why data. It details the steps necessary to carry out the test, including roles, functions, education needed, how data will be collected, and how long the test will last. Based on analysis of data, which identifies a problem, the team plans and implements a strategy/intervention to improve. In Step 2, Do, the pilot plan is tested on a smaller scale such as on only one unit. Execution of the test is carried out. In Step 3, Study, the team collects and analyzes data to evaluate the outcomes. The outcomes are compared with the predictions. Results are measured and analyzed to evaluate whether outcomes have been met. In Step 4, Act, the modifications are implemented based on the outcomes. Then the next pilot test is planned and implemented on a larger scale, and the process continues until the desired outcomes are achieved. Once desired outcomes are achieved, the strategy/intervention is standardized and disseminated.

Lean Approach

The lean approach focuses on value to the customer, the patient, by decreasing waste in time, effort, and cost; doing more with less (Litvak & Bisganon, 2011). Toyota originally developed the approach as a compo-

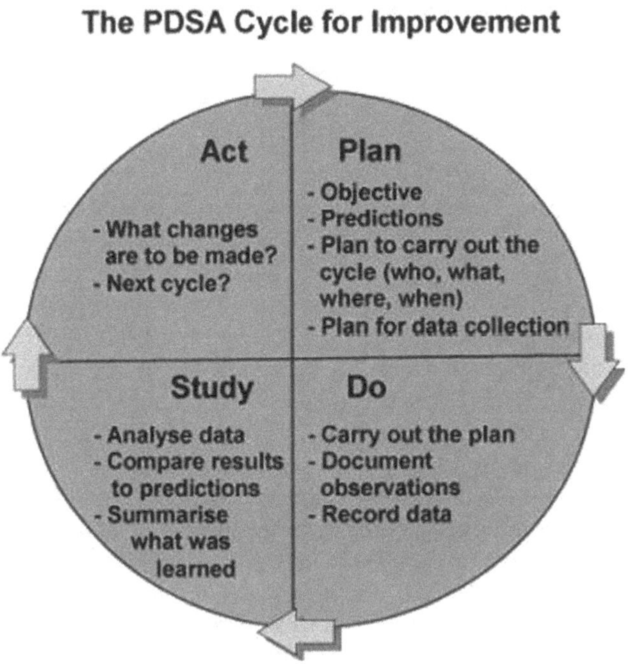

The PDSA Cycle for Improvement

Plan
- Objective
- Predictions
- Plan to carry out the cycle (who, what, where, when)
- Plan for data collection

Do
- Carry out the plan
- Document observations
- Record data

Study
- Analyse data
- Compare results to predictions
- Summarise what was learned

Act
- What changes are to be made?
- Next cycle?

FIGURE 6.6. *PDSA Cycle.*

nent of its process improvement system for inventory management and waste reduction (Black & Miller, 2008). Due to Toyota's success with this approach, health care organizations have adopted it as well. A five-step process includes the following: (1) Evaluating the current situation, (2) identifying areas of opportunity, (3) Modifying the existing process, (4) Substantiating and enumerating improvements, and (5) Implementing new work standards (Lean Enterprise Institute, 2011). Initially, to assess the current state, the team collects data that, through analysis, identifies processes that are not providing any value to the patient. Then, the team develops new or revised processes to eliminate the nonvalue ones. Lean tools such as the 5S system—sort, simplify, standardize, sweep, and selfdiscipline—facilitate identification of the new processes. For example, cleaning and organizing an area equates to sorting and simplifying. Using such a technique may identify how to reduce time for completion of a task. Following modification, the team pilot-tests the new processes and measures the impact, including savings whether in terms of cost or time. Finally, if the new processes are successful, they are standardized and disseminated. The focus on cost raises a concern with this approach, because overemphasis on cost may result in failure to view the QI initiative from a larger perspective. Nonetheless, such an approach demonstrates effectiveness in addressing QI initiatives focusing on waste, e.g., overproduction, duplication of services, processing delays, and nonproductive staff hours (Belter *et al.*, 2012; Hummer & Daccarett, 2009; Mazzocato *et al.*, 2012).

Six Sigma

Six Sigma offers a measurement strategy to reduce variation and eliminate deviations or deficits in processes. It includes three key elements: "(1) Measure work output, (2) Apply the process throughout all departments in the organization, until it eventually becomes part of the organization, and (3) maintain a goal of no more than 3.4 errors per 1,000,000,000 operations" (Fallon, Beguin, & Riley, 2013, p. 265). Six Sigma focuses on statistical methods to identify errors and process variability to reduce defects and achieve the goal. "Sigma is a statistical measure of variability in the process" (Pyzdek, 2003, p. 59).

Define and measure-analyze-design-verify (DMADV) represents a method used by Six Sigma. Using this method, the team defines project goals and outcomes, analyzes the process, and then verifies performance (Finkelman, 2018). *Define and measure-analyze-improve-control* (DMAIC) represents another available method (Finkelman, 2018). Although DMAIC is similar to DMADV for the first two steps, in the third step, the process improves by removing defects so that future performance is controlled. DMADV is typically used when a new process or product needs to be developed or when there is a process or product that has been changed but needs more improvement. The combination of the lean approach with Six Sigma is referred to as Lean Six Sigma.

Just-in-Time

Originated by the founder of Toyota, just-in-time means "only what is needed, when it is needed, and in the amount it is needed" (Toyota Motor Corporation, 2018). Developed for management, the method focuses on inventory. Basically, supplies and equipment are not stored; they are available and provided only when needed. The method eliminates the need for maintenance of inventory. However, for this process to be successful, several factors, such as timing, availability of the item, and transport processes, need to be considered. Therefore, application of the method to other sectors failed to demonstrate effectiveness in terms of management of supplies and equipment needed for certain products. For example, in health care organizations, items must be readily available to provide delivery of care for unexpected and acute conditions. Therefore, a consistent and ready inventory of items is required to meet this need.

However, businesses have recognized the value of this method in application to other systems such as staffing and teaching. Just-in-time staffing provides the needed amount of labor when required. Today, many human resource agencies provide a variety of temporary employees. For health care, agencies provide nurses, non-licensed medical technicians, and medical administrative support for placement, as needed, in health care organizations. Just-in-time teaching provides the needed education when it is needed. This concept has been applied in in health care organizations for a variety of patient care procedures, such as lumbar punctures, tracheal intubation, and splinting (Cheng, Liu, & Wang, 2017; Kessler *et al.*, 2015; Nishisaki *et al.*, 2010). In addition, due to limited opportunities for formalized teaching inclusive of lectures or seminars, just-in-time teaching has proved valuable as an alternative opportunity. In a study of 147 medical residents in a pediatric residency program, a supplemental e-learning program 2 weeks prior to and during their 4-week service block was useful for meeting the evolving learning needs of the residents (Mangum, Lazar, Rose, Mahan, & Reed, 2017).

Chapter Takeaways

1. Appraisal of evidence and implementation of evidence-based practice projects requires command of research methods.
2. Collaborations with academic institutions will greatly facilitate the DNP nurse's acquisition of research process competencies, close the gap between research and translation into practice, and promote focus on addressing clinical issues.
3. Implementation of health care reform and scrutiny on quality care mandates that DNP nurses possess quality improvement knowledge and skills.
4. Active engagement in the monitoring and reporting of quality metrics required by regulatory, credentialing, and other national agencies, as well as in the identification, development, monitoring, and reporting of health care facility designated metrics, broadens the DNP nurse's effect on nursing practice.
5. Knowledge, skills, and experience in multiple quality improvement methods maximizes approaches to examine variations in care to include evidence-based practices with consideration of service delivery support systems and organizational structures.

Chapter Summary

In health care organizations, research and quality improvement function as systemwide entities, in that they interface with all aspects of the organization. Evidence-based practice does not stand alone and is influenced by research and quality improvement. To analyze and improve practice, address clinical problems, and develop, implement, and sustain evidence-based practice, the DNP nurse must be proficient in the research process and quality improvement strategies. This chapter offered a description of the relevant research and quality improvement competencies along with presentation of a collaborative research approach and quality improvement metrics and methods. The goal for the DNP nurse is not only to apply the best evidence, but also to engage in the discovery of evidence and to facilitate innovation, quality, safety, and value in health care through research and quality improvement.

Chapter Reflection Questions

1. What research process knowledge and skills are relevant to your evidence-based practice projects? How would you acquire such competencies outside of your DNP curriculum?
2. How could collaborations between academe and your health care organization be initiated and sustained?
3. What are the quality metrics being measured in your health care organization and how do they compare to national standards?
4. What approaches for evaluating processes of care are present in your health care organization?
5. How would your acquisition of research and quality improvement competencies benefit your health care organization?

References

American Association of Colleges of Nursing (AACN) (2006). *The essentials of doctoral education for advanced nursing practice*. Washington, DC: AACN.

American Nurses Association (ANA) (2010). *Nursing-sensitive indicators*. Retrieved from http://www.nursingworld.org.

American Nurses Credentialing Center (2014). *Application manual: Magnet recognition program*. Silver Springs, MD: American Nurses Credentialing Center.

American Nurses Credentialing Center (2018). *Magnet recognition program*. from https://www.nursingworld.org/organizational-programs/magnet/magnet-model/.

Belter, D., Halsey, J., Severtson, H., Fix, A. Michelfelder, L., Michalak, K., . . . De Ianni, A. (2012). Evaluation of outpatient oncology services using Lean methodology. *Oncology Nursing Forum, 39*, 136–140.

Berwick, D. M., Nolan, T. W., & Whittington, J. (2008). The triple aim: Care, health, and cost. *Health Affairs, 27*, 759–769.

Bodenheimer, T., & Sinsky, C. (2014). From triple aim to quadruple aim: Care of the patient requires care of the provider. *Annals of Family Medicine, 12*, 573–576.

Boland, M. G., Kamikawa, C., Inouye, J., Latimer, R. W., & Marshall. S. (2010). Partnership to build research capacity. *Nursing Economics, 28*, 314–321, 336.

Burstin, H., Leatherman, S., & Goldmann, D. (2016). The evolution of healthcare quality measurement in the United States. Journal of Internal Medicine, 279, 154–159.

Centers for Medicare and Medicaid Services (2005). *Hospital quality improvement* (Deficit Reduction Act. Section 5001). Retrieved from https://www.cms.gov/Medicare/Medicare-Fee-for-Service-Payment/HospitalAcqCond/Statute_Regulations_Program_Instructions.html.

Centers for Medicare and Medicaid Services. (2018a). *CMS measures inventory tool.* Retrieved from https://cmit.cms.gov/CMIT_public/ListMeasures?Q=&filters=MeasureGroup_untok%7Cd%7CACO&RemoveFilterField=MeasureGroup_untok&RemoveFilterValue=ACO

Centers for Medicare and Medicaid Services. (2018b). *Consumer Assessment of Healthcare Providers and systems.* Retrieved from https://www.cms.gov/Research-Statistics-Data-and-Systems/Research/CAHPS/index.html

Centers for Medicare and Medicaid Services (2018c). *Hospital-acquired conditions.* Retrieved from https://www.cms.gov/medicare/medicare-fee-for-service-payment/hospitalacqcond/hospital-acquired_conditions.html

Centers for Medicare and Medicaid Services. (2016). *CMS quality strategy.* Retrieved from https://www.cms.gov/Medicare/Quality-Initiatives-Patient-Assessment-Instruments/QualityInitiativesGenInfo/Downloads/CMS-Quality-Strategy.pdf

Centers for Medicare and Medicaid Services. (2011, June 27). *Hospital value-based purchasing.* Retrieved from http://www.cms.gov/Hospital-Value-Based-Purchasing.

Cheng, Y. Liu, D. R., &Wang, V. J. (2017). Teaching splinting techniques using a just-in-time training instructional video. *Pediatric Emergency Care, 33*, 166–170.

Committee on the National Quality Report on Health Care Delivery, Institute of Medicine (2001). *Envisioning the national healthcare quality report.* Washington, D.C.: The National Academies Press. doi:10.17226/10073.

Cronenwett, L., Sherwood, G., Barnsteiner, J., Disch, J., Johnson, J., Mitchell, P. . . . Warren, J. (2007). Quality and safety education for nurses. *Nursing Outlook, 55*, 122–131

Donabedian, A. (1980). *Explorations in Quality Assessment and Monitoring Vol. 1. The Definition of Quality and Approaches to Its Assessment.* Ann Arbor, MI: Health Administration Press.

Finkelman, A. W. (2018). *Quality improvement: A guide for integration in nursing.* Burlington, MA: Jones & Bartlett Learning.

Gallagher, R., & Rowell, P. (2003). Claiming the future of nursing through nursing-sensitive quality indicators. *Nursing Administration Quarterly, 27*, 273–284.

Gettrust, L., Hagle, M., Boaz, L., & Bull, M. (2016). Engaging nursing staff in research: The clinical nurse specialist in an academic-clinical partnership. *Clinical Nurse Specialist, 30*, 203–207.

Hatfield, L. A., Kutney-Lee, A., Hallowell, S. G., Del Guidice, M., Ellis, L. N., Verica, L., & Aiken, L. H. (2016). Fostering clinical nurse research in a hospital context. *The Journal of Nursing Administration, 46*, 245–249.

Hendrix, C. C., Matters, L., West, Y., Stewart, B. & McConnell, E. S. (2011). The Duke-

NICHE program: An academic-practice collaboration to enhance geriatric nursing care. *Nursing Outlook, 59*, 149–157.

Hummer, J., & Daccarett, C. (2009). Improvement in prescription renewal handling by application of the Lean process. *Nursing Economics, 27*, 197–201.

Institute of Medicine. 1990. *Medicare: A Strategy for Quality Assurance* (Vol.1). Washington, DC: National Academies Press.

Institute of Medicine. 1999. *To Err is Human: Building a Safer Health System*. Washington DC: National Academy of Sciences.

Institute of Medicine. 2001. *Crossing the Quality Chasm: A New Health System for the 21st Century*. Washington DC: National Academy of Sciences.

Institute of Medicine. 2001. *Envisioning the national healthcare quality report*. Washington, DC: Committee on the National Quality Report on Health Care Delivery

Institute of Medicine. 2010. *The Future of Nursing: Leading Change, Advancing Health*. Washington, DC: National Academy of Sciences.

Institute for Healthcare Improvement (IHI). (2012). How to improve. Retrieved from http://www.ihi.org/knowledge/Pages/HowtoImprove/default

Institute for Healthcare Improvement. (2017). *QI essentials toolkit: Failure modes and effects analysis*. Retrieved from www.ihi.org/resources/Pages/Tools/FailureModesandEffectsAnalysisTool.aspx

Kessler, D., Pusic, M., Chang, T. P., Fein, D. M., Grossman, D., Mehta, R. …Auerbach, M. (2015). Impact of just-in-time and just-in-place simulation on intern success with infant lumbar puncture. *Pediatrics, 135*, e1237–e1246.

Kirschling, J. M., & Erickson, J. I. (2010). The STTI practice-academe innovative collaboration award: Honoring innovation, partnership, and excellence. *Journal of Nursing Scholarship, 42*, 286–294.

Kroch, E., Vaughn, T., Koepke, M., Roman, S., Foster, D., Sinha, S., & Levey, S. (2006). Hospital boards and quality dashboards. *Journal of Patient Safety, 2*, 10–19.

Langley, G., Moen, R., Nolan, K., Nolan, T., Norman, C., & Provost, L. (2009). *The improvement guide: A practical approach to enhancing organizational performance* (2nd ed.). San Francisco, CA: Jossey-Bass Publishers.

Lauver, L., & Phalen, A. G. (2017). An example of a statistics course in a Doctor of Nursing Practice (DNP) program. Nurse Educator, 37, 36–41.

Litvak, E., & Bisganon, M. (2011). More patients, less payment: Increasing hospital efficiency in the aftermath of health reform. *Health Affairs, 30*(1),76–80.

Magyary, D., Whitney, J. D., Brown, M.A. (2006). Advancing practice inquiry: Research foundations of the practice doctorate in nursing. *Nursing Outlook, 54*, 139–151.

Mazzocato, P., Holden, R. J., Brommels, M., Aronsson, H., Backman, U., Elg, M., & Thor, J., (2012). How does Lean work in emergency care? A case study of a Lean-inspired intervention at the Astrid Lindgren Children's Hospital Stockholm, Sweden. *BMC Health Services Research, 12*. Retrieved from http://www.bmchealthservres.biomedcentral.com/track/pdf/10.1186/1472-6963-12-28

Montalvo, I. (2007). The National Database of Nursing Quality Indicators (NDNQI). *OJIN: The Online Journal of Issues in Nursing, 12*.

National Committee for Quality Assurance. (2018). *Healthcare effectiveness data and information set (HEDIS) and performance measurement.* Retrieved from https://www.ncqa.org/hedis/

National Quality Forum. (2011). *Fact sheet: Serious reportable events.* Retrieved from file:///C:/Users/user/Downloads/SRE%20fact%20sheet%20121411.pdf

Nishisaki, A. Donoghue, A. J., Colborn, S., Watson, C., Meyer, A., Brown, C. A. ... Nadkarni, V. M. (2010). Effect of just-in-time simulation training on tracheal intubation procedure safety in the pediatric intensive care unit. *Anesthesiology, 113*, 214–223.

Polancich, S., James, D. H., Miltner, R. S., Smith, G. L., & Moneyham, L. (2018). Building DNP essential skills in clinical data management and analysis. *Nurse Educator, 43*, 37–41.

Press Ganey. (2018). *National database of nursing quality indicators.* Retrieved from http://www.pressganey.com/solutions/clinical-excellence/nursing-quality

Pyzdek, T. (2003). *The six sigma handbook.* New York: McGraw-Hill.

Sollecito, W. A., & Johnson, J. K. (2013). The global evolution of continuous quality improvement: From Japanese manufacturing to global health services. In W. A. Sollecito & J. K. Johnson (Eds.), *McLaughlin and Kaluzny's continuous quality improvement in health care* (4th ed., pp. 4–5). Burlington, MA: Jones & Bartlett Learning.

Soltani, S. N., Kannaley, K., Tang, W., Gibson, A., Olscamp, K., Friedman, D. B... .Hunter, R. H. (2017). Evaluating community-academic partnerships of the South Carolina healthy brain research network. *Health Promotion Practice, 18*, 607–614.

The Joint Commission. (2018). *2018 national patient safety goals.* Retrieved from https://www.jointcommission.org/standards_information/npsgs.aspx

The Joint Commission. (2018). *Specifications manual for national hospital inpatient quality measures* (version 5.4). Retrieved from https://www.jointcommission.org/specifications_manual_for_national_hospital_inpatient_quality_measures.aspx

The Joint Commission. (2017a). *Joint Commission measures.* Retrieved from https://www.jointcommission.org/assets/1/18/The_Joint_Commission_Measures_Effective_January_1_2018.pdf

The Joint Commission. (2017b). *Sentinel event policy and procedures.* Retrieved from https://www.jointcommission.org/sentinel_event_policy_and_procedures/

Toyota Motor Corporation. (2018). *Just-in-time—Philosophy of complete elimination of waste.* Retrieved from https://www.toyota-global.com/company/vision_philosophy/toyota_production_system/just-in-time.html

U.S. Department of Health and Human Services (HHS), Agency for Healthcare Research and Quality (AHRQ). (2017). *About the national quality strategy.* Retrieved from https://www.ahrq.gov/workingforquality/about/index.html

U.S. Department of Health and Human Services, Agency for Healthcare Research and Quality. (2018). *AHRQuality indicators.* Retrieved from https://www.ahrq.gov/cpi/about/otherwebsites/qualityindicators.ahrq.gov/qualityindicators.html

Zinn, J., Reinert, J., Bigelow, A., Ellis, W., French, A., Milner, F., & Letvak, S. (2011). Innovation in engaging hospital staff and university faculty in research. *Clinical Nurse Specialist, 25*, 193–197.

JOYCE E. JOHNSON

7
Health Policy Development, Critical Analysis and the DNP-Prepared Nurse Executives

Chapter Objectives

- Describe the role of government in defining and advancing health and health care.
- Define policy, policy analysis, and the role of the policy analyst.
- Describe the steps in the policy analysis process.
- Analyze the impact of hidden assumptions, stakeholders, and transparency.
- Create an alternative criterion matrix to select best-fit policy options.
- Describe the steps in conducting a SWOT and a cost-benefit analysis.
- Describe the structure and modes of policy arguments, and evaluate policy arguments based on logic.
- Discuss policy implementation, outcome monitoring, and the consequences of policies and information source subsets.
- Discuss the role of nursing in policy analysis, formation, and advocacy challenging nursing's traditional internally focused approach.

KEY WORDS: problem identification, policy analysis, health policy, policy options, transparency, evidenced-based analysis, argumentation, authorizing environment, policy implementation, policy evaluation

Introduction

Most doctor of nursing practice—(DNP-)prepared nurses in leadership roles believe that devotion to health and well-being underpins administrative practice. There is general agreement that health is a basic requirement to live a full, vibrant life and that good health focuses on the maximum level of well-being that an individual can enjoy (World Health Organization, 2005). Good health is necessary to engage in our social and political systems and to work and support ourselves and those for whom we care.

Without good health, "life, liberty, and the pursuit of happiness" ring hollow to those struggling with poor health and disease.

In 2006, the American Association of Colleges of Nursing (AACN) articulated eight *Essentials of Doctoral Education that support the DNP degree* (AACN, 2006). In this chapter, *Essential* number five (Health Care Policy for Advocacy in Health Care) and *Essential* number two (Organizational and Systems Leadership for Quality Improvement and Systems Thinking) come together in policy analysis and formation. C-Suite (where all chief executives reside) nurse executives advance health policy and must understand the policy formation process and develop proficient analytic skills that enable them to set the policy agenda vs. simply advocating for policy approval.

This chapter discusses the formation of health policy from an analytic perspective that is grounded in the theories and models of classic policy analysis. Key elements that drive policy development are relevant to the successful C-Suite nurse executive's practice and align with American Organization for Nursing Leadership (AONL) (formerly the American Organization of Nurse Executives) Nurse Executive Competencies (AONE, 2015). Nurse executives ensure safe, effective, and equitable patient-centered care through policy development that guides practicing nurses and ancillary personnel in their daily practice. Understanding the policy analysis process enables C-Suite nurse leaders to influence decision-making at the highest level of the organization. Although AONL's common core set of competencies provide guidance for leadership development, it is policy analysis that provides the important tools that ensure the nurse executive's success in achieving all components of the Quadruple Aim: improving clinical outcomes, reducing the cost of health care, and improving both patient and care provider satisfaction (Bodenheimer & Sinsky, 2014).

Definition of Health Policy

What is policy? The simplest definition is that policy is a course or a principle of action (Dunn, 2008). There are government policies that define actions the government initiates to address an issue. Corporate policy defines corporate actions, whereas personal policies are actions taken by individuals. According to Dunn (2008), policies guide action and tell us what to do in a defined circumstance.

The definition of health policy depends on an individual's appreciation of the role of health and health care in the policy environment. Health policy requires an understanding of health, health care and the role of government, corporations, individuals, and families in health and health care. Gill and colleauges (2008) suggest that health policy attempts to define the interrelationship between individuals and institutions such as the government. This suggests that health policy is a multidimensional concept that can include an individual's beliefs about health and health care, the description of the policy, ownership of the policy, and the role of that policy (McLaughlin & McLaughlin, 2015).

A good example is employer-sponsored health care. American employers care about health. In the modern workplace, employers want employees to access health care in order for them to come to work and be productive. During World War II, companies faced labor shortages, as well as wage and price freezes (Rook, 2015). Employers who were unable to raise salaries during war-time wage control used health care to enrich employee benefits and attract desirable employees. Although providing health care and other benefits has helped small and large companies to recruit employees, today's employers now realize that providing health care as an employee benefit is an open-ended commitment that may have grown too expensive to offer (McLaughlin & McLaughlin, 2015).

The Government and Health Care

What is government's role in health care? The government desires a productive society and a good economy. Individuals who are employed and productive pay taxes, whereas products made and sold in the United States (U.S.) and other countries solidify the affluence of American society. This requires healthy, productive citizens who pay taxes. McLaughlin and McLaughlin (2015) suggest that this premise is the basis of every government that seeks an affluent citizenry.

In addition, there is a *social compact* in our society that includes health care for those in need. For example, if someone falls in the street and is seriously injured, we expect an ambulance to come. Failure to do so means that the government failed to fulfill its responsibility to citizens. The American social compact suggests that the government must provide help for citizens. However, the issue is complicated by the American belief in the *responsibility of the individual* (McLaughlin & McLaughlin 2015). Valid points exist on both sides of this difficult debate.

The relationship between health and health care is an important, but complicated, government issue. For example, the government provides health care to members of the military and, if injured during duty, the government has a clear responsibility to provide health services. However, the issue is less clear about the responsibility of caring for veterans. Some citizens believe that the government has the clear responsibility to create a healthy environment for all citizens and to provide clean water, safe pharmaceuticals, and the regulation of foodstuffs (Frieden, 2013; Resnik, 2007). Although there is general agreement about the government's responsibility, there is less enthusiasm about the government's involvement in individual choices, such as the consumption of high sugar drinks or tobacco products.

The U.S. government pays for almost 50% of all health care spending via Medicare (20%), Medicaid (16%), and other federal, state, and local programs (14%). Private insurers pay for 33% of all health care spending, whereas out-of-pocket payments account for approximately 15% (Morone & Ehlke, 2013). Thus, the government has a significant involvement in health and health care. Given our aging boomer population and the increase in access to health care services as Americans grow older, projected government expenditures justify the government's interest and concern about health care. In 2016, Eberstadt suggested that government has the most to lose in the health care cost proposition, especially with the significant expansion of entitlement programs and a debt ceiling that will soon exceed 23 trillion.

The Social Compact and the Federalist Model

The social compact in the U.S. is driven by the Federalist model—an affiliation of voluntary states. The model provides for state sovereignty, with the states enjoying singular rights (McLaughlin & McLaughlin, 2015) such as succeeding from the Union, a right clarified during the Civil War. States are not lesser partners with the government, but are full partners in the enterprise of U.S. society. States enjoy significant rights, responsibilities, and fewer restrictions than the Federal Government. It is the Federal Government that has delegated powers in the Constitution, with "all powers not delegated to the Federal Government belonging to the states" (Longley, 2017). The states are charged with ensuring the health of their citizens, and the Federal Government effectively has no role in health care.

A significant belief in American society is individual responsibility. In our society, each person is a responsible for achieving their dreams. However, those who are born into a poor family and live in a disadvantaged environment can only be as responsible as possible and may not have advancement opportunities. As a result, social mobility may be non-existent and the individual will inevitably be "poor at birth and poor at death" (Alexander, Entwisle, & Olson, 2014).

Americans also embrace the concept of social justice, in which we have some duty to the poor. The concept of social justice remains as a principle with only the degree of duty in question (McLaughlin & McLaughlin, 2015). Americans also believe in the right to seek wealth through hard work, innovation, invention, and entrepreneurship, but not through dishonesty such as stealing, cheating, lying, and engaging in unlawful acts. We believe in free and open markets and market competition. The Federal Government invests resources to keep markets open, restrains trade to enable individuals to enter the market, and ensures that those individuals can sell their products without impediment (McLaughlin & McLaughlin, 2015)

Americans also believe in public safety and the role of the government in ensuring public safety and decreasing risk from poorly designed roads and unsafe bridges. Today, there are escalating concerns about America's crumbling infrastructure and the government's clear role in maintaining or replacing that infrastructure. Aligned with AONL's executive leadership competency, business skills and principles (AONE, 2015), Americans believe in corporate responsibility, which means that corporations are responsible for producing safe products and are responsible for any harm from those products.

The Impact of Health Politics

Politics

Although politics is associated with political functions such as government, O'Bryne and Holmes (2009) suggest that politics involves all individual actions that result in individual behavior. In essence, it is through a political process that individuals make decisions for our entire society by setting an agenda and codifying regulations and laws. A policy that is drafted, adopted, and implemented can alter the political landscape. One example is the 2010 Patient Protection and Affordable Care Act (ACA) (Patient Protection and Affordable Care Act, 2010), which was designed to increase the number of Americans with health insurance. The controversy about the ACA divided our nation due to the many difficulties associated with providing affordable coverage for all Americans.

Political Influence

Politics are embedded in policy agendas, adoptions, and implementation. One example is the 1965 effort by President Harry S. Truman to provide a comprehensive national health insurance plan. The effort failed to secure sufficient support and devolved into a national health insurance plan for the elderly, which was further distilled to hospital coverage for the elderly in the form of Medicare. The major political influence that stimulated repeated modification of the original bill was the American Medical Association (AMA). This was one of the greatest victories for the AMA as member's wives and supporters contacted neighbors and friends and wrote letters of opposition to members of Congress. This effort succeeded despite the lack of support for the government during this time (Morone & Ehlke, 2013).

Another example from the 1970s occurred when members of Congress attempted to offer great patient care at a lower price (Morone & Ehlke, 2013). Opposition forces added so many burdensome amendments that the final bill hardly resembled the original. However, the bill gave rise to

HMOs and, in doing so, limited costs through market competition. In 1983, the prospective payment legislation introduced the diagnostic-related group (DRG) concept in an attempt to stabilize health care prices. Despite intense lobbying by the AMA, the legislation changed the practice of medicine by shifting power from physicians to administrators, who continue to have authority over physicians (Hervis, 1993).

Another example is the 2003 Bush Prescription Drug Plan Part D legislation (Morone & Ehlke, 2013). This prescription plan for the elderly resulted from a failed attempt to move the costly Medicare program into a new market framework. Amid mounting opposition to privatization, the only part of the original bill that passed was Medicare Part D.

The most recent example that illustrates the complexity of the political process in the U.S. is passage of the ACA. With the requirement of the 60th vote to pass in Congress, Nebraska won a 100 million dollar "cornhusker kickback" that brought the final Democrat vote to pass the legislation (Morone & Ehlke, 2013). Although hurdles remain, the ACA has weathered a myriad of storms, such as repeated partisan attempts to "repeal and replace" the Act. In addition to providing health care coverage to over 30 million Americans, the ACA aims to foster wellness and preventive care and to increase the number of nurses and physicians in minority communities (Sanger-Katz, 2017).

Health Policy and the Government

Government Concerns

Understanding the government's concerns about the health care system aligns with AONL's nurse executive competency, knowledge of the health care environment (AONL, 2015). In the American health care system, the government functions as a payor, insurer, employer, regulator, and/or provider (McLaughlin & McLaughlin, 2015). Given the multiplicity of roles, government policies seem contradictory, especially when aligned with our Federalist system of government. However, the government's interest focuses on sustaining a productive society centered on the health of its citizens who work and pay taxes to the government.

The government has major concerns about health policy. First, the type and amount information provided to the consumer by corporations, combined with the complexity of the health care systems and its products, places the consumer at risk. Consumers are at the mercy of providers, drug companies, medical device manufacturers, and regulated and non-regulated experts (McLaughlin & McLaughlin, 2015). A simple example is the hospital bill given to a patient after a hospital stay. The patient has little recourse in disputing the charges given the system complexities, lack of familiarity with billing, and inability to verify item usage attributed to his or her inpatient hospital visit.

Second, the reality is that providers do not act solely in the interests of the patient. Providers may order unnecessary tests or medication that increase revenues for the provider and company research efforts, both of which stem from self-interest and not the best interest of patients. Third, the American market-based system promotes the consumption of products that are marketed by companies. Fee-for-service medicine is an excellent example of incentivizing consumption, although there appears to be a shift away from providing health care services and toward advancing health.

Government's Response

The government can respond to these concerns in a variety of ways. One way is advancing the provision of universal coverage to all citizens, such as in Canada, the United Kingdom, and other countries where clinical outcomes compare with the U.S. (McLaughlin & McLaughlin, 2015). The government can also attempt to eliminate provider self-interest by developing a single payor system in which providers are expected to act in the best interest of the insurers. This is potentially fraught with risk that the providers will act in the best interest of the government, although it remains an option (McLaughlin & McLaughlin, 2015). Germany, the United Kingdom, and some Asian companies have government programs in which captive payors adhere to strict and prescriptive government controls in managing the payor approach (The Guardian, 2017). With this model, the government is the insurance provider for most citizens. The U.S. continues with a market-oriented approach in which market competition is encouraged. Faced with government options such as these, American providers invest heavily in public relations campaigns, massive marketing and education efforts, and endless, expensive lobbying in Congress. Every American hospital has a public relations department; drug companies continuously promote products on television 24 hours a day, and lobbyists hover around members of Congress at every turn.

ACA Update

The ACA changed the approach of American health care from a fee-for-service model to a value-driven purchasing approach (McLaughlin & McLaughlin, 2015). Mandatory participation reflects the notion of a care continuum in which disease management occurs across episodes of care, and providers share reliable and clear information through electronic health care record systems that support bundled care (Fontenot, 2013). The intent is to promote population health (not necessarily health care), quality of care, and efficiency. The experience of receiving care must meet rigor-

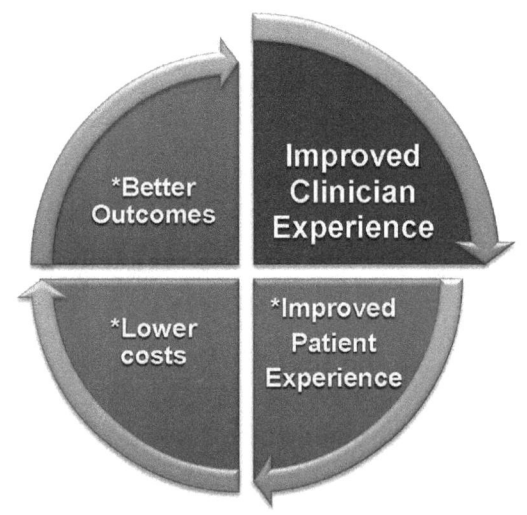

Figure 7.1. *The Quadruple Aim. Adapted from Bodenheimer & Sinsky, 2014. Courtesy of Diane B. Stoy*

ous standards, as seen in The Institute of Healthcare Improvement's Triple Aim initiative (Berwick, Nolan, & Whittington, 2008). Within the ACA mandates, health care organizations were challenged to pursue improvements in three dimensions: the patient experience with care, improvement in health populations, and reducing the per-capita cost of health care. A fourth dimension has enriched this initiative by adding an additional component to improve "the work life of health care providers," which includes clinicians and staff (Bodenheimer & Sinsky 2014).

The four Quadruple Aim components are important elements of any health care system. Specific interest in the experience of care components that focus on the Institute of Medicine's (IOM's) report, *To Err is Human: Building a Safer Health System*, underscores that individuals should not be harmed when receiving their care (Kohn, Corrigan, & Donaldson 2000).

Defining Characteristics of Public Policy and Policy Analysis

Definition of Policy

Policy is a principle that guides our action and effectively tells us what to do in a defined circumstance (Dunn, 2008). Public policy is a purposeful government action designed to deal with a matter of public concern (Anderson, 1975) and guide political decisions on programs that achieve goals valued by a society (Cochran & Malone, 2014). Policy determines what action promotes the good society (Vining & Weimer, 2010). Dunn

(2018) describes policy analysis as an applied social science that employs numerous research methods and models to argue, debate, create, forecast, and communicate information that supports policies. According to Dunn (2018), a "good analysis or even a good decision does not guarantee that the best solution will be selected or implemented" (p. 4). Policy analysis can assist leaders in selecting the best course of action from the available alternatives. Policy analysis cannot substitute for defective decision-making or bad judgment by policymakers. Although the job of the policy maker is "not to do what is right," but "to know what is right" (Dunn, 2008, p. 7), accurate analysis can assist leaders in understanding all aspects of policy options.

The Role of Policy Analysis

Policy analysis addresses five questions: What exactly is the problem that needs a solution? What is the best course of action or option to address the problem? What outcomes occur as a result of selecting the best course of actions? Will these outcomes solve the problem? If other options are selected, what are the projected outcomes? The most important component of policy analysis rests in defining the problem and accurately defining the problem may be easier said than done because, as Dunn (2018) suggested, "a fatal error in policy analysis is defining the wrong problem" (2004, p. 6).

Kingdon (2011) suggested that there is a difference between a condition and a problem, in that a concern or issue only becomes a condition when social values and judgment determine that something should be done to address it. After that, the condition becomes a problem. Dunn (2008) said that the problem need not get any worse or better for society to place sufficient value on the problem and to ultimately require a solution in the form of a public policy. Examples include addressing highway deaths due to high speeds by enacting the 55 mph speed limit and enforcing Joint Commission security procedures to mitigate the risk of hospital nursery infant abduction.

Role of the Policy Analyst

Policy analysts work in formal roles such as a legislative analyst and in informal situations such as a subject matter expert assigned to develop a policy that addresses a problem in a health care institution. The work of analyst is simply determining if a new policy needs to be developed to address an identified problem, or if an existing policy's revision or termination will address the issue.

Although the role may be similar, each policy analyst may view the process from a different perspective (Dunn, 2018). For instance, a policy analyst with a scientific background may view a problem from a theoretical perspective and will search for theory and truth by using a scientific and purely analytic approach. A political policy analyst may favor advocacy of policy positions and develop policies by using rhetoric to maximize policy value. A professional policy analyst may focus on problem design and target improvement of policy and policymaking through cost-benefit analysis, simulations, and traditional decision analytics (Dubnick & Bardes, 1983).

In addition, policy analysts may engage in a process approach by examining a part of the policy process. Another might assess the causes and effects of policy using scientific methods and a logical-positivistic approach. Still another might utilize the phenomenological approach and analyze experiences by using intuitive research techniques. One of the most engaging approaches is the participatory approach in which the policy analyst examines the role of multiple actors in policy making (Lester & Stewart, 2000).

Policy analysts may conduct a prospective policy analysis in developing a new policy or a retrospective policy analysis in determining the value of an existing policy (Dunn, 2018). The retrospective policy analysis answers the question: What happened with the policy now in force and what difference did it make? Was the problem corrected and the underlying condition improved or eliminated? The retrospective policy analysis process studies the impact of a policy and describes intended or unintended consequences (Dunn, 2008). The intent of the prospective form of policy analysis is to answer what might happen and what needs to be done to correct the problem and positively improve the underlying condition. According to Dunn (2008), prospective policy analysis requires the collection of enormous amounts of data, managing and sorting that information, and ultimately reducing the data to usable sound bites prior to developing a new draft policy.

Looking at Problems from Multiple Perspectives

An example of assessing multiple perspectives is evaluation of the increasing rates of breast cancer among women who drink more than two alcoholic beverages per day. The problem can be framed as a failure of women to heed research findings and limit their drinking. The problem could also be related to stress and fulltime employment, single parenthood, or caring for elderly parents. Other considerations could be the government's lack of regulations for alcohol consumption and/or the failure of the government and others to fund research and apply taxes to alcoholic beverages in an effort to diminish alcohol consumption.

Another current example is the rising number of individuals with Type II diabetes. The problem could be a result of a concomitant rise in obesity among children and adults, the failure of parents to encourage exercise and good food selection, the failure of health care providers to provide adequate and timely health education, or the failure of the government to eliminate high fructose in prepared, processed food products. Since each of these perspectives requires a different policy or solution, it is important to examine the multiple perspectives of a problem prior to developing policy. Nurse leaders know that organizational problems require a systems approach to advance an effective solution. Understanding a problem's multiple perspectives is a first step in the policy analysis process that requires considerable research and engagement.

Evidenced-Based Analysis

Today's C-Suite nurse executives must understand the transformation of problem-solving into evidence-based policy making. Similar to evidenced-based medicine (EBM), the policy analyst searches for relevant data about the clinical issue, assesses the validity of the data, selects the best corrective option, implements the option, and evaluates the results. C-Suite nurse executives are keenly aware of the impact of EBM and the struggle to maintain high evidence quality and validity, given political and economic interests (McLaughlin & McLaughlin, 2015). Big Pharma represents an excellent example of corporate interest that attempts to secure high quality evidence related to problem-solving through policy development. Another example is the ACA's inclusion of EBM that established the Patient-Centered Outcomes Research Institute (PCORI) with the Center for Medicare and Medicaid Studies (CMS) (PCORI, 2013). The rich, robust research generated by the PCORI never found its way into policy at the U.S. Department of Health and Human Services (HHS) due to concerns that the data may be included in the Medicare Advisory Payment Commission's rule and regulations (McLaughlin & McLaughlin, 2015). In the end, a myriad of political processes, societal norms, and intervening factors affected the policy's success by being hidden from the policy analyst and the analytic process.

Hidden Assumptions

Increased proficiency in evidenced-based policy processes eventually reveal the presence of interfering ideological or political assumptions that are largely hidden from policy analysts until their presence exerts an effect that harms the policy analysis process (Kingdon, 2011). These hidden assumptions, which are believed to be caused by a lack of transparency in the policy development process, may exert a "harmful effect on policy making in areas ranging from health, education, and welfare to national security and the environment" (Dunn, 2016, p. 41)

An example of hidden assumptions that complicate the evidenced-based policy making process is found in the proposed policy to develop patient-centered medical homes for aging baby boomers (Morrell, 2017). In this model, primary medical services are provided to the patient at home, which is a more efficient, accessible system, especially for seniors in rural communities where the distance to health care facilities is problematic. There are several hidden assumptions. First, the effort may be based on the belief that society has an obligation to provide accessible, high-quality, cost-effective care to residents, regardless of residential status or age. Second, others may believe that current health care practices inadequately coordinate care in a patient-centered, interprofessional manner. Third, the general population might agree that quality care improves patient care outcomes. Any of these hidden assumptions affects the policy process and, in particular, the stakeholders.

Stakeholders

Stakeholders are parties who affect or can be affected by a proposed policy. Each party has a stake in the formation and implementation of policy and will bring to that process individual goals and objectives that they want to maximize during the policy development process (Dunn, 2008). Early identification of stakeholders—in health care venues and state and local government settings—is key to successfully advancing policy. An example of stakeholder impact can be seen on Capitol Hill at any given moment and on any given policy when lobbyists work to influence congressional perspectives and votes for policy approval or failure. The repeated attempts to repeal and replace the ACA are a recent example of stakeholder influence.

Methods to successfully manage stakeholders include first identifying each party and their ranking and then prioritizing their importance in the policy making process (Dunn, 2018). Ranking and prioritizing is completed by determining the degree to which the policy affects the identified stakeholder and the degree to which the stakeholder can either promote or derail the policy analysis process.

The Policy Analysis Process

Dunn's approach to policy analysis rests on the definition of policy analysis as an "applied social science discipline that employs multiple methods of inquiry to solve practical problems" (Dunn, 2016, p. xvii). The underlying premise is based on the belief that policy analysis cannot be reduced

Table 7.1 Six Steps in the Policy Analysis Process.

Step 1: Confirm, Define, and Describe the Problem
Step 2: Assemble the Evidence
Step 3: Search for Alternative Policy Options
Step 4: Select the Best-Fit Option
Step 5: Make the Recommendation
Step 6: Implement, Monitor, and Evaluate

to a formula, because everyday problems, regardless of venue, typically require multiple, different analyses. Table 7.1 illustrates the six traditional steps in the policy analysis process based on Bardach's eight-step path (Bardach, 1996; Bardach & Patashink, 2016). The following steps offer a sensible way for nurse executives to engage in the policy analysis process and ensure the development of a sound policy.

Step 1: Confirm, Define, and Describe the Problem

How to identify the problem. Although there are endless ways to look at a problem, time, resources, and energy limit all efforts (Dunn, 2008). It is important to understand how a condition gives rise to problem identification. But, how would a nurse executive know that the problem is exactly the right problem? For example, if the problem is the high cost of medications, could the problem be corrected through drug importation? Could the same solution apply to state Medicaid programs even if quality might be a problem depending on the country manufacturing the drug? Could the problem be related to the freedom of each individual to purchase his or her drugs from whatever source he or she wishes? Or, could the problem be related to each state's right and the ability to make this decision for its citizens?

Consider the potential resolution of the problem. Political, operational, and financial aspects often magnify the challenges of resolution. Some believe that it is not in their best interest to resolve the problem. A classic example is Congress, with one side resistant or obstructing the other side's potential success. Inadequate resources can also thwart problem resolution despite agreement of all stakeholders. Today's opioid crisis is a good example. There is a national consensus that the government must address the crisis, but given the massive scope of the problem, there are inadequate resources that have been allocated to address the issue (McLaughlin & McLaughlin, 2015).

Table 7.2 identifies components that might be considered in the problem identification process. The list is not exhaustive, but provides useful options for nurse executives to consider (Bardach & Patashink, 2016; Musso, Biller, & Myrtle, 1999).

According to Bardach (1996), the first problem definition provides a sense of direction for evidence-gathering and a reason for the research. The analyst must reduce the problem definition to one that can be managed through analysis and which makes common sense (Bardach, 1996). Quantifying the perception of the problem, which might involve introducing a weighting methodology, can clarify any areas of confusion.

Writing the problem in one clear, concise sentence forces the nurse leader to distill the problem components. This step can be difficult. For example, stating that "Excess opioid synthetic street drugs is the cause of rising overdose-related deaths" implies that eliminating the excess of the

Table 7.2 How to Identify the Problem.

Steps to Consider
1. State the problem clearly and concisely in one sentence. 2. Determine the seriousness of the condition to be addressed. 3. Do NOT hesitate to redefine the problem as more information surfaces. 4. Discard unrelated or useless data. 5. Always question the "accepted thinking" about the issue. 6. Use ONLY evidence-based data. 7. Locate comparable policies in force. 8. Answer the question: Can this problem be solved? 9. Identify stakeholders. 10. Determine stakeholder power. 11. Estimate required resources. 12. Restate the problem periodically and do NOT offer a solution.

synthetic drug is the cause of the problem and that a simple elimination of the excess amount is the best solution. Such thinking overshadows the real cause of the problem—rising deaths due to opioid use. Stating the problem as "rising deaths due to opioid use" narrows the focus and opens the opportunity to identify alternative approaches that can address the issue of concern (Bardach & Patashink, 2016). After the problem is clearly defined, the analyst can begin developing solutions. If the problem is the high cost of drugs, the solution might include price controls on costly domestic drugs, pharmaceutical programs that provide vouchers for those unable to pay, or the creation of government or insurance company purchasing plans that can negotiate for lower drug costs. Each problem requires different solutions.

One final word of advice is ensuring that the scenario is correct. This refers to researching information related to the problem and ensuring its accuracy (McLaughlin & McLaughlin, 2015). The net evidence enables the executive to produce evidence-based policies.

Step 2: Assemble the Evidence

How to assemble evidence. At this point, most of a policy analyst's time focuses on searching for solid evidence (Bardach & Patashink, 2016; Dunn, 2018). Accessing data that can constitute evidence becomes critical to advance policy solution alternatives. Busy executives appreciate the challenges of data mining and statistical analyses. The importance of solid evidence cannot be understated.

Bardach and Patashink (2016) identified three purposes for gathering data. First, the nature of the problem must be defined to quantify its depth and breadth. Second, the data must help explain the unique features of the problem that must be understood and categorized for problem clarity. Third, data gathering can reveal similar policies that may help the analyst appreciating any potential policy outcomes.

A word about transparency. Transparency is an issue on the national and global stage in politics and government (Moi, 2010). Disclosing information in any area of political analysis suggests that the public's right-to-know takes precedence over other values embraced by a democratic society that values the protection of its citizens. In the policy analysis process, gathering credible evidence takes time and disclosing small amounts of unconfirmed data to potential stakeholders can create serious political furor, from which the analytic process may never recover. Transparency functions as a political advantage and a personal practice for the policy analyst and stakeholders. Thus, in the policy analytic process, decisions about information disclosure can represent ethical and moral dilemmas that must be carefully considered.

Step 3: Search for Alternative Policy Options

Use only evidence-based data. After problem identification and evidence-based research efforts have created a clear problem statement, the next step is to identify policy options. Searching for feasible options initially involves a wide range of options that should always include a no-action alternative (Bardach & Patashink, 2016; Musso, Biller, & Myrtle, 1999). The no-action alternative is important because some change occurs with or without encouragement and may correct the identified problem over time.

The SWOT analysis. One common situational analysis technique that can clarify multiple options is the SWOT analysis, depicted in Table 7.3 (Baker & Baker, 2014; Paterson, 2014). This technique is helpful after the analyst has identified options from consulting experts, brainstorming, Delphi methods, or scenario writing. The analysts can then identify the three or four best options and then conduct a situational analysis for each.

Table 7.3 SWOT Analysis Chart for a National Electronic Healthcare Record Policy.

Strengths	Weaknesses
• Improvements in data accuracy. • Reduction in ha-copy medial record storage. • Care coordination improvements through interoperability.	• Costly with long-term ROI. • Training requirements significant. • Implementation disruption significant. • Coordination between providers dependent on data-sharing.
Opportunities	Threats
• Improved coordination of care. • Creation of improved and robust national data base. • Link with insurers for episodic are and focus-on-health initiatives.	• IT vendor software product hoarding. • Congressional oversight requirements. • Insurance company information gathering on providers and consumers affecting privacy.

With a SWOT analysis, each option's internal strengths and weaknesses, and external opportunities and threats eventually narrow the choices to a best-fit option. The outcome clarifies components of each option, helps to eliminate options, and prepares accumulated data for weighting in a decision-making matrix such as the Alternative-Criterion Matrix (Musso, Biller, & Myrtle, 1999).

Step 4: Selecting the Best-Fit Option

Constructing an alternative-criterion matrix. Underlying each policy alternative are values that can be categorized into evaluative criteria such as effectiveness, adequacy, equity, responsiveness, appropriateness, and efficiency (Dunn, 2008). Effectiveness refers to achieving the expected effect. Adequacy determines if the alternative truly addresses the problem. Equity, equality, and justice suggest that policy development determines if the policy option can be fairly distributed to all equally regardless of social group. A policy option that solves the problem is appropriate particularly if it addresses the needs of those it intends to satisfy are and is responsive to the needs of the people.

Efficiency involves determining the cost-effectiveness of all options and conducting costbenefit analyses (Bardach, 1999). A cost-benefit analysis requires cost estimating and forecasting. An example of massive cost-benefit analysis is the work completed on many congressional bills by the Congressional Budget Office (CBO). The CBO must determine the cost-benefit impact of proposed policies in financial terms (CBO, 2017).

A cost-benefit analysis enables policy analysts to compare and contrast policy options by quantifying total monetary cost and total monetary benefits. By doing so, the policy analyst measures all costs and benefits to society or those affected by the policy option alternative. An option is deemed efficient if net benefits are greater than zero. However, the analyst must assure that all costs and all benefits are accurately reduced to monetary terms. This includes all direct, indirect, variable, fixed, and semi-variable costs. The more difficult analysis is the translation of expected direct and indirect benefits into accurate monetary values.

The steps in a cost-benefit analysis for each policy option include defining the outcome threshold as Cost/Benefit ≤ 1, determining the total cost by adding all direct and indirect costs, determining the total benefits of the policy, translating those benefits into a monetary value, and dividing the total costs by the total benefits. If the result is ≤ 1, then the benefits outweigh the costs and the option should likely be considered (Paterson, 2014). The accompanying Policy example in Appendix A illustrates the cost-benefit calculation of a proposed new health care policy entitled "Transforming Georgia's Rising Demand for Healthcare Coordination" (Weaver, 2017).

After each option includes an accurate cost-benefit calculation, the next step is determining the best-fit option that addresses the identified problem by constructing an alternative-criterion matrix (ACM). Today's health care executives access enormous amounts of data and must analyze multiple options and a myriad of variables. An ACM can clarify options and highlight key attributes that factor into the final decision (Fabian, 2017). This can remove emotion and confusion from the process. An ACM enables numerous alternative comparisons. When factors are believed to be more or less important, a weighted ACM can rank alternatives based on a fixed-point priority (Fabian, 2017; Musso, Biller, & Myrtle, 1999).

Selecting and weighting the criteria. Constructing an ACM involves creating a table as depicted in Table 7.4. The left-hand vertical row lists each policy option under consideration, whereas the top horizontal row shows the evaluative criteria, which can be identified through brainstorming to ensure criterion clarity, unmistakable meaning, and ready observability (Bardach, 1999; Dunn, 2018).

Table 7.5 illustrates commonly considered evaluative criteria, although the list does not include all options (Bardach, 1999; Dunn, 2016).

After all criteria are identified, the analyst can narrow the options to 4 to 6 and then weigh each on a scale of 0 to 5. Calculating the scores is a matter of multiplying each alternative rating or weight with each respective criteria rating or weight and adding all scores for each alternative. The alternative with the highest score represents the best-fit policy option. Table 7.6 is an ACM from a policy analysis involving access to health care providers for patients located in rural areas. As illustrated, the second policy alterna-

Table 7.4 Alternative Criterion Matrix Chart.

Criteria	Policy Alternative I: State Policy Here Rank:	Policy Alternative II: State Policy Here Rank:	Policy Alternative III: State Policy Here Rank:
State Criterion Here Weight:	Score: Multiply Rank & Weight	Score: Multiply Rank & Weight	Score: Multiply Rank & Weight
State Criterion Here Weight:	Score: Multiply Rank & Weight	Score: Multiply Rank & Weight	Score: Multiply Rank & Weight
State Criterion Here Weight:	Score: Multiply Rank & Weight	Score: Multiply Rank & Weight	Score: Multiply Rank & Weight
Total Weighted Score	Total All Scores for Policy Alternative I	Total All Scores for Policy Alternative II	Total All Scores for Policy Alternative III

Table 7.5 Optional Criteria for Consideration.

Optional Criteria	
Lowest Risk	Complexity Level
Cost	Implementation Time
Implementation Ease	Required Political Support
Quickest to Implement	Implementation Disruption
Resource Use Efficient/Effective	Problem correction timeline
Political Impact	Stakeholder engagement
Required Resources Accessibility	Stakeholder resistance
Degree of Control Required	Feasibility

tive (Interactive Hospital Portal Expansion) appears as the best-fit option with the highest score of 69.

Step 5: Make the Recommendation

Developing the argument. Given the back and forth at Congressional policy sessions where bills are either amended or presented on the floor for final vote, nurse executives can see the importance of arguments in the policy development process. Successful C-Suite executives appreciate the importance of effective communication in relationship building, an AONL executive leadership competency (AONE, 2015). Dunn (2018) suggested that argumentation enables analytic results to be communicated, discussed, and evaluated as part of the critical thinking component of information processing and active debate. One of the most effective ways to understand and prepare for winning arguments is through argument mapping. Toul-

Table 7.6 Alternative-Criterion Matrix for Addressing Rural Health Care in Missouri.

Criterion for "scoring"	Policy Alternative I: Home-Centered Telemedicine	Policy Alternative II: Interactive Hospital Portal Expansion	Policy Alternative III: Rural Healthcare Clinic Expansion
	Rank: 4	Rank: 5	Rank: 3
Feasibility Weight: 4	Score 16	Score 20	Score 12
Cost Weight: 4	Score 16	Score 20	Score 12
Efficiency Weight: 5	Score 20	Score 25	Score 15
Total Weighted Score	52	69	39

min's (2000) structural model of argument mapping is an effective way to investigate structures and processes of practical reasoning, particularly when logic lacks [for the most part] mathematical certainty (Dunn, 2018).

The first step to effective argument mapping is understanding the components of the structure: Information (I), claim (C), warrant (W), backing (B), rebuttal (R), and qualifier (Q). I represents the evidenced-based data to prove the argument; C is the statement that is being actively argued; W is a logical statement that provides a bridge between the evidenced-based information and the claim; B refers to statements from stakeholders or supporters who back the warrant but cannot prove the truth of the warrant; R is rebuttal or counterarguments that refute the data in the information or the claim; and Q, the qualifier, indicates that the claim is accurate or plausible. Nurse executives may find this model helpful when preparing to present and subsequently argue the worth of a proposed policy. Such preparation can make a real difference in winning or losing the argument.

Consider the following examples. In Table 7.7, the policy analyst suggests that the ACA implementation disrupted long-standing physician-patient relationships and contributed to the successful Republican bid to win the 2016 presidential election. The accompanying Policy example in Appendix A contains a second example.

This process will enable C-Suite nurse leaders to develop arguments that address the anticipated resistance from stakeholders who may be less inclined to support change in a new policy. The process also requires that nurse executives complete the required data gathering and analysis that will strengthen the position of subject matter expert on the debated topic.

Interpreting arguments and addressing key elements. Dunn (2018) suggests that policy argumentation generates debate that improves the soundness and efficacy of policy and offers the most valid or sound conclusions.

Table 7.7 ACA Revision Argumentation Scenario.

Information I: The Republicans have won the White House in the 2016 election. The new President, backed by congressional Republicans, supports a revision to the ACA that would allow individuals to keep their own physicians.
Qualifier Q: Considering the public backlash during ACA implementation regarding this cogent point, this revision seems like a "no-brainer." This is the same conclusion many consumer groups have reached such as the powerful AARP.
Claim C: Enabling individuals to retain their physician keeps a campaign promise and secures and/or improves care coordination—a hallmark of the ACA healthcare transformation.
Rebuttal R: Realignment of ACA regulatory design requires major shifts in insurance company physician provider panels disrupting newly created business models.
Backing B: Both the President and congressional Republicans understand the preference of the conservative base.
Warrant W: Maintaining the provider-patient relationship promotes improved outcomes and care coordination.

Most important, policy argumentation persuades others to agree with the proposed policy option, which is the aim of the entire process.

When interpreting policy arguments, a policy analyst must consider hidden meanings. Dunn (2018) suggests that arguments may conceal underlying nuances that can derail stakeholder understanding and ultimate support of the policy. Dunn advises analysts to look for words designed to discredit a person, stakeholders, or the target audience that policy is design addresses.

Policy analysts and policy proponents must understand the political environment to develop strategies that enable policy adoption (Dunn, 2008). Since policies are developed in subjective, complex, and dynamic political environments, irrational arguments can emerge when the discussion of policy feasibility fails to take place. Dunn (2008) suggests that actors, or those engaged in supporting or thwarting proposed policy, are influenced by other actors or inputs and can emerge as a substantial and powerful cohort. Policy proponents must understand the motivation of potential adversaries to mitigate their influence on the proposed policy. Key stakeholders are critical, and analysts must consider their views early and often in the policy development process.

An interesting phenomenon occurs routinely as attempts to modify or reverse existing policy periodically surface. For example, the hint of changes to Medicare or Social Security stimulates passionate resistance. Although these programs have existed for many years, the ACA "repeal and replace" effort stimulated the same angry response. After a change to the status quo is suggested, individuals are more likely to oppose the change because they prefer the "devil they know" rather than the "devil they don't know." This phenomenon, identified in 1978 by Starr, a sociology professor at Princeton, is called *Starr's Policy Trap*.

The importance of actors in the political arena cannot be underrated. Nurse executives must be aware of the stakeholders who can easily derail policy development efforts. These key actors comprise the authorizing environment for policy approval (Starr, 1978). The agendas of each key actor vary. Some may represent the regulation and resource bureaucracy, whereas others may represent the courts, government, powerful organizations, and lobbying groups. A clear understanding of the key actors can be advanced by creating an authorizing environment chart (Dunn, 2018). This simple exercise forces the policy analyst to identify every key actor whose motive must be fully understood. Figure 7.2 illustrates an authorizing chart. A second example is found in Appendix A.

Transforming policy approval into policy action requires alignment of key actors who appreciate the original problem and value at least a portion of the proposed solution (Dunn, 2016). When these three components converge, a window of opportunity opens and the policy may advance to serious consideration, as shown in Figure 7.3.

Step 6: Implement, Monitor, and Evaluate

Successful policy implementation requires that actors, organizations, procedures, and techniques work together to adopt policies that achieve specific goals (Dunn, 2018). Social and behavioral science research provides approaches for addressing implementation challenges (McLaughlin & McLaughlin, 2015; Milstead, 2013). The Consolidated Framework for Implementation Research (CFIR), which was developed primarily to advance implementation science, identifies potential influences that affect implementation (CFIR, 2017). According to Tummers (2011), the inclination of professionals to implement new policies correctly falls short at times and traditional resistance to change emerges when professionals feel comfortable in demonstrating their unwillingness to engage in the adoption of new policies. Some causes of implementation failure, such as resistance to change, unrealistic implementation plans, failure to execute critical plan

Authorizing Environment

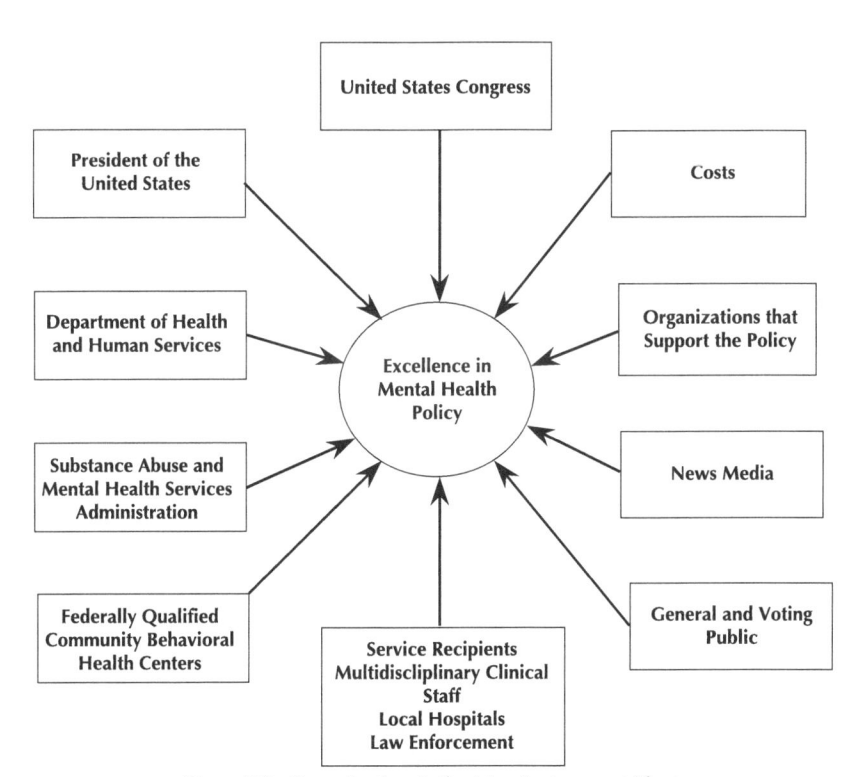

Figure 7.2. *Example of an Authorizing Environment Chart.*

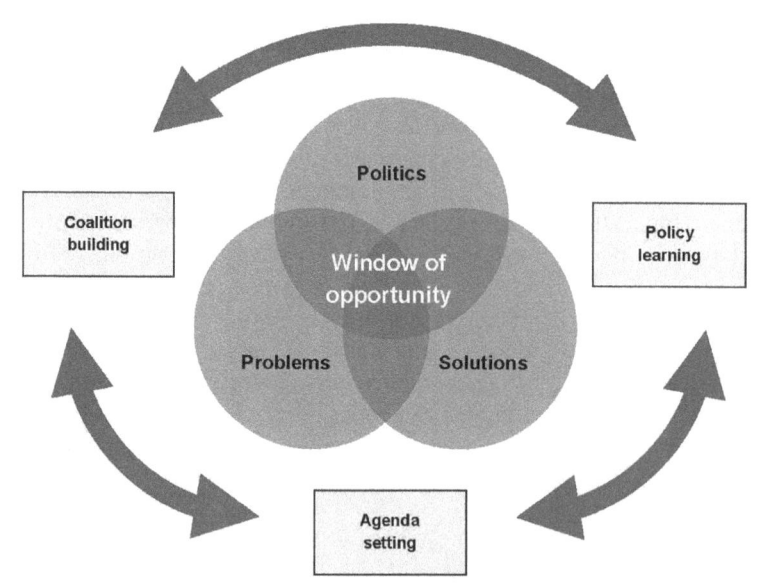

Figure 7.3. *The Kingdon Policy Streams Model. Adapted from Kingdon, 2011. Courtesy of Diane B. AStoy*

elements, competing organizational challenges such as a budget crisis, and technological, leadership, or government changes, are familiar to experienced C-Suite nurse leaders. Such failures reflect negatively on the AONL executive leadership Competencies™, relationship management, and the ability to influence behaviors (AONE, 2015).

One example that occurred in the 1970s and is still relevant today is the deinstitutionalization of psychiatric patients. The implementation plan required that government funds be transferred from psychiatric institutions to community-based facilities to support discharged patients struggling with mental illness. Unfortunately, sufficient fund transfer did not occur and the result was an entirely new population of homeless citizens.

Developing an implementation plan. Successful policy implementation requires the development of a plan that follows key stages (Bardach & Patashink, 2016; Centers for Disease Control and Prevention, 2018; McLaughlin & McLaughlin, 2015), as shown in Table 7.8.

Defining the scope of the project, which is so critical to overall policy success, demands a clear understanding of policy details. A clearly written policy with appropriate definitions alerts planning experts to policy nuances and the policy intent. In this early phase of the process, policy analysts who assisted in developing the policy are best suited to offer clarification, correct misconceptions, and refine the project scope definition (Bardach & Patashink, 2016). The second, more detailed step includes a list of project policy activities that includes all information and control systems, priori-

Table 7.8 Stages of Implementation Planning.

1. Define the project scope
2. Identify project activities
3. Define and secure all required resources
4. Develop step-by-step timeline target(s)
5. Establish controls
6. Identify and orient implementers
7. Secure plan buy-in from all implementation stakeholders
8. Implement

tization and schedule development, task requirements for implementation, performance monitoring and risk mitigation, and stakeholder management (Bardach & Patashink, 2016). Most important is Step 3, noted in Table 7.8, which identifies all costs and essential funding requirements.

A step-by-step timeline provides much needed structure in any policy implementation process. This step involves classic tools such as the Gantt, PERT, Pareto Charts, or Responsibility Assignment Matrix, as depicted in Figure 7.4.

The traditional Gantt chart requires that project tasks and related tasks are defined with start and stop dates that are useful to the implementation team. This enables project leaders to plan and visually communicate planned activities (Bright Hub Project Management, 2017). The PERT chart, which is appropriate for complex policy implementation, displays all implementation activities (Office Timeline, 2017; Bright Hub Project Management, 2017). Tracking or managing quality aspects of policy implementation can be supported with a Pareto chart, in which the points on the chart depict quality measurements at selected points in time (Office Timeline, 2017; Bright Hub Project Management, 2017). The Responsibility Assignment Matrix specifies each individual who is assigned to project implementation segments and the expected deliverables (Bright Hub Project Management, 2017).

Designing a monitoring system. Despite best implementation efforts, the consequences of policies cannot be known in advance. To ensure success, there must be a monitoring system that ensures policy implementation (Dunn, 2018). Monitoring produces an appreciation of a policy's impact and the situational effect experienced by affected parties. Implementation consequences of the ACA, for example, are well-known, including the early problems with the website, the inability of consumers to retain their preferred physicians, and the dramatic increase in personal insurance costs in the marketplace. Monitoring effectively identifies causes and consequences of the policy, which are then transformed into policy problems that may initiate the policy analysis process all over again (Bardach & Patashink, 2016; Dunn, 2018). If adequately designed, immediate remedial measures can help leaders adjust policies and remain accountable for the originally expected outcomes.

Task Name	Q1 2009 (Dec '08, Jan '09, Feb '09, Mar '09)	Q2 2009 (Apr '09, May '09, Jun '09)	Q3 2009 (Jul '09, Aug)
Planning	▓▓▓▓▓		
Research	▓▓▓▓		
Design	▓▓▓		
Implementation		▓▓▓▓▓▓▓	
Follow up			▓▓

Gantt Chart
Retrieved from http://www.gantt.com/

A Gantt chart depicts activities, tasks or events against time. A list of the activities resides at the left of the chart and a time scale is placed at the top. Bars represent each activity with its length reflecting the start-to-completion timeline denoting what has to be completed and by the schedule for completion.

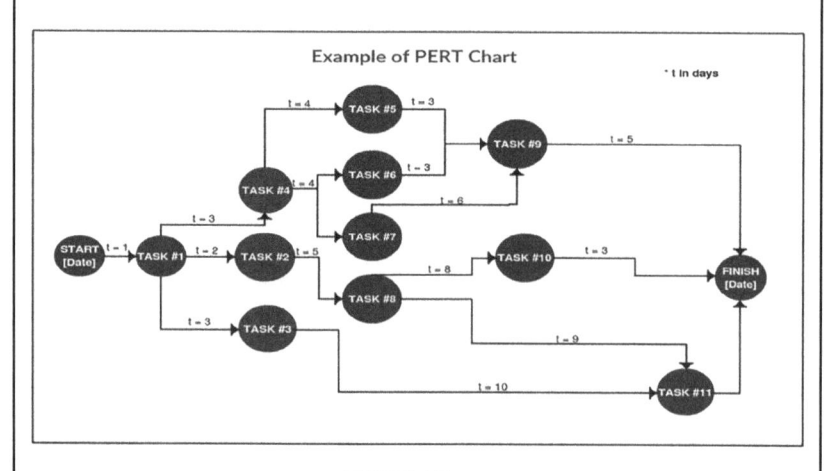

PERT Chart
Brenda Berg, December 6, 2017. The Benefits of Using a PERT Chart for Project Planning. Retrieved from https://creately.com/blog/project-management/pert-in-project-management/

A PERT chart assists in developing a realistic project timeline that simply specifies the series of steps necessary to complete the identified project. Each step includes a defined measure related to the length of time required for completion, thus ultimately providing a reality-based visual schedule.

Figure 7.4. *Gantt, PERT, Pareto Charts, or Responsibility Assignment Matrix.*

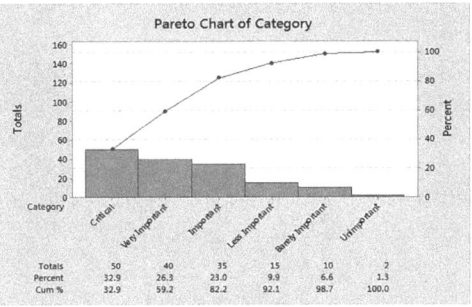

Pareto Chart

Eston Martz, September 14, 2016 The Minitab Blog retrieved from http://blog.minitab.com/blog/understanding-statistics/when-to-use-a-pareto-chart

A Pareto chart arranges category metrics from the greatest to the lowest, from left to right. The greater components beginning on the left are considered more critical than the components on the far right. A Pareto chart assists in better identifying factors that are most important, the "vital few," and those which are considered least important, the "trivial many."

WBS Element	Project Team Members				Other Stakeholders		
	I.B. You	M. Jones	R. Smith	H. Baker	F. Drake	Sponsor	Clnt Mgt	Func Mgt
1.0.1.1 Activity A	N				R			
1.0.1.2 Activity B		R	C					
1.0.1.3 Activity C	R		S			A		G
1.0.2 Activity D			R		S			A
1.0.3.1 Activity E			R			N		
1.0.3.2 Activity F				R				
1.0.3.3 Activity G	R		S			A	A	
1.0.4 Activity H		R			C	N		

Key: R = Responsible, S = Support Required, C = Must Be Consulted, N = Must Be Notified, A = Approval Required, G = Gate Reviewer

Responsibility Assignment Matrix

2020 Project Management retrieved from http://2020projectmanagement.com/2013/10/the-responsibility-assignment-matrix-ram/

A Responsibility Assignment Matrix defines who in the organization is responsible for individual project components and deliverables. By forming a template with the detailed project structure and identifying who in the organization assumes responsibility, lower level task assignment easily occurs. Each task is assigned as a work breakdown structure (WBS) element and as an organizational breakdown structure component, including the department responsible, the person responsible, and the scope of work required.

Figure 7.4 (Continued). *Gantt, PERT, Pareto Charts, or Responsibility Assignment Matrix.*

According to Dunn (2008), standard monitoring tools do not exist for policy monitoring. Policy administrators can select an activity monitoring report approach or a record review. Some may focus on stakeholders and beneficiary groups by conducting interviews to obtain feedback. Others may use qualitative research methods to measure attitudes, knowledge, behavior, and experience with the new policy (Dunn, 2018). The information enables policy administrators to ensure policy compliance, conduct resource and service audits, account for social and economic changes that result from policy implementation, and explain the reasons that policy outcomes differ from the original policy's intent (Bardach & Patashink, 2016; Dunn, 2018)

Monitoring processes also requires an understanding of policy action, such as policy impacts and processes (Dunn, 2008). Policy impacts are the resources, time, and money required to produce the expected policy effect, such as the policy budget. Policy processes refer to organizational, administrative, political activities, and attitudes that create the policy. Table 7.9 provides examples of policy actions, outcomes, processes, outputs, and impacts.

According to Dunn (2008), monitoring can easily be confused with research. The common features include an emphasis on policy-relevant outcomes, a focus on goals, and change-oriented outputs that permit cross-classification of outputs and impacts by any variable in the implementation plan (Dunn, 2018). Monitoring involves facts searching for the problem that generated the policy while evaluation focuses on determining the actual value of the outcome (Dunn, 2018).

Developing an evaluation design. Evaluation achieves several major

Table 7.9 *Examples of Policy Actions and Outcomes.*

Issue Area	Policy Actions		Policy Outcomes	
	Inputs	Processes	Outputs	Impacts
Healthcare	ACA	# of new subscribers as a percentage of total covered population	Preventive care for at risk pre-diabetics	Reduction in diabetes growth rate
Nursing	IOM	# of BSN graduates as a percentage of total RN workforce	Growth in RN-BSN programs, both brick and mortar and distance-learning	Steep growth toward 2020 IOM target
Physicians	ACA-EHRs requirement	# of practices achieving "meaningful use" deadlines	Care coordination and clinical outcome improvement	Healthier population; Reduced hospitalizations

Table 7.10 Criteria for Policy Evaluation.

Type of Criterion	Question
Efficacy	Has a valuable outcome been achieved?
Efficiency	What effort was necessary to produce the valuable outcome?
Adequacy	Does achievement of the valued outcome fix the problem?
Equity	Do different groups share the costs & benefits?
Responsiveness	Do the outcomes meet the needs of specific groups?
Appropriateness	Are the outcomes of real value?

functions in policy analysis and development (Dunn, 2008). First, evaluation can generate reliable, valid data about policy performance and the success of the policy as realized by the affected group. Second, evaluation reconsiders the operationalized goals and objectives and critiques them based on the perceived policy values.

Dunn (2008) offers criteria for policy evaluation as noted in Table 7.10. The components add a robust dimension to the construction of an evaluative design.

Values considered worthy within the health care arena and that distinguish the industry include equity in the access to care regardless of ability to pay (McLaughlin & McLaughlin, 2015). These values include an appreciation of the AONL's nurse executive competency, diversity, wherein cultural competency is a value and workforce attribute in creating an environment conducive to idea exploration and outcome achievement (AONE, 2015). Patient privacy takes on a new dimension in the age of information technology. The Health Insurance Portability and Accountability Act of 1996 (HIPPA) protects patients and health care providers and ensures confidentiality. Federal regulations govern research with human subjects in mandatory informed consent requirements. Since lifestyle choices affect the cost of health care; encouraging personal responsibility in maintaining health emerged as a primary ACA component. Malpractice reform efforts to limit the size of awards to plaintiffs are challenged, with placing a value on a lost life. A code or statement for each profession drives truthfulness, respect of patients, and patient safety in the form of professional ethics. Economic considerations of the impact of health care on our gross domestic product (GDP) buttresses value considerations of lives saved and avoiding pain and suffering in underwriting welfare. Finally, rationing of care and ensuring equity and fairness at times conflicts with the right of consumers to make personal health care decisions that affect clinical outcomes (McLaughlin & McLaughlin, 2015, pp. 342–345). These criteria enable C-Suite nurse executives to support critiques with the vision, mission, and values of health care organizations that operationalize the AONL leadership competencies (AONE, 2015).

Healthcare Policy and the Role of the DNP-Prepared C-Suite Nurse Executive

The American Nurses Association (ANA) social policy statement was originally written in 1980 and subsequently revised in 1995 (ANA, 2010). One of the most important early points in the policy suggests that nursing is responsible to society, because its professional interests must be perceived as serving the interests of society. This social contract acknowledges nursing commitment to ethical core values that ground health care in the U.S. As a result, nursing is obligated to provide care to citizens and non-citizens, regardless of economic or societal position or culture. The elements of nursing's social contract include the relationship of the nurse and the patient experiencing health and illness; public policy, the systems designed for the delivery of health care; and the ability of these to affect population health and professional nursing (ANA 2010). As a result, C-Suite nurse executives must appreciate that the primary goal of nursing is not to serve its own interest since nurses do not own nursing. Society has a claim on nursing, and we as nurses honor that claim by providing health care to our citizenry.

Dr. Mary Paterson, Professor Emeritus at The Catholic University of America School of Nursing, suggests that in many instances, our focus has largely been lost. This may be because many nurses view nursing as a beleaguered profession—that nurses have been trivialized, diminished, or treated unfairly. This message has caused many nursing colleagues to become angry because many believe that our primary job is to better nursing, and the patient—while important—is secondary to that overarching goal. This thinking is the kind that will make nursing irrelevant. We have witnessed this happening as physician assistants filled gaps created by physician shortages when these gaps should have been filled by advanced practice nurses. This also happened when chief operating officers were selected from our male hospital administration colleagues and not chief nursing officers (CNOs). If we want to become a proud profession trusted by society, maintenance of that trust means *working for the good of society* (Paterson, 2015). Knowing how to do that in a sensitive and sensible way requires understanding policy and its development—the policy analysis process.

What does the social policy statement say about nursing leadership? It reminds every CNO that nursing leaders must be concerned with the organization, and the delivery and financing of quality health care. The ANA (2010) has declared that health care is a human right and all nurse executives must address the increasing costs of health care, the ongoing concern about health disparities, and the continuing lack of safe and accessible care, given that medical errors are the third leading cause of death in the U.S. health care system (Cha, 2016). Nursing—the largest health care profession—certainly shoulders a portion of the responsibility. The provision of care simply falls short if a C-Suite nurse executive, an educator, or a researcher focuses solely on a narrow nursing field. The nurse executive has the responsibility to educate society in making the environment safe and addressing infectious disease prevention and the historical increase in opioid-related deaths. This is the C-Suite nurse executive's responsibility.

What are the policy responsibilities of nurse leaders who occupy the highest positions in health care organizations? First, invest in yourself as leaders and secure your terminal degree if you have yet to do so. Academia offers the grounding substantive experience and content so critical to full professional achievement and operational success. Second, establish a national nursing policy presence by conducting research designed to benefit communities. Base your work on the 2010 IOM recommendations, the population health initiatives, or the Quadruple Aim components, which were advanced by the ACA. Better yet, partner with nursing organizations such as AONL or the ANA to develop or promote initiatives designed to improve society's health. Your research findings may prove critical to developing and advancing institutional and public policy. Finally, C-Suite nurse executives must help young nurses focus outward on serving our communities and the nation, and not inward and solely on our profession (Paterson, 2015).

In the coming years, our country will struggle to continue supporting health care costs, which are projected to reach 20% of our GDP by 2025 (Advisory Board, 2017). The ACA's strong focus on population health is an attempt to decrease the increasing health care costs. Nurse executives must be involved with, if not leading, this process. Given the increasing resistance to employing interventions not supported by evidence, rational care strategies now take on new meaning as proven affordable results begin to emerge (Martinez, King, & Cauchi, 2016). All of these findings contribute to the modification of or the development of new policies, with each one following the policy analysis process. This chapter includes the tools for nurse executives to successfully contribute to and independently develop health care policy. C-Suite nurse executives must engage in crafting policy agendas and fully appreciate the analytic dimensions inherent in policy formation. In the end, it will be nurse executives who are defining where nursing is going, what their role will be, and how they will lead.

Chapter Takeaways

1. The initial challenge in policy development is accurately identifying the problem; understanding and articulating the conditions that gives rise to the problem is crucial to effective problem resolution.
2. Nurse executives should seek disparate views of a problem, seeking to

amass *multiple perspectives* that frame the problem and uncover basic *hidden assumptions* regarding the problem.
3. Creating an authorizing environment graphic requires the identification of key policy development *stakeholders* and enables nurse executives to advance policy agendas through consensus-building.
4. Nurse executives seeking problem resolution through policy development should engage in a search for *alternative policy options* as part of the decision-making process
5. Constructing and conducting *SWOT* and *cost-benefit* analyses enables C-Suite executives to build arguments based on data-driven evidence.
6. Nurses executives who master the art of *argumentation* can enhance their ability to advance policy agendas.
7. Successful C-Suite leadership includes detailed plans for policy implementation, monitoring and evaluation.

Chapter Summary

The content of this chapter will enable the DNP-prepared C-Suite nurse executive to excel in policy development and implementation. From correctly identifying a problem and gathering supportive evidence, identifying multiple options for problem correction, and winning policy approval through successful argumentation, this chapter has described significant C-Suite competences. The administrative environments in which today's nurse leaders find themselves are intense and political, and political figures will attempt to diminish leadership strengths to secure their preferred outcomes. This chapter is intended to advance the nurse executives skill set well beyond that expected of C-Suite administrators. The nurse executive who has elected to prepare their professional practice armed with the doctor of nursing practice academic degree must practice, refine, and utilize these concepts. Only then, does knowledge become integrated into practice and change the way in which the nursing profession defines what is required to become a successful C-Suite nurse executive and an unchallenged health care leader who advocates for the patients we serve.

Chapter Reflection Questions

1. In the policy analysis process, what component surfaces as most important? How does the C-Suite nurse executive ensure that this component receives adequate oversight in the policy analysis process?
2. In developing an alternative criterion matrix, what work must be completed prior to engaging in the mathematical calculation the produces the "best-fit" option?

3. How can the policy analyst manipulate the "best-fit" option outcome selections? Where are the pitfalls in the policy analysis process?
4. What are the policy positions of four of the major nursing organizations? Are they focused on "nursing" or are they focused on the patient's nursing services?

References

Advisory Board (2017). *CMS: US healthcare spending to reach nearly 20% of GDP by 2025*. Retrieved from https://www.advisory.com/daily-briefing/2017/02/16/spending-growth.

Alexander, K. L., Entwisle, D. R., & Olson, L. S. (2014). *The long shadow: Family background, disadvantaged urban youth and the transition to adulthood.* American Sociology Association Rose Series in Sociology. New York: Russell Sage Foundation.

American Association of Colleges of Nursing (2006). *The essentials of doctoral education for advanced nursing practice.* Washington, DC: American Association of Colleges of Nursing.

American Nurses Association (2010). *Nursing's social policy statement: The essence of the profession.* Silver Spring, MD: American Nurses Association.

Anderson, J. E. (1975). *Basic concepts in political science.* Westport CT: Praeger Publishers.

American Organization of Nurse Executives (2015). *AONE Nurse Executive Competencies.* Chicago, IL: American Organization of Nurse Executives. Retrieved from www.aone.org.

Baker, J. J., & Baker, R. W. (2014). *Health care finance: Basic tools for non-financial managers.* (4th ed.) Burlington, MA: Jones & Bartlett Learning.

Bardach, E. (1996). *The eight-step path to policy analysis.* Berkeley, CA: University of California Press.

Bardach, E., & Patashink, E. M. (2016). *Practical guide for policy analysis: The eightfold path to more effective problem solving.* (5th ed.) Los Angeles, CA: Sage Publications, Inc.

Berwick, D. M., Nolan, T. W., & Whittington, J. (2008). The triple aim: Care, health, and cost. *Health Affairs, 27*(3), 759–69.

Bodenheimer, T., & Sinsky, C. (2014). From triple to quadruple aim: Care of the patient requires care of the provider. *Annals of Family Medicine, 12*(6), 573–576.

Bright Hub Project Management. (2017). *Common project management charts.* Retrieved from http://www.brighthubpm.com/project-planning/53691-common-project-management-charts/.

Centers for Disease Control and Prevention (2018). *Brief 4: Evaluating policy implementation.* Retrieved from https://www.cdc.gov/injury/pdfs/policy/Brief%204-a.pdf.

Cha, A. E. (2016). Researchers: Medical errors now third leading cause of deaths in the United States. *The Washington Post.* Retrieved from https://www.washingtonpost.

com/news/to-your-health/wp/2016/05/03/researchers-medical-errors-now-third-leading-cause-of-death-in-united-states/?utm_term=.103c66aaf8e7.

Cochran, C. L., & Malone, E.F. (2014). *Public policy: Perspectives and choices.* (5th ed.) Boulder, CO: Lynne Rienner Publishers.

Consolidated Framework for Implementation Research (CFIR) (2017). Retrieved from http://www.cfirguide.org/

Congressional Budget Office (2017). *Introduction to the CBO.* Retrieved from https://www.cbo.gov/about/overview .

Dubnick, M.J., & Bardes, B.A. (1983). *Thinking about public policy: A problem-solving approach.* Hoboken, NJ: Wiley Publishers.

Dunn, W.N. (2004). *Public policy analysis.* (2nd ed.) Upper Saddle River, N.J.: Pearson Prentice Hall

Dunn, W.N. (2008). *Public policy analysis.* (4th ed.) Upper Saddle River, NJ: Prentice-Hall.

Dunn, W.N. (2016). *Public policy analysis.* (5th ed.) New York: Routledge.

Dunn, W.N. (2018a). *Public policy analysis: An integrated approach.* (6th ed.) New York.

Dunn, W.N. (2018b) *Public policy pnalysis: An introduction.* Retrieved from https://www.slideshare.net/nida19/public-policy-analysisdunn

Eberstadt, N. (2016). *America's entitlements explosion: Evidence and implications.* American Enterprise Institute. Retrieved from https://www.aei.org/wp-content/uploads/2016/07/Prepared-Statement-Eberstadt-July-6-2016-final.pdf

Fabian, K. (2017). Decision matrix: What it is and how to use it. *Business News Daily.* Retrieved from http://www.businessnewsdaily.com/6146-decision-matrix.html

Fontenot, S. (2013). The Affordable Care Act and electronic health care records. Retrieved from http://sarahfontenot.com/wp-content/uploads/2015/04/5-Dec-2013-Will-EHRs-Improve-Quality-Article.pdf

Frieden, T.R. (2013). Government's role in protecting health and safety. *New England Journal of Medicine, 368*, 1857–1859. doi: 10 1056/NEJMp130819

Gill, W., Shiffman, J., Schneider, H., Muray, S., Brugha, R., & Gilson, L. (2008). Doing health policy analysis: Methodological and conceptual reflections and challenges. *Health Policy and Planning, 23*(5), 308–317.

Goudreau, K.A. & Smolenski, M.C. (2014). Health policy and advanced nursing practice: Impact and implications. New York: Springer Publishing Company.

Hennessey, K. (2010). Dr. Gruber's honesty about lying. Retrieved from https://keithhennessey.com/2014/11/10/honesty-about-lying/ .

Hervis, R.M. (1993). Impact of DRGs on the medical profession. *Clinical Laboratory Science, 6*(3), 183–185.

Hoffman, M. (2008). *Methods of argument analysis and construction in public policy.* Retrieved from http://www.prism.gatech.edu/~mh327/PUBP-8803_argument-syllabus.pdf.

Kingdon, J.W. (2011). *Agendas, alternatives, and public policy.* New York: Pearson Publishers.

Knickman, J. R. & Kovner, A.R. (2015). *Healthcare delivery in the United States.* New York: Springer Publishing Company.

Kohn, L. T., Corrigan, J., & Donaldson, M. S. (Eds.). (2000). *To err is human: Building a safer Health System.* Washington, DC: National Academy Press.

Lester, J.P., & Stewart, J. (2000) *Public policy: An evolutionary approach.* Stamford, CT: Wadsworth Thomson Learning.

Longley, R. (2017). Federalism: A government system of shared powers. Retrieved from https://www.thoughtco.com/federalism-powers-national-and-state-governments-3321841

Martinez, J.C., King, M.P., & Cauchi, R. (2016). Improving the health care system: Seven state strategies. *National Conference of State Legislatures.* Retrieved from http://www.ncsl.org/Portals/1/Documents/Health/ImprovingHealthSystemsBrief16.pdf

Mason, D.J., Gardner, D.B., Outlaw, F.H., & O'Grady, E.T. (2016). *Policy & Politics in Nursing and Healthcare.* (7th ed.). St. Louis, MO: Elsevier.

McLaughlin, C, P., & McLaughlin, C.D. (2015). *Health policy analysis: An interdisciplinary approach.* Burlington, MA: Jones and Bartlett Publishers.

Milstead, J.A. (2008) *Health policy and politics: A nurses' guide.* Sudbury, MA: Jones and Bartlett Learning.

Moi, A.P. (2010). The future of transparency: Power, pitfalls, and promises. *Global Environmental Politics, 10*(3), 132-143.

Morone, J. A., & Ehlke, D. C. (2013). *Health politics and policy.* (5th ed.). Stamford, CT: Cengage Learning.

Morrell, B. (2017). *Patient-centered medical homes for baby boomers.* (Doctoral dissertation). The Catholic University of America School of Nursing. Washington, D.C.

Musso, J., Biller, B., & Myrtle, B. (1999, February). *The tradecraft of writing for policy analysis and management.* University of Southern California School of Public Policy, Planning, and Development. Retrieved from file:///C:/Users/joyce/Downloads/Tradecraft_of_Writing_Effective_Policies%20(4).pdf

Navigating Accounting. (2017). The Toulmin model of argumentation. Retrieved from http://www.navigatingaccounting.com/sites/default/files/Posted/Common/Resources_webbook/Toulmin_Model_of_Argumentation.pdf.

Nickitas, D.M, Middaugh, D.J., & Aries, N. (eds.). (2011) *Policy and politics for nurses and other health professionals.* Sudbury, MA: Jones and Bartlett.

O'Byrne, P., & Holmes, D. (2009). The politics of nursing care: Correcting deviance in accordance with the social contract. *Policy, Politics & Nursing, 10*(2), 153–162.

Office Timeline. (2017). *Visual project management.* Retrieved from https://www.officetimeline.com/project-management

Paterson, M.A. Personal communication, October 20, 2015.

Paterson, M. A. (2014). *Healthcare finance and financial management: Essentials for advanced practice nurses and interdisciplinary care teams.* Lancaster, PA: DEStech Publications Inc.

Patient Protection and Affordable Care Act, 42 U. S. § 18001. (2010). Retrieved from https://www.hhs.gov/healthcare/about-the-law/

Patient-Centered Outcomes Research Institute. (2013). *Cooperative agreement funding announcement: Improving infrastructure for conducting patient-centered outcomes research*. Retrieved from https://www.pcori.org/assets/PCORI-CDRN-Funding-Announcement-042313.pdf

Porche, D. J. (2012). *Health policy: Applications for nurses and other healthcare professionals*. Sudbury, MA: Jones and Bartlett Learning.

Resnik, D.B. (2007). Responsibility for health: personal, social, and environmental. *Journal of Medical Ethics, 33*(8), 444–445.

Rook, D. (2015). How we got to now: A brief history of employer-sponsored healthcare. Retrieved from https://www.griffinbenefits.com/employeebenefitsblog/history-of-employer-sponsored-healthcare

Rosdahl, C.B., & Kowalski, M.T. (2012). *Textbook of basic nursing*. (10th ed.). Philadelphia, PA: Lippincott Williams & Wilkins.

Sanger-Katz, M. (2017). Grading Obamacare: Successes, failures and "incompletes." Retrieved from https://www.nytimes.com/2017/02/05/upshot/grading-obamacare-successes-failures-and-incompletes.html

Starr, P. (1982). *The social transformation of American medicine*. New York: Basic Books.

Starr, P. (2011). *Remedy and reaction*. New Haven, CT: Yale University Press.

Strether, L. (2014). *Jonathan Gruber, ObamaCare, and "stupid voters:" It couldn't happen to a Nicer Shill*. Retrieved from https://www.nakedcapitalism.com/2014/11/jonathan-gruber-obamacare-stupid-voters-couldnt-happen-nicer-shill.html.

The Guardian. (2017). *How does the US healthcare system compare with other countries*? Retrieved from https://www.theguardian.com/us-news/ng-interactive/2017/jul/25/us-healthcare-system-vs-other-countries

The Toulmin Model of Argumentation. Retrieved from http://www-rohan.sdsu.edu/~digger/305/toulmin_model.htm

The Toulmin Model of Argumentation. Retrieve November 13, 2017, from http://commfaculty.fullerton.edu/rgass/toulmin2.htm

Toulmin, S. (1958). *The uses of argument*. Cambridge, UK: Cambridge University Press. p. 127.

Tummers, L.G. (2011). Explaining the willingness of public professionals to implement new policies: A policy alienation framework. *International Review of Administrative Sciences, 77*(3), 55–581.

University of Cambridge Institute for Manufacturing. *Decision support tools: Criteria rating form, weighted ranking*. Retrieved from https://www.ifm.eng.cam.ac.uk/research/dstools/criteria-rating-form/ .

Van Delinder, S. (2017). How much transparency is too much? How to find the right balance. *Visibility*. Retrieved from https://www.visibilitymagazine.com/much-transparency-much-find-right-balance/.

Vining, A.R., & Weimer, D.L. (2010) Policy analysis: Concepts and analysis. New York: Routledge. Retrieved from http://www.aspanet.org/public/aspadocs/par/fpa/fpa-policy-article.pdf

Washoe County, NV. (2017). Evaluating alternatives: Criteria Rating (grid analysis). Retrieved from https://www.washoecounty.us/.../Evaluating%20Alternatives%20%20Criteria%20rating.

Weaver, B. S. (2017). Transforming and meeting Georgia's rising demand for health care coordination. Doctoral dissertation, Unpublished manuscript. The Catholic University of America School of Nursing. Washington, D.C.

Weimer, D., & Vining, Aidan. (1992). Policy analysis: Concepts and practice. (2nd ed.). Englewood Cliffs, NJ: Prentice-Hall.

World Health Organization. (2005). Constitution of the World Health Organization. Retrieved from http://www.who.int/governance/eb/who_constitution_en.pdf

Appendix A—Policy Example
Transforming and Meeting Georgia's Rising Demand for Health Care Coordination
by Barbara S. Weaver PhD(c)
April 26, 2017

Executive Summary

The state of Georgia faces a health care crisis of great proportion related to a lack of care coordination tragically impacting access to care and negatively impacting population health. As the population in Georgia continues to grow, combined with a worsening deficit of primary care physicians, and the decision to reject the Medicaid expansion, the rapidly expanding lack of access intensifies.

Advanced practice registered nurses (APRNs) currently constitute the fastest growing segment of the professional workforce in Georgia and offer a means to transform and improve care coordination (Advanced Practice Registered Nurses of Georgia, 2017). The literature reveals Georgia laws unduly restrict APRNs practice and lag behind the rest of the country (Advanced Practice Nurses of Georgia, 2017; Stephens, 2015). Health care falls under state's rights granting legislators the authority to make decisions in the best interest of its citizens.

This new health care policy entitled *Transforming and Meeting Georgia's Rising Demand for Health Care Coordination* used a six-step analytical framework and a professional, logical-positivist approach to analyze the new policy development, selection process, implementation, monitoring and evaluation techniques, ending with recommendations and conclusions. The analysis revealed the need for improved access and the removal of barriers to care coordination. The process identified and examined three policy alternatives to address the issue including a) no change alternative, b) removal of barriers to APRNs and c) the use of telehealth to reach rural and disadvantaged areas. Based on several qualitative and quantitative analyses techniques (SWOT, cost-benefit analysis and calculation, alternative-criterion matrix) the newly developed health care policy selected removal of barriers to APRNs as the best fit option. The analysis details a two-year implementation plan including frequent monitoring and the evaluation processes exemplified in tables. This policy analyst advocates for proactive state reform aligned with the objectives of the Patient Protection and Affordable Care Act (ACA) and recommendations of the Institute of Medicine (IOM) to support full practice authority for APRNs leading to reduced cost, improved outcomes and increased access to care (Institute of Medicine, 2010; Patient Protection and Affordable Care Act, 42U, S, § 18001, 2010).

Introduction

This new health care policy analysis examines the original problem identified by the Georgia legislature involving a lack of care coordination affecting population health. The new health care policy entitled *Transforming and Meeting Georgia's Rising Demand for Health Care Coordination* calls for state action to address and resolve the crisis Georgia now faces to deliver coordinated health care by removing barriers to APRN practice.

Key terms associated with this policy include advanced practice nurse, full practice authority, restrictive practice, scope of practice, and telehealth. In Georgia, APRNs include medical professionals with an advanced nursing degree "in one of four areas; certified registered nurse anesthetist, certified nurse midwife, clinical nurse specialist, and certified nurse practitioner" (Stephens, 2015). Full practice authority in other states entails the collection of state practice and licensure laws that permit APRNs to practice independently and autonomously "upon successful completion of a formal academic program and demonstration of competency in that profession" (National Council of State Boards, 2017). Restrictive practice refers to Georgia's law restricting the ability of an APRN "to engage in at least one element of APRN practice" (National Council of State Boards of Nursing, 2017). Georgia currently requires supervision, delegation, or team management by a physician for an APRN to provide patient care (Stephens, 2015). Scope of practice refers to the legislatively defined rules and regulations in which a fully qualified practitioner practices. Telehealth refers to the use of "electronic telecommunications to deliver and support health care using technology with distance separating the patient and provider" (Henderson, Davis, Smith, & King, 2014).

Stakeholders pertain to those interested in the outcomes, affected by or with an effect on the new healthcare policy. Key stakeholders include; Georgia legislators, Governor, Secretary of State, American Medical Association (AMA), Georgia State Board of Nursing, National Nursing organizations, Department of Health and Human Services (DHHS), Healthcare facilities, citizens of Georgia, academia, American Association of Retired Persons, physician assistant groups, and the media (See Appendix J, Authorizing Environment Chart).

The social dilemma in this policy involves social inequities in access to a primary care provider that put many Georgians at a further disadvantage from a lack of care coordination limiting health and wellness. A lack of health equity creates disparities in health between more and less socially advantaged Georgia citizens. Solution alternatives to the problem include (a) Alternative I a no change alternative, (b) Alternative II removing barriers to APRN practice including eliminating physician regulatory oversight and direct reimbursement for services, and (c) Alternative III the expansion of the technical infrastructure to support telehealth in underserved areas in Georgia. From a novice professional policy analyst approach this policy analysis incorporates a policy analyst type and approach.

Description of Policy Development & Selection Process

The over-reaching policy goal is to remove barriers to qualified health care providers to broaden access to medically underserved Georgia residents. This policy seeks significant state reform aligned with the objectives of the ACA and recommendations of the IOM to support improved care coordination through strategies leading to improved population health, reduced cost, and improved access to care. Objectives include (a) increase the number of primary care providers in Georgia, (b) increase access to primary care providers to support disease prevention, promotion, and health education and maintenance, and (c) reduce health care costs related to emergency room misuse and lack of preventative health care. The measurement plan includes evaluating the quality of care and health outcomes, access, health care costs, and satisfaction.

Stakeholders include the Georgia legislators, Governor Deal, APRNs, healthcare facilities, consumers, payers and state agencies, APRNs, physician and physician assistant groups, and supporters (See Appendix J Authorizing Environment Chart). Political backers include a bipartisan group of Senators including Senators Unterman, Burke, Kirk, and Orrock, lobbyists, and special interest groups at the national and local level (Advanced Practice Registered Nurses of Georgia, 2017). Adversaries include Sharon Cooper who chairs the House Health and Human Services committee and opposes full autonomy and expansion (Advanced Practice Registered Nurses of Georgia, 2017). The damage from this opposition further aggravates the validity of the legislation as she earned a Master's Degree in Nursing and taught nursing. The Georgia Medical Association supports multiple lobbyists and frequently point out the years of medical education, superiority of the medical, and the risks of permitting full authority to APRNs. Apathy towards political involvement on the part of APRNs in Georgia further harms the movement (Advanced Practice Registered Nurses of Georgia, 2017).

To identify and search for alternative policies an alternative-criterion matrix considered and evaluated each option for cost, quality, and accessibility to ascertain the best fit option (See Appendix A, Alternative-Criterion Matrix). The alternative-criterion matrix identified alternative II probably leads to the outcome judged as the best possible outcome, therefore judging Alternative II as the best (See the Alternative-Criterion Matrix Appendix A). A SWOT analysis functioned as a strategic tool to narrow down best fit options (See Appendix B, C, and D SWOT analyses). The outcome of the SWOT analyses clarified and enabled weighting criterion assisting in eliminating alternative I and III and revealing Alternative II as option providing the best possible fit (See Appendix E Decision-Making Matrix). Alternative II ranked the highest for the most important criteria justifying the option as the preferred alternative. The preferred option selection removes laws restricting the autonomy of APRNs and heralds full practice authority without requirements for physician supervision including direct reimbursements for services. The cost-benefit analysis, a key method to determine the best option, indicated the positive economic benefits of each of the health policy alternatives (See Appendix F, G, and H for the Cost-Benefit Analysis for the Health Policy Alternatives). The alternative cost-benefit calculation analysis set the critical outcome threshold ratio at less than 1 and indicated alternative II provides positive economic benefits (ratio = .0064) (See Appendix I Alternative Cost-Benefit Calculation Analysis). Groups impacted by alternative II include the Georgia legislature, APRNs, physician and physician assistants, consumers, health care facilities, state and local agencies, payers, academia, state board of nursing, other major nursing organizations, and Joint Commission Starr's review of the tortuous evolution of health care and the unintended policy trap applies in that state and federal level funding for healthcare as a universal right remains an expectation entangling many Georgians (Starr, 2011). The current fragmented, health care system demands full transparency as a desirable condition in the political process to advance public policy. Transparency enhances accountability, informs, and attracts a collaborative public.

The policy addressed legality by appropriately recommending legislative changes to the state statutes that impact APRNs scope of practice, reimbursement, and state practice and licensure laws. The policy addressed political feasibility by identifying the problem, identifying critical key interest groups, stakeholders, and actors, identifying the current political environment in Georgia, gathering and organizing information on policy alternatives, and analyzing the data. This analyst estimates a high level of support for the proposed alternative. Factors supporting political feasibility include bipartisan supporters, APRNs, National Organizations, supporters such as American Association of Retired Persons and public support. Obstacles to political feasibility include opposition from within the legislative body and through the power and financial backing of the AMA. An increasing shortage of primary care providers, escalating costs, and poor population health in Georgia lends support to counter-balance the political

Appendix A: Alternative Criterion Matrix
Transforming and Mettin gGeorgia's Rising Demand for Health Care Coordination
Note: Highlighted cells indicate best performance on resprctive criteria.

Health Policy Alternatives	Criterion A—Cost	Criterion B—Quality of Care	Criterion C—Accessibility
Health Policy Alternative I: No change alternative continues to restrict APRN practice	1.6 Million initial cost and 1 million annual cost • Continue current forgiveness incentives to assist physicians with medical school costs • Maintain support to office spaces for new physicians in disadvantaged areas • Continue lobbyist support • Costs of medical school far exceed cost of APRN education	• The policy alternative provides a high level of quality care with a neutral impact on the current state • Decreasing numbers of primary care physicians impacts quality of care with crisis projected for 2025	• Alternative I offers no change and sustains the current accessibility problem • Projected :increase in the numbers of APRNs increasing the number of inner city primary care providers and improving access to urban areas • Continues to restrict APRNs in the face of an increasing aging population, growing number of under served Georgians, and decreasing number of primary care physicians decreasing access
Health Policy Alternative II: State mandates allow APRNs to practice autonomously without physician regulatory oversight including direct reimbursement	2.3 Million annual cost/1.65 Million annual cost • Lobbyist support • Committee member daily expense allowance to oversee enactment of new legislation to include members of the committee who are not legislators, state officials, or state employees • Marketing and education costs for legislative brief, public brochure, APRN awareness and value video, posters, travel expenses for promotion, branded items i.e. tee shirts, cups, pencils, stress balls • Decreased costs to consumers secondary to current reimbursement laws • Decreased cost to the state from decreased emergency room visits and health promotion and prevention	• The policy alternative improves the quality of care by removing barriers to practice increasing care coordination and improved quality of care • Robust evidence suggests that APRNs positively impact quality of care and in several reports improve quality outcomes in comparison to physicians • Risk of large numbers of currently employed nurses leaving the bedside to improve earning potential as APRN s straining the current nursing shortage and reducing quality of care	• Alternative II transforms law at the state level providing increased access of qualified healthcare providers to all Georgians • The policy alternative increases accessibility improving access in underserved areas • Currently more APRNs provide primary care services than physicians with projections for increasing numbers of APRNs • More than half of surveyed currently practicing APRNs in Georgia responded with willingness to work in rural areas with the removal of practice barriers improving access to disadvantaged Georgians

(continued)

197

Appendix A (continued): Alternative Criterion Matrix
Transforming and Mettin gGeorgia's Rising Demand for Health Care Coordination
Note: Highlighted cells indicate best performance on resprctive criteria.

Health Policy Alternatives	Criterion A—Cost	Criterion B—Quality of Care	Criterion C—Accessibility
Health Policy Alternative III: Expansion of the technical infrastructure to support telehealth applications in underserved areas in Georgia	18.6 Million initial cost/7.65 Million annual cost • Hardware and software initial and maintenance costs • Licensing costs per Telehealth application • Vendor assistance and contracts • Development of educational programs • Initial eight hour and annual four hour training costs • Information technology salaries, wages, benefits and after hours support contract	• The policy alternative benefits rural areas by providing accessibility and level of care currently nonexistent. • Some evidence suggests that waiting to talk to a telehealth provider reduces some patients and healthcare providers perception of quality • Limited evidence on impact on quality	• The policy alternative :increases the number of primary care providers in disadvantaged areas • The lack of a current infrastructure creates delays in implementation

Appendix B: SWOT Analysis: Health Policy Alternative I—No Change Alternative
Note: In each box below, list the alternative's strengths, weaknesses and the associated external opportunities and threats.

Strengths	Weaknesses
• Physician satisfaction with current system • Clear boundaries for services with no competition or overlap in services from non-physicians • Well established and comfortable infrastructure to deliver healthcare • Geographical location in highly suitable locations in major Georgia cities • Esteemed reputation in the community • Strong physician relationships with other area physicians and hospitals	• Fragmented care that in turn depletes financial reserves • Inadequate number of primary care providers especially to underserved areas • Unfair disadvantage in method of care to Georgia citizens with increasing numbers of APRNs • Promotes unfair and questionably deceptive methods of competition affecting commerce and consumer choice
Opportunities	**Threats**
• Growing metropolitan communities • Population increase and changes in Georgia's population profile or need (aging, chronic illness and disability)	• Economic instability without Medicaid expansion and increasing numbers of uniinsured • Workforce vulnerability from APRN dissatisfaction potentially leading to the practitioner leaving Georgia for less restrictive practices • Financial vulnerability from a sensitive market • Current lack of medical practitioners and projected deficit by 2025 • Decreasing government reimbursement • Health care reform and ACOs with increasing pressures to reduce healthcare costs

*Appendix C: SWOT Analysis: Health Policy Alternative II—
State Mandates allow APRNs to practice at autononmously without physician
regtulatory oversight including direct reinbursment.*

*In each box below, list the alternative's strengths, weaknesses and the
associated external opportunities and threats*

Strengths	Weaknesses
• Increased consumer choice • Deploys highly skilled practitioners to promote population health • Large APRN resource in Georgia • Strong public trust • Promotes timely, cost effective and accessible health care • Several studies demonstrate efficiency, accessibility, quality, and satisfaction as equal to or better than care under a physician • Reduced stress for obstetric (midwives) and pediatric patients with stable primary care provider	• Lack of public and medical education and recognition in Georgia on the role of APRNs • Overlapping scopes of practice and fear of financial impact on medical practices and from physician assistants due to lower market share • Requires restructuring of current APRN workforce currently under physician regulatory oversight
Opportunities	**Threats**
• Enormous opportunities with the fragmented and dysfunctional current system to enhance Georgia's efforts to support the redesign the workforce to provide high quality, cost effective health care • Healthcare reform in line with the recommendations of the Institute ofMedicine and the ACA • Globalization with increased possibility to network and reach new markets • Procompetitive improvement in health care services likely to spur innovation in care delivery and increase competition i.e. opening weekend or extended evening hours or in-home visits	• Regardless of alternative without the Medicaid expansion the current system is unsustainable • Lack of acceptance in Georgia from the elderly and medicine • Potential for adversarial breakdown with physicians secondary to competition • Increased number of APRNs causing drops in wages secondary to increased supply • Potential for destabilization of current nursing workforce with nurses leaving the bedside for higher earing potential • Strong resistance from medicine and some legislators

Appendix D: SWOT Analysis: Health Policy Alternative III—Telehealth

In each box below, list the alternative's strengths, weaknesses and the associated external opportunities and threats

Strengths	Weaknesses
• Access to health services for Georgians living in underserved and remote areas reducing disparity • Permits rural residents to receive expert diagnosis and treatment from distant experts and medical centers • Reduction in medical costs through early prevention and treatment and the avoidance of hospitalizations and costly emergency room visits Improves administrative efficiency and coordination • Eliminates risk of transmitting infectious diseases between health care facilities, providers and patients • Reduction is costs to provider and patient for travel	• Cost • Distrust and a lack of patient awareness and acceptance • Lack of specialized education by the clinician • Difficulty incorporating into the community and existing practice • Lack of infrastructure to support the technology in rural • Fear of loosing existing jobs when deployed • Need for workflow reengineering to synthesize telehealth
Opportunities	**Threats**
• Competitive cost advantage to managed care plans and large health systems which potentially driving leverage with legislators Potential to radically reshape and restructure health care in Georgia • New trends in providing preventive and personalized care for the new generation of clinicians • New careers requiring new skills Mechanism to expand new regional, national and international market Attractive technology to the Gen-Y (millennials) and Gen-Z generations	• Rapid advances in technology making system obsolete • Lack of education on technology in the medical and nursing educational system • Complex interface to the existing or non-existent infrastructure • Lack of cross cultural and multilingual user friendly platforms • External threats from viruses, malware, and essential loss of power from weather (Georgia hurricane season) • Competition and need for secure internet clouds and lines for privacy, confidentiality, and security • Resistance from the burgeoning older generation • State funding changes and the inability to sustain the functionality, training, and necessary upgrades financially

Appendix E: Decision-Making Matrix

Transforming and Meetings Georgia's Rising Demand for Health Care Coordination

Criterion for "scoring" Score on a scale of 1–5; 5 = most important	Health Policy Alternative I No Change Alternative Score on a scale of 1–5; 5 = most important **RANK: 1**	Health Policy Alternative II State mandates allow APRNs to practice autonomously without physician regulatory oversight including direct reimbursement Score on a scale of 1–5; 5 = most important **RANK: 5**	Health Policy Alternative III Technical infrastructure to support Telehealth applications for physician services in the state of Georgia Score on a scale of 1–5; 5 = most important **RANK: 3**
Criteria 1 Cost Weight: 3	Score: 3	Score: 15	Score: 9
Criteria 2 Quality Weight: 4	Score: 4	Score: 20	Score: 12
Criteria 3 Access Weight: 5	Score: 5	Score: 25	Score: 15
Total Weighted Score	12	60	36

Appendix F: Cost-Benefit Analysis for Health Policy Alternative I

Transforming and Meeting Georgia's Rising Demand for Health Care Coordination
Health Policy Alternative I: No Change Alternative

Cost			Benefit		
Element	Initial Cost	Annual Cost	Element	Initial Benefit	Projected Annual Benefit
Continue forgiveness incentives to assist physicians with medical school costs in exchange for practice in disadvantaged areas for 5 years with initial bonus and yearly stipends for 5 years	1 Million	400K	Taxable salary expenditure per primary care physician	100K	150K
Maintain support to office spaces for new physicians in disadvantaged areas	400K	400K	Labor income to the state for office staff to support the physician	150K	150K
Maintain current lobbyist	200K	200K	Average annual net revenue generated by a primary care physician for their affiliated hospitals	400K	400K
Total Costs	1.6 Million	1 Million	Total Savings	650K	700K

203

Appendix G: Cost-Benefit Analysis for Health Policy Alternative II

Transforming and Meeting Georgia's Rising Demand for Health Care Coordination

Health Policy Alternative II: State legislation for full practice authority for APRNs including direct reimbursement

Cost			Benefit			
Element	Initial Cost	Annual Cost	Element	Initial Benefit	Projected Annual Benefit
State legislative and committee expenses to oversee new legislation enactment including travel expenses, support personnel and lobbyist	1 Million	500K	Reduction in health care costs stemming from increased use of APRNs in Georgia	4 Million	8 Million
Marketing and public awareness campaign of redesign and the expanded role of APRNs	300K	150K	Increased labor income APRNs (5,000 jobs)	200K	500K
Technology for data management and research, APRN awareness, support, and education	1 Million	1 Million	Economic benefits to the state and local government	150 Million	250 Million
Total Costs	2.3 Million	1.65 Million	Total Savings	154.2 Million	258.5 Million

Appendix H: Cost-Benefit Analysis for Health Policy Alternative III

Transforming and Meeting Georgia's Rising Demand for Health Care Coordination Health Policy Alternative III: Telehealth

Cost			Benefit		
Element	Initial Cost	Annual Cost	Element	Initial Benefit	Projected Annual Benefit
Capital purchase of platforms and infrastructure including access to high speed internet rural Georgia, hardware, software license costs, network, workstations, maintenance costs and vendor assistance	18 Million	7 Million	Improved accessibility of health care translating to a reduction in overall spending per Georgia citizen	500K	3 Million
Information systems department team of-fice space, salaries, wages, and benefits	400K	350K	Decreased costs of emergency room visits	5 Million	7 Million
Development of educational programs, initial, ongoing training and system upgrade training	200K	300K	Decreased costs to consumer and provider in travel	65K	65K
Total Costs	18.6 Million	7.65 Million	Total Savings	5.565 Million	10.65 Million

Appendix I: Alernative Policy Cost-Benefit Calculation Analysis

Transforming and Meeting Georgia's Rising Demand for Health Care Coordination

Critical Outcome Threshold colt/Benefit ration < 1

Policy Alternative	Total Annual Cost	Total Annual Benefit	Annual Cost-Benefit Ratio
Health Policy Alternative I No change alternative	1 Million	700K	1 Million/700K = 1.43
Health Policy Alternative II State legislation grants APRNs full practice authority without physician oversight including direct reimbursement	1.65 Million	258.5 Million	1.65 Million/258.5 Million = < 1 or .0064
Health Policy Alternative III Expansion of the technical infrastructure to support telehealth applications in underserved areas in Georgia	7.65 Million	10.65 Million	7.65 Million/10.65 Million = < 1 or 0.72

survival test. The new health care policy addresses equity and the equal right to health care for all Georgians with an emphasis on the disadvantaged, vulnerable and marginalized groups. Hidden assumptions of the new policy involve the belief that Georgians readily trust, accept, and utilize the redesign to a new APRN primary care model from the well-established medical model.

Co-creating value and sustainability of the new policy requires lobbying, marketing, and education to engender ongoing stakeholder support and partnership. Lobbying efforts include bringing the issue to the attention of policymakers during meetings, finding champions, and creating a policy brief with explicit key information legislators require. Early and often statewide advocacy through marketing and public education become essential to get the health care policy position solidified. Because of economic and social invisibility of APRNs in Georgia, the benefits and value of the role of APRNs require clarification and visibility through public events, television, radio, and social events. Additional marketing and education efforts include social medias, policy news on the Georgia Board of Nursing and State website, and the development of a brochure to provide education on the value of redesign on health promotion and prevention, accessibility, and outcomes.

The environment surrounding the policy alternative displayed in the authorizing environment chart outlines the authorizing entities that enable the policy to move forward (See Appendix J Authorizing Environment Chart). Relevant actors include government and nongovernment actors, including but not limited to the Governor, Georgia legislators, elected state officials, federal agencies, consumers, healthcare facilities, national and state or-

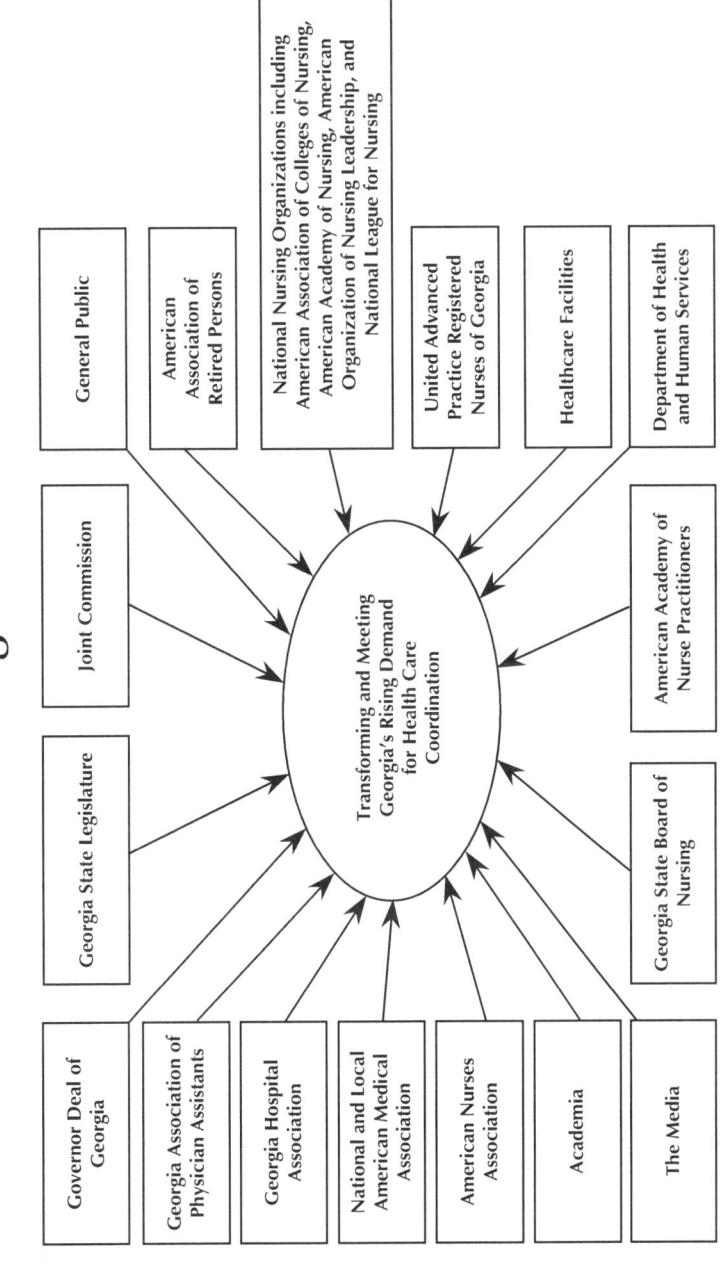

Appendix J: Authorizing Environment Chart.

Authorizing Environment

Central focus: **Transforming and Meeting Georgia's Rising Demand for Health Care Coordination**

Authorizing entities:
- Governor Deal of Georgia
- Georgia State Legislature
- Joint Commission
- General Public
- Georgia Association of Physician Assistants
- American Association of Retired Persons
- Georgia Hospital Association
- National Nursing Organizations including American Association of Colleges of Nursing, American Academy of Nursing, American Organization of Nursing Leadership, and National League for Nursing
- National and Local American Medical Association
- United Advanced Practice Registered Nurses of Georgia
- American Nurses Association
- Healthcare Facilities
- Academia
- Department of Health and Human Services
- The Media
- Georgia State Board of Nursing
- American Academy of Nurse Practitioners

ganizations, interest groups, media, and APRNs. For economic viability the new health care policy requires financial sustainability. The economic analysis concerned with the value for Georgians highlights the costs and benefits of services. Cost-benefit analysis measures economic viability and highlights changes needed to ensure present and future financial viability. Evidence plays a large role in arguing the importance of the proposals viability for decision making or taking action. Empirical representations that operationalize economic or financial viability through description such as cost effectiveness, quality of care, lives saved, accessibility or sustainability become necessary to frame the policy proposal and share relevant data with stakeholders. The analysis used Toulmin's Model to structurally reveal both the strengths and limits of the policy argument and present valid and robust conclusions (See Appendix K Argumentation Flow Chart).

Implementation

The projected implementation process plans a top-down structure to operationalize the policy into practice and action. The creation of subcommittee for strategic and operational planning and authority chaired by the DHHS serves to formalize and execute the implementation. Tasks include developing an implementation plan, public relations campaign, advisory group, and policy champions within the healthcare system, academia, and public health division (See Appendices L, M, and O). The monitoring system through the state and DHHS assists with policy monitoring and evaluation. Initial costs estimated at 1.6 Million support the necessary resources to support associated oversight, marketing, technology and education. Stakeholders located at the state, local and micro-levels include the state subcommittee, APRNs, health care administrator, media, Georgia residents, physicians, state and federal payer programs, professional groups, and universities supporting analysis. Other needed resources affecting implementation include marketing and education, and legal counsel to manage risk.

The projected policy monitoring process evaluates connections between the policy implementation and short and long-term health-related indicators prior to policy approval and unfolds overtime (See Appendix N Monitoring and Evaluation Plan and Appendix O Implementation Plan). The monitoring process utilizes existing website based programs and monthly meetings to evaluate the data and identify opportunities for improvement. The evaluation processes include a) the direct link between mandating full practice authority for APRNs and effects on specific preventable diseases and health outcomes and b) the evaluation of health care redesign and the effects on population determinants of health and inequalities in access, health care cost, and quality (Weiland, 2016). Alternative II reflects a distributive policy allocating benefits to the larger Georgia population. An

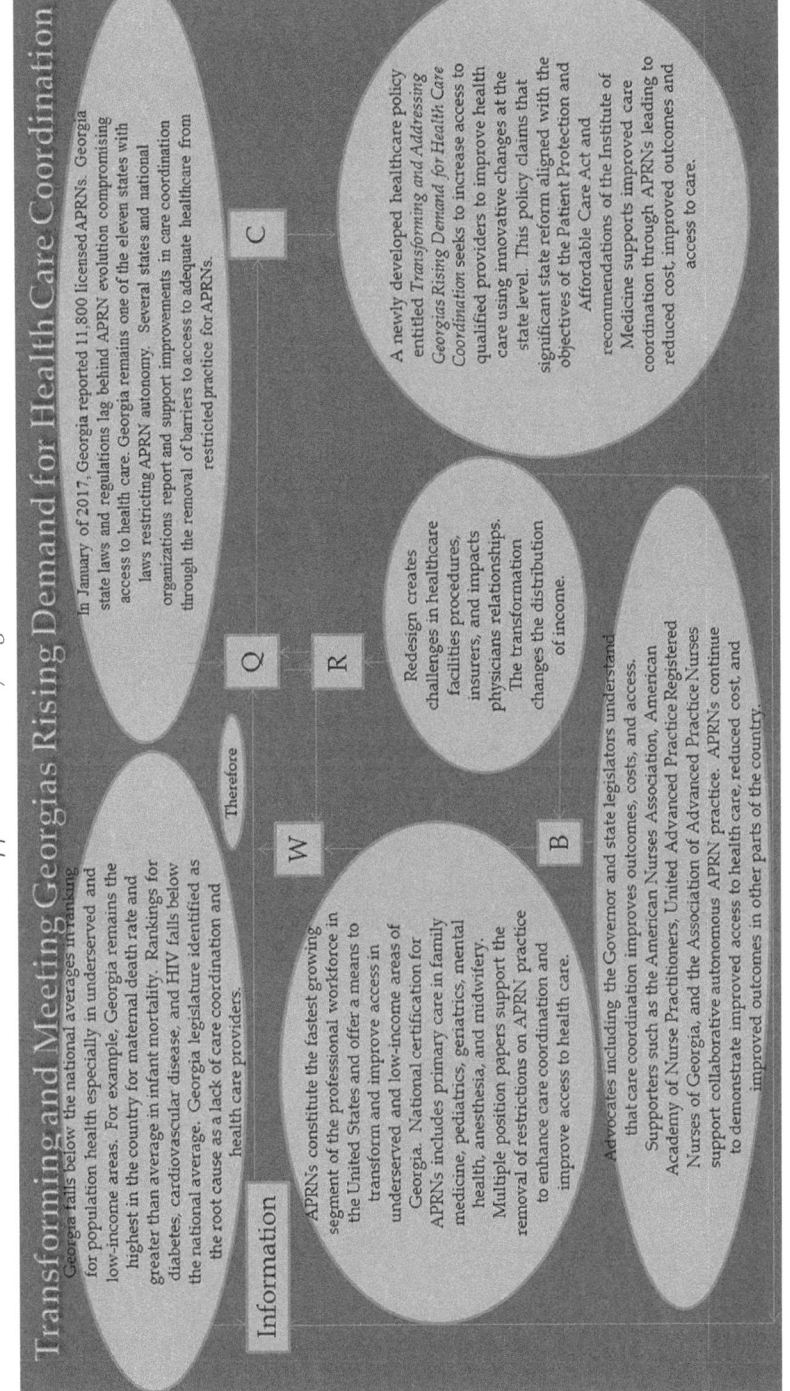

Appendix K: Policy Argument Chart.

Transforming and Meeting Georgia's Rising Demand for Health Care Coordination

Information

Georgia falls below the national averages in ranking for population health especially in underserved and low-income areas. For example, Georgia remains the highest in the country for maternal death rate and greater than average in infant mortality. Rankings for diabetes, cardiovascular disease, and HIV falls below the national average. Georgia legislature identified as the root cause as a lack of care coordination and health care providers.

APRNs constitute the fastest growing segment of the professional workforce in the United States and offer a means to transform and improve access in underserved and low-income areas of Georgia. National certification for APRNs includes primary care in family medicine, pediatrics, geriatrics, mental health, anesthesia, and midwifery. Multiple position papers support the removal of restrictions on APRN practice to enhance care coordination and improve access to health care.

Therefore

W

Q → **C**

R

B

In January of 2017, Georgia reported 11,800 licensed APRNs. Georgia state laws and regulations lag behind APRN evolution compromising access to health care. Georgia remains one of the eleven states with laws restricting APRN autonomy. Several states and national organizations report and support improvements in care coordination through the removal of barriers to access to adequate healthcare from restricted practice for APRNs.

A newly developed healthcare policy entitled *Transforming and Addressing Georgia's Rising Demand for Health Care Coordination* seeks to increase access to qualified providers to improve health care using innovative changes at the state level. This policy claims that significant state reform aligned with the objectives of the Patient Protection and Affordable Care Act and recommendations of the Institute of Medicine supports improved care coordination through APRNs leading to reduced cost, improved outcomes and access to care.

Redesign creates challenges in healthcare facilities procedures, insurers, and impacts physicians relationships. The transformation changes the distribution of income.

Advocates including the Governor and state legislators understand that care coordination improves outcomes, costs, and access. Supporters such as the American Nurses Association, American Academy of Nurse Practitioners, United Advanced Practice Registered Nurses of Georgia, and the Association of Advanced Practice Nurses support collaborative autonomous APRN practice. APRNs continue to demonstrate improved access to health care, reduced cost, and improved outcomes in other parts of the country.

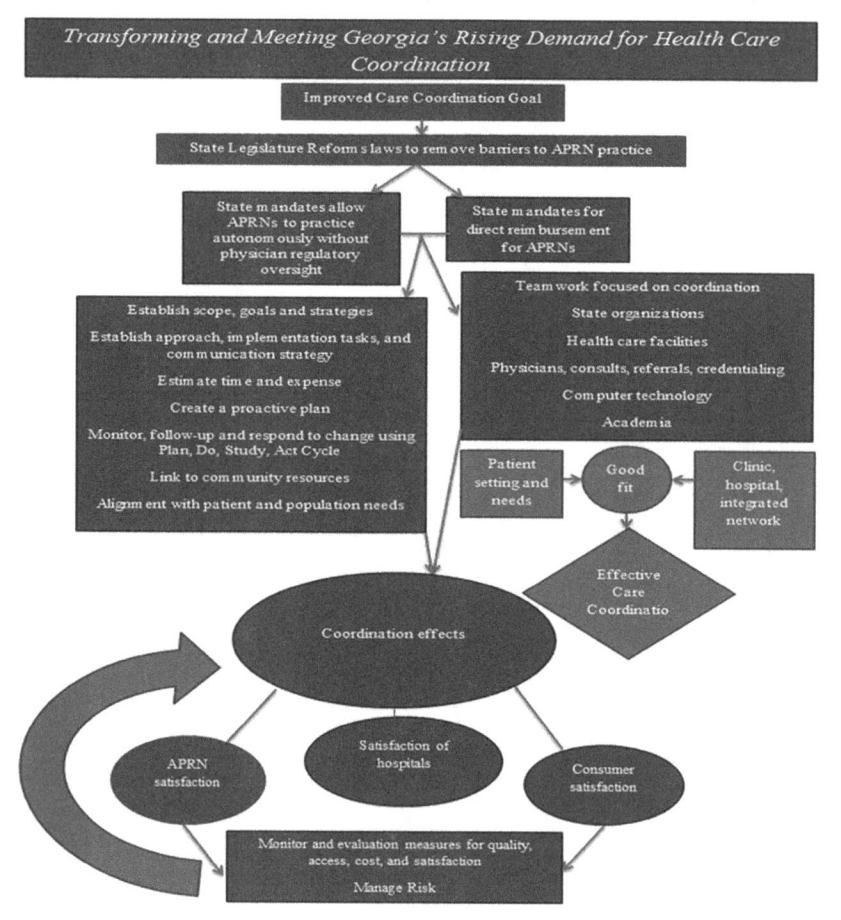

Appendix L: Conceptual Framework.

envisioned distributive consequence relates to competition and the reality that APRNs overlap in scope of practice with primary care physicians changing the distribution of patients.

Measurements used to determine the effectiveness of the policy include indicators of quality, access, costs, and satisfaction (Agency for Healthcare Research and Quality, 2011). Poorly coordinated care increases hospital readmissions and length of stay, emergency room visits, reduces indicators of population health and increases costs. Actual measurements include a decrease in the number of medically underserved areas in Georgia, increased access to primary care providers, decreases in health care costs and emergency room visits. Outcomes performance measurements include mortality, morbidity, length of stay, number of clinicians per 100,000 residents, number of emergency room visits and the patient experience.

Appendix M: Selected Policy Option Implementation Process.

Selected Policy Option Implementation Process New Health Care Policy Transforming and Meeting Georgia's Rising Demand for Health Care Coordination
Goals and Strategies
Members and Officers: Creation of a committee with members and officers from stakeholders including a chairperson from the DHHS Committee, two state legislators, President of the Georgia Nurses Assooiation, a member ofilie Georgµ Board of Nursing, representatives from the United Advanced Practice Registered Nurses of Georgia, fulltime physician and physician's assistants fulltime APRNs, Dean or Director from a sohool of nursing, member of the public, Georgia Hospital Association, and Accreditation.
Powers and Duties: To study and evaluate the conditions, needs and barriers to successful implementation and develop an action plan. Set up regular meetings, reporting, and duties. Creation of clear goals and strategy. If the committee makes recommendations to revise the legislation the chairperson is responsible for filing a report with the Secretary of State.
Allowances expenses and fundng: Allowances provided for in Code Section 28-1-8 ofthe Official Code of Georgia Annotated.
Funds appropriated from Senate to the committee and respective agencies.
Approach
Top-down. Creation of project teams with clear roes and responsibilities.
Implementation Stage
Based on assessrnent tasks indude purchase, forms, marketing techniques, data collection responsibilties and any training required. Creation of implementation plan, policies, procedures and anticipated timeline.
Communication Strategy
Process for meetings, regulr communication, minutes, and structuring of who needs to know what information.
Estimated Time and Expenses
Estimated number of hours for implementation including the role, name, number of hours, number of weeks, and total hours.

Table 1 : Template for Estimated Number of Hours for Implementation

Role	Name	Number of Hours	Number of Weeks	Total number of hours

Table 2: Template for Resourses Needed for Implementation

Resource	Estimated Expenditure (costs)
State legislature and committee expenses to oversee new legislation enactment including travel expenses, support personnel and lobbyists to assist with adversaries.	1 Million
Marketing and public awareness campaign of redesign and the expanded role of APRN's	300K
Technology for data management and reasearch, awareness, support, and education	1 Million

Table 3: Approvals Needed

Name	Issue for Approval	Date Requested	Estimated Expenditure (costs)
State government	Budget		

Performance Measures
PDCA Cycle

Monitor Performance (monthoy) x 1 year, evolving to every 3 months, quarterly, and annually) **and Magage Risk**

Appendix N: Monitoring and Evaluation Plan.

Monitoring and Evaluation Plan	
Monitoring Plan: Chairperson from the DHHS Committee to work with state and local government, Georgia Nurses Association, and the Jian Ping Su School of Public Health and Epidemiology under the direction of Dr. Robert Vogel to manage collection, communication, and documentation on policy outcomes. Baseline data supports benchmarks set by committee. The House of Representatives releases and controls funding.	
Evaluating the quality of care through health outcomes. Increased access to primary care provider focused on health promotion and prevention.	Evaluates the quality of care measured through health outcomes data. Captures data to identify annual health outcome indicators for mortality from diabetes, cardiovascular disease, maternal and infant morbidity data currently captured through Georgia Oasis.
Evaluating access to care. Decrease in the number of underserved areas in Georgia.	Evaluate the number of clinicians (Primary care physicians and APRNs) per 100,000 residents in Georgia by county and urban and rural averages captured through Georgia DHHS.
Evaluating health care costs. Decreased health care costs related to access to primary care provider and decreased use of emergency room services for primary care.	Evaluate the differences in length of stay, number of emergency room visits, readmissions and cost in dollars per episode of illness using Georgia Hospital Association, DHHS, and Georgia Oasis data.
Evaluating perceptions of patients, APRNs and physicians.	Evaluate how patients rate their physical and psychological wellness and their level of satisfaction through gallop polling already in place by the DHHS and the Georgia Hospital Association data. Captures numerical level of satisfaction of clinicians per survey through gallop.

Potential conflicts with implementation include overlapping scope of practice with physicians and conflicts over turf. The envisioned cause relates to financial competition and lack of focus on the benefits to society. A potential conflict relates to changes in the state budget priorities impacting funds required for redesign. Next year represents an election year for state Governor increasing the chance of differing ideologies and priorities. Potential problems with implementation involve resistance to redesign by health care organizations and uncertainty. Envisioned causes include communication breakdown, lack of consensus, and unclear goals. Potential contradictions arise when hospitals, APRNs and physicians remain separate and unable to work together to create innovations in the current system for consumers. Medicines preference for innovation and change contradicts their continued resistance to health care reform and APRN autonomy.

A potential political issue relates to maneuvers by some physicians or adversaries to stall, undermine or derail full practice authority and direct reimbursement. A potential bargaining point relates to the reduced rate of reimbursement of APRNs for equal services or the need for staged implementation to minimize the impact of a mass exodus of APRNs rocking the stability of the current system. Although not anticipated, in the event of the need for bargaining or deal making the vast experience of the American Nurses Association, a professional lobbyist, or the support of other national organizations offers powerful support (Yox & Stanik-Hutt, 2016). Potential policy revisions include supervisory hours for new graduate APRNs or a residency program to transition from academia to practice. If the committee makes recommendations to revise the legislation, the chairperson is responsible for filing a report with the Secretary of State. Solutions to political issues include a well prepared and united campaign, lobbyist, and efforts to educate physicians, consumers, and legislators on the value and roles of APRNs and the ultimate over-arching state-wide goal of improving care coordination as a team for society. Forecasted technology requirements include enhanced cyber security to protect privacy, greater connectivity and speed between platforms and hardware to bring things together, and the ability to deliver more data to consumers in the name of transparency (Henderson, Davis, Smith, & King, 2014).

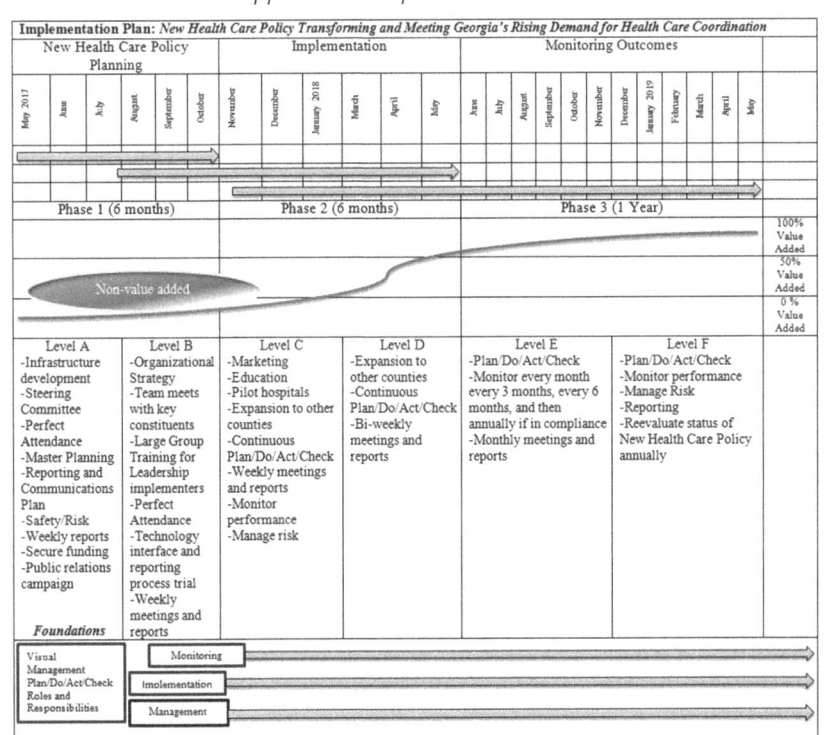

Appendix O: Implementation Plan.

Level A	Level B	Level C	Level D	Level E	Level F
-Infrastructure development	-Organizational Strategy	-Marketing	-Expansion to other counties	-Plan/Do/Act/Check	-Plan/Do/Act/Check
-Steering Committee	-Team meets with key constituents	-Education	-Continuous Plan/Do/Act/Check	-Monitor every month every 3 months, every 6 months, and then	-Monitor performance
-Perfect Attendance	-Large Group Training for Leadership implementers	-Pilot hospitals	-Bi-weekly meetings and reports	annually if in compliance	-Manage Risk
-Master Planning		-Expansion to other counties		-Monthly meetings and reports	-Reporting
-Reporting and Communications Plan	-Perfect Attendance	-Continuous Plan/Do/Act/Check			-Reevaluate status of New Health Care Policy annually
-Safety/Risk	-Technology interface and reporting process trial	-Weekly meetings and reports			
-Weekly reports	-Weekly meetings and reports	-Monitor performance			
-Secure funding		-Manage risk			
-Public relations campaign					
Foundations					

Monitoring & Evaluation

The envisioned evaluation criteria include qualitative and quantitative methodologies, continuous system feedbacks during implementation and the effectiveness of the policy change. The envisioned plan for monitoring tools for rapid and proactive dissemination include the use of activity monitoring reports, existing databases, statistical review from Georgia data bases (OASIS), stakeholder and beneficiary interviews, and qualitative techniques for electronic satisfaction surveys. Cogent values include equal access to a qualified health care provider regardless of geographic location or social status, quality health care, choice, and health prevention and promotion. A two-year anticipated evaluative timeline, implemented by members of the steering committee, report directly to the Governor Deal and Secretary of State B. Kemp who oversees licensure (See Appendix M Implementation Plan). The DHHS, acting as the chairperson, calls committee meetings in suitable locations and times to enable it to fully and effectively perform assigned duties and accomplish the objectives and purposes of the policy. The reporting structure is managed by the chairperson who distributes electronic minutes including findings, recommendations, and action to all members of the committee, state or local entities, consumers, or groups involved or needing to know or use the information (See Appendix M Implementation Plan Levels).

Conclusions and Recommendations

Evidence from the analysis of three viable health policy alternatives revealed alternative II resulted in the ideal change option with the best cost-benefit to address the problem of care coordination in Georgia. Policy implementation problems that surface require remedial measures to address the problem and get back in line with the objectives. Corrective recommendations include tightening control, realigning the goals, improving or changing methods of communication, visibility, enlisting champions, and clarifying understanding.

The development and implementation of Alternative II grants full practice authority to APRNs, freeing over 10,000 qualified practitioners to broaden access to medically underserved Georgia residents solving the original problem of care coordination and leading to reduced costs, improved outcomes, and access to healthcare. This policy analyst urges and recommends Georgia's distinguished legislature to eliminate barriers to practice for APRNs. By facing these important barriers, the state allows reformation and the implementation of strategies allowing APRNs to provide health care services in a manner consistent with their level of training and education to protect and promote the health and welfare of all Georgians. The ACA and IOM support improved care coordination through APRNs leading to reduced costs, improved outcomes, and access to care and constitutes the best option with the potential of reaching the goals outlined. The development and implementation of this policy grants full practice authority for a growing number of Georgia's APRNs to provide health care to underserved areas. The government exists to protect the welfare of the people and the decision rests in the hands of state legislators to deem what is best for the health of the Georgia's people.

References

Advanced Practice Registered Nurses of Georgia. (2017). *United advanced practice registered nurses political action committee*. Retrieved from https://uaprn.enpnetwork.com/page/21501-united-advanced-practice-registered-nurses-political-action-committee-uaprn-pac

Agency for Healthcare Research and Quality (AHRQ). (2011). *National strategy for quality improvement in health care*. Retrieved from https://www.ahrq.gov/workingforquality/index.html

Henderson, K., Davis, T. C., Smith, M., & King, M. (2014). Nurse practitioners in telehealth: Bridging the gaps in healthcare delivery. *Journal of Nurse Practitioners, 10*(10), 845-850. doi: 10.1016/j.nurpra.2014.09.003

Institute of Medicine. (2010). *The future of nursing: Leading change, advancing health*. Washington, DC: The National Academies Press.

National Council of State Boards of Nursing. (2017). Retrieved from https://www.ncsbn.org/Georgia.htm

Patient Protection and Affordable Care Act, 42 U. S. § 18001. (2010). Retrieved from https://www.hhs.gov/healthcare/about-the-law/

Starr, P. (2011). *Remedy and reaction: The peculiar American struggle over health care reform*. New Haven, CT: Yale University Press.

Stephens, B. (2015). Perspectives on advanced practice registered nursing in Georgia. Retrieved from http://www.georgiawatch.org/wp-content/uploads/2015/01/APRN-01072015WEB.pdf

Weiland, S. A. (2015). Understanding nurse practitioner autonomy. *Journal of the American Association of Nurse Practitioners, 27*(2), 95-104. doi: 10.1002/2327-6924.12120

Yox, S. B. & Stanik-Hutt, J. (2016). APRNs versus physicians: Outcomes, quality, and effectiveness of care according to the evidence. Retrieved from https://www.medscape.com/viewarticle/865779

MARY A. PATERSON

8
Health Care Finance and the DNP Nurse Executive

Chapter Objectives

- Define and discuss current strategic financing problems in the U.S. health care financial markets with an emphasis on the interaction of state and federal government regulation with free market concepts, financial risk, and the impact of regulation and risk on health care delivery.
- Compare and contrast macro- and micro-level health care financing strategies appropriate for a given regulatory environment at the corporate and program level.
- Develop an organizational health care financial strategy, operational financing plan, and budget compliant within a specific regulatory environment.
- Define and apply financial monitoring strategies consistent with the developed financial strategy, and plan such as cost-benefit, variance, and financial risk analyses.
- Identify and discuss methods of shaping financial strategy at the corporate level, including government advocacy, operational stakeholder consultation and management, and feedback mechanisms based on quantitative finance.

KEY WORDS: macrofinancing, microfinancing, free markets, financial risk, business risk, strategic financial management, operational financial management, cost-benefit analysis, and variance analysis

Introduction

A working knowledge of the principles of health care finance is important for nurse executives. The required financial skills depend on the organization's mission, goals, and the executive management structure. In large organizations, a DNP prepared nurse executive is usually supported by an executive team that includes finance and accounting specialists. In smaller organizations or independent practice settings, a nurse executive will typically work with specialized professionals who are hired as financial consultants on an as-needed basis. This approach requires management skill in selecting the best consultant for the job. In either situation, nurse executives need knowledge of the principles and the historical basis of the United States (U.S.) system of health care financing, as well as the leadership skills needed to ensure organizational survival.

This chapter introduces basic health care system (macro) level financial principles, as well as basic operational (micro) level skills. The discussion begins with a review of the health care financing environment within an organization. Understanding this environment, trends in health care financing, and regulation at the systems level is important for strategic planning, advocacy, operational management, and evaluation of organizational performance. The chapter concludes with brief cases for discussion and practice with both macro- and micro-level health care financing principles and concepts.

Health System Financing and Regulation

This section addresses three fundamental questions about the U.S health care system: (1) Who pays for health care services? (2) Who regulates health care services? (3) How should the health care organization respond to payers and regulators?

Who Will Pay

The question of who pays for health care services in the U.S. is complex. Payment for these services is based on the assumption that health care is not a constitutional right but is an important service that should be available at some level for all citizens and legal residents of the United States. The U.S. health care system is a market-driven system based on free market principles that are basic to all U.S. markets. The principle characteristics of a free market are shown in Table 8.1.

Much regulatory effort at the state and federal level focuses on keeping U.S. markets open and competitive, avoiding large monopolies, and removing barriers to price and wage competition among market suppliers. Health care markets present significant challenges to the free market model in part because of the purchasing arrangements for health care in the U.S. Most consumer health care is purchased by third-party payers, such as insurers or selfinsured employers, or by the state or federal government health insurance plans, such as Medicare or Medicaid. Acting as the consumer's agent, these third-party payers make many purchasing decisions that are fundamental to the health care market. The presence of third-party payers that make pur-

Table 8.1 Characteristics of a Free Market.

- Many buyers and sellers—each participant is small in relation to the market and cannot affect the price through its own actions
- Neither consumption nor production generate externalities (spillover benefits or costs)
- Free entry and exit from the market—new firms can open and existing firms can leave the market without costs as conditions change
- Symmetric information—all market participants know the same things so that no one has an informational advantage over others
- No transaction cost—the buyers and sellers incur no additional cost in making the transaction, and the complexity of decisions has no effect on choices
- Firms maximize profits and consumers maximize well-being

Reproduced from Austin & Hungerford, 2010.

chasing decisions complicates the provider/consumer relationship by introducing conflicts of interest that arise because the consumer is not the only party involved in a given health care transaction. This variation of the usual seller/buyer relationship in a market complicates situations for service providers, because the consumer is rarely the principal payer for the service, and providers are accountable to several stakeholders who have different objectives. This creates conflicts that are often very difficult to resolve.

For example, the consumer may wish to access an expensive service (e.g., a private hospital room) when the insurer does will not pay for this level of service. The consumer may also wish to consult with a specific specialist or hospital that is not part of the preferred provider panel that the insurer will reimburse. Such conflicts must be adjudicated, which requires additional effort from all parties, increases bureaucracy, raises costs for everyone involved in the transaction, and promotes overall dissatisfaction with the complexity of the system that requires negotiation.

Regulatory strategies to mitigate payer problems or expand consumer access can sometimes help, although they can also increase the system's complexity. One example is the requirement that insurers must sell insurance to individuals with pre-existing and often costly conditions, which is socially important but increases the cost of insurance coverage for everyone in the insurance pool. The regulation benefits some consumers while it disadvantages others, and it increases the costs of managing health insurance that arise from costly claims and the complex health needs of consumers with pre-existing health conditions. Thus, payment for services in the U.S. market-driven health care system is not a simple issue despite the apparent simplicity of the free market approach.

There have been national efforts to remove the barriers between the consumer in need of care and the potential providers of that care. Health Savings Accounts (HSA) is a savings approach to financing health care that allows the consumer to place tax-free dollars in a dedicated savings account that can be used to purchase health care services. These HSA accounts accumulate from year to year, which allows the consumer to save a significant amount of pre-tax dollars to pay for needed health care over their lifetime. Tax law and regulations govern the amount that the consumer may sequester each year in an HSA, as well as the mechanisms and documentation required when the HSA funds are used to pay for the consumer's care (U.S. Internal Revenue Service, 2016). The benefit of HSAs is the removal of the third-party payer from the health care transaction. Consumers who pay for care with their own funds are able to engage in a direct transaction with the care provider without the need for the insurer's approval.

There are two major problems with this approach. First, most elderly consumers do not have enough time to accumulate sufficient HSA funds before they need them. Second, all consumers face the problem of *information asymmetry* between the care provider and the consumer. Information asymmetry is a difficult problem because few consumers are knowledgeable enough to understand exactly what their purchasing needs are for a complex health care service. Information may also not be available for consumers. This asymmetry results in risk and additional costs for the consumer, who is attempting to make a wise purchase of health care directly from a provider. Efforts to remedy information asymmetry include consumer purchasing guides such as quality ranking systems, provider certifications, and standardized outcomes reporting. Educated consumers may be able to use these tools effectively to purchase care, although their effectiveness in emergencies or with low-education or impaired consumers presents challenges that can result in less than optimal care.

The question of who pays for health care is shaped by four major stakeholders in the transaction: the consumer, insurer, regulator, and provider. Purchasing health care requires the availability of complex information that may not be easily understood by the consumer of the service. In addition, stakeholders emphasize different aspects of the health care transaction to which the provider must respond. Consumers are most interested in optimal outcomes and consumer-focused care; insurers prioritize cost and risk control; regulators have varying interests depending on their constituent base, political orientation, and stakeholder influence; and providers focus on optimizing outcomes for their patients and meeting their revenue expectations given the substantial investment they have made in education and training. With the diversity of stakeholder interests, it is not surprising that health care payment systems are complex and costly.

Since third-party payers are an intrinsic part of the health care market, payer arrangements are an important consideration in any provider's organizational approach to health care delivery. Health care executives must be aware of the payer mix for the services they offer and shape their strategic plans and financing accordingly. This requires an understanding of the payer's service delivery requirements and the market entry, as well as the reimbursement and performance reporting requirements defined by the payer.

Revenue analysis and planning are the typical approaches for managing the payer mix. Revenue analysis gathers information for each prospective payer in five areas: (1) beneficiaries insured by the payer, (2) services that are reimbursed, (3) procedures necessary to request and receive reimbursement, (4) the incentive and penalty structure, and (5) the qualifications for payment. Revenue planning supports revenue management by analyzing revenue by payer accounts and setting revenue projections based on evidence of payer behavior with payment and payment adjudication. Accurate revenue planning assures accurate budgeting by helping health care executives know what funds are expected and when they will be received. The other important consideration for strategic and operational financing planning is the regulatory environment that surrounds the health care organization.

Who Regulates

Health care regulation in the United States is a fragmented, complex endeavor with the major regulators responsible to different stakeholders, such as government, insurers, employers, and provider groups that are interested in control over health care delivery. To understand health care regulation in the United States, it is important to understand the underlying social compact that exists between American citizens and their government. This social compact is expressed in the Declaration of Independence:

> We hold these truths to be self-evident, that all men are created equal, that they are endowed by their Creator with certain unalienable Rights that among these are Life, Liberty and the pursuit of Happiness. That to secure these rights, Governments are instituted among Men, deriving their just powers from the consent of the governed.

The important principles articulated in this passage are derived from ideas expressed by philosophers of the Enlightenment period (1650–1800). This influential period of philosophical thought was an influential force for the founders of the United States and is seen in many of the founding documents of this country including the Declaration of Independence and the Constitution (Wood, 2009). Unlike many European governments that evolved from a monarchical structure where a strong central authority held power and eventually ceded some power to the people, the agreement in the United States was different in that power belonged to the people who then ceded limited power to the government. This fundamental difference in political philosophy influenced the social compact between the American people and their government and continues as a major influence on the government's approach to health care regulation. Constitutional scholars and the courts agree that health, welfare, and domestic safety are clearly within the powers reserved to the individual or the states. In the early days of the U.S., the individual and their provider were the only parties to health care transactions unless the state had good reason to become involved, such as with individuals who served in the military or were wards of the state.

These early arrangements shaped the orientation of the individual to the government and provided a historical basis for the current resistance of many American citizens and states to a centrally financed health care system. Historically, U.S. citizens viewed health care as a private matter and did not expect federal government involvement in health care unless circumstances made individual citizens unable to provide for themselves. In such cases, the state in which the person resided, and not the federal government, was expected to act. The only basis for federal involvement in health care is found in the Commerce Clause of the Constitution, which provides for the federal right to tax and spend for the general welfare and to regulate commerce across state lines (Leonard, 2010). This is the reason states regulate much of the health care today—from licensing health care professionals and facilities to instituting programs for those who are below the poverty line or dependent. When President Johnson signed the amendment to the Social Security Act in July 1965, which established the Medicare and Medicaid program, the federal government for the first time became a major payer for individual health care financing for private citizens. Prior to this act, the role of the federal government was minimal compared to the states and private health care enterprises, although the U.S. military and veterans care were historically a federal responsibility.

A direct result of this social compact and division of responsibility is the current complex mix of private, state, and federal regulation of health care. Much of the health care system is firmly in private hands, which emphasizes the agreement that health care is a private matter between the citizen and the provider. This is the reason that much of health care quality regulation is the responsibility of private organizations, such as the Joint Commission (TJC) formally referred to as the Joint Commission on the Accreditation of Hospitals and Healthcare Organizations (TJCAHO) or The National Committee for Quality Assurance (NCQA) (Pawlson & O'Kane, 2002). Payer regulations are part of the regulatory landscape, and since Medicare is one of the largest payers for care, the federal government benefit and quality regulations for Medicare beneficiaries are an important consideration for health care providers. However, it is important to appreciate that Medicare and many other payers delegate part of their regulatory authority, such as with the TJCAHO accreditation, as a requirement for participation as a provider for Medicare beneficiaries.

The result of the public/private payer mix for health care, together with the general orientation to regulation of care at the state rather than federal level, is that health care executives must be aware of the regulatory requirements for general entry into a given health care market, as well as the regulations specific to each payer in their payer mix. The federal government becomes a regulatory agent primarily through their presence as a payer in the Medicare market, whereas the state government has a larger share of the health care regulatory landscape that applies, regardless of the beneficiary base.

Some areas of state regulation include provider licensure and practice definitions through professional practice acts, regulation of provider educational institutions within the state, licensure of hospitals and other venues of care, and regulation of health care insurance markets and protection of consumers within the state. However, emerging areas of regulatory concern, such as the management of sensitive consumer information and the nation-wide implementation of electronic health records, have become federal initiatives. It is unclear if federal involvement in these areas will continue or may be delegated to the states.

How Should The Health Care Organization Respond?

The organizational arrangements that deliver health care largely depend on payment and regulatory strategies. Most payments for health care services are the responsibility of third-party payers (insurers), which are organizations that provide health care services and must serve two masters at a minimum: the consumer and the insurer. When the insurer is a government entity (e.g., Medicare and Medicaid) the providers of health care services also need to consider government regulations that define participation in the program. Insurers and the government may directly regulate quality of care or they may delegate such regulation to private sector organizations, such as the JCAHO or NCQA.

The resulting complexity of the U.S. health care market is a force that favors market consolidation since small providers of health care cannot afford the infrastructure necessary to comply with the complex requirements of the consumer and their insurer, as well as state and federal regulations. Historical market analysis of the U.S. system supports the market consolidation trend, which consistently rewards larger providers of care and discourages smaller providers from entering or remaining in the market. As a result, health care services violate the theoretical assumptions of a free market and present a formidable array of challenges to consumers, providers, and payers. To be effective, health care executives must be aware of market principles and the challenges presented by the current, complicated mixed approach to health care financing and regulation. Tools that are important to manage this complex environment include revenue planning and management, as well as stakeholder mapping to enhance understanding of the regulatory environment. The following case provides practice in focused regulatory mapping.

Mini-Case #1: Heartland Memorial Hospital

Heartland Memorial is a 100-bed rural hospital in Nebraska. The hospital does not have an emergency room, and 25% of its beds are allocated to skilled nursing care. The majority of the residents in the catchment area of 450,000 individuals who are spread over 41,000 square miles are engaged in small farming and small business rural services, such as tractor repair and agricultural products and services. There is one "Big-Box" store that employs 150 people who have employer-provided health insurance, whereas the rural small employers in the area do not usually offer health care benefits. There is an agricultural co-op that offers a group insurance plan with an HSA option for some farm families. There are also a small number of federal employees in the catchment area covered by the Blue Cross federal employees' program. The population of the catchment area is classified as a middle-income population with 3% of the population below the poverty line. The restrictive state Medicaid program extends coverage to women and children below the federal poverty line with very strict limitations. This means that 10% of the population is uninsured.

The largest services at Heartland Memorial are maternity and pediatric care, skilled nursing care for the elderly Medicare population, and orthopedic care focused on simple joint repair, uncomplicated back and neck surgery, and rehabilitation. The hospital has one operating room used by the general surgical practice in the area that focuses on uncomplicated elective surgical cases and refers specialized surgical cases to the University Hospital in Lincoln. The hospital has entered into a "swing-bed" agreement with the U.S. Department of Health and Human Services that allows it to allocate beds to skilled rehabilitation care, as needed. Occupancy rate in the hospital is usually above 90% and demand projections continue to be strong. The payer mix is 60% Medicare, 10% state Medicaid, and 30% private insurance. Nebraska has consistently rejected Medicaid expansion, which makes uncompensated care a significant problem for all Nebraska hospitals.

As a strategic manager and a DNP prepared nurse executive at Heartland Memorial, you have been asked to provide a patient care regulatory stakeholder map with the above payer mix. Your map should consider the regulations focused on direct patient care only. You do not have to consider engineering or architectural standards, general health workforce regulations, or accessibility regulations. You may also disregard provider entry requirements, general hospital accreditation regulations, and HIPPA regulations. You may assume that Heartland Memorial is accredited by the Joint Commission (JC), and is considered a critical access hospital under Nebraska state definitions. The private insurers active in your market are Blue Cross, Medica, and Celtic. There is a federally facilitated Nebraska health exchange that uses the marketplace plan management model. This means that the state oversees some aspects of the plans offered on the exchange. The details you need to include on your map should focus on the direct patient care regulations mandated by each payer. This will require some research. Remember that the federal government's role as a regulator of direct patient care is largely due to its status as the Medicare insurer for 60% of your patient base. Your case analysis should reference the regulatory body and the general focus of the regulation. For example, because you have swing skilled nursing beds, the body of regulation on skilled care for Medicare patients would be one of the entries in your map. You do not have to consider the specifics of the regulation in this map. Your goal should be to compile as complete of a list as possible of the regulatory stakeholders and the general focus of the regulation. For example, Medicare requires skilled nursing facilities to file reports on the quality of patient care. Since your hospital has swing beds, you would need to include this item on your stakeholder map. You would enter Medicare as a stakeholder and quality of SNF care as a one of the regulatory areas for this stakeholder. Here is a sample entry:

Stakeholder	Focus
Medicare	Quality of skilled nursing facility care—annual report required by stakeholder

Appendix B provides an overview and brief example of stakeholder mapping. Creating such a map provides practice in building strategic planning tools that provide health care executives with methods to delegate reporting and monitoring tasks. These are helpful in controlling business risks and understanding the staffing requirements and costs related to regulatory compliance. There will be entries in your map that require information that you cannot immediately locate. For these entries, indicate the stakeholder and focus area that needs further investigation. As an executive, these are focus areas for stakeholder consultations that you may undertake or delegate to one of your employees.

Business and Financial Risk in Health Care Organizations

Managing any health care enterprise in the United States requires that executives at the strategic management level, the C-Suite executives, consider risk and return at both the system (macro) and organizational (micro) financial level. The challenge of aligning the organizational goals and strategic plan with the environment surrounding the organization is significant given the number of stakeholders who must be considered. Since understanding and managing both business and financial risk is a daily challenge for any C-Suite team, every executive must be familiar with concepts of business and financial risk to position their organization to achieve its goals and survive.

A convenient way of considering risks is to separate risks into those inherent in the business of health care and those from specific financial management strategies, such as the use of debt or capital chosen by the organization to finance and deliver health care. These risks are interdependent, although the strategies to manage them are essentially different. Complex payer arrangements and the regulatory environment surrounding health care introduce additional costs and risks. These environmental challenges are referred to as macro-financial challenges, while those within the organization itself are called micro-financial challenges. The macro-financial challenges faced by a health care organization must be as clearly defined as possible given the dynamic health care environment. The stakeholder regulatory map created in the first case is an example of a risk management tool for macro-financial risks. In general, C-Suite executives must know the stakeholders and the stakeholder management strategies and reporting required to succeed. Large health care organizations usually have government liaison positions or paid lobbyists whose assist with state and federal stakeholder management and influence these stakeholders in the organization's best interest. Smaller organizations may ask their top executives to assume this task directly, in addition to their usual leadership duties. In either case, managing business risks posed by governments or private payers is essential for organizational survival. The skills required for executives include focused information access and management, effective negotiation and conflict management, political awareness, and influence management at the appropriate government level.

The many advocacy groups available to health care organizations are also a valuable risk management resource for the strategic executive. Developing a working relationship with the advocacy organizations that have the most impact on the organization requires an investment of time and money. This relationship activity is a vital part of the strategic executive's role. Those new to the C-Suite role must form positive, productive relationships not only with organizational staff and consultants involved in government and insurance outreach, but also with professional organizations relative to their management area. The influence gained by outreach to appropriate professional and advocacy organizations is a critical business risk management strategy that can help insure organizational survival.

The more familiar area for the strategic executive is management of micro-financial business risk. C-Suite executives must understand and manage internal business risks within their area of responsibility. DNP prepared nurse executives, for example, will typically focus on the specific organizational requirements for nurses, local nursing labor markets, staffing, quality of care, and other regulatory issues that affect both the cost and supply of the organizational nursing workforce. Nursing is usually the largest professional staff within the health care organization, and as such poses a significant business and financial risk to the organization if not well-managed. Careful management of the nursing staff, together with expert recruitment and training, can make the difference between organizational survival and failure.

Another area of micro-financial business risk is patient care management. Managing this risk requires an understanding of the organizational effects of payer requirements, the general characteristics of those insured by each payer, and the regulatory requirements for direct care of the patient population. The importance of population-level data to this task cannot be over-emphasized. Population demographics including educational level, literacy rate, household composition, and income level provide a health care executive with an indication of the type of services that will be needed to assure a good outcome for the patient population served. For example, a health care organization that serves an aging population with lower incomes and smaller household size will need specialized discharge planning services that are focused on the needs of such a population. If the population is younger, services that support families with children, maternity care, and employment-related injuries should be included in the risk management strategy.

In general, business risk management required a clear understanding of the payer base, a specific focus on the consumers likely to need the health care services offered, and the health workforce available to the organization. A systematic analysis of each of these components, together with an accurate analysis of the regulations that are pertinent to the care provided, is the optimal risk management tool. Information is a vital resource for business risk management and each executive must ensure that the information they use to make business risk management decisions is accurate, timely, and pertinent to the need.

Financial risk management generally refers to the risks the health care enterprise assumes as a result of the its financing decisions. For example, the assumption of debt increases the financial risk profile of an organization as measured by the proportion of debt to total equity within the organization (the debt/equity ratio). The higher the organizational debt, the higher the financial risk. Assuring that the revenue earned is adequate to service the organization's debt is the fundamental risk management strategy that is required. It is easy to appreciate that expert organizational management of business risk contributes to good management of financial risk. For example, a hospital that assumes debt to start a new service must depend on its executive managers to assure that the service is appropriately staffed, delivers care of acceptable quality, and is compliant with the regulations that pertain to the service. Each of these business factors contributes to the decisions of how much debt to assume, as well as to assure that the funds provided will result in sufficient revenue to service the debt. Financial risk is usually managed by in-house financial staff or by financial consultants. However, the decisions they make must be informed by the executive team, which focuses on the management of the health care enterprise and understands the business risk profile of their particular area of responsibility. The following case is designed to develop an appreciation of the interaction between executive teams as they work together to manage business and financial risk.

Mini-Case #2: Suburban Family Practice Associates LLC

Suburban Family Practice Associates LLC (SFPA) is located in an upper-middle class suburb in St. Louis, MO. It is a large multi-disciplinary primary care practice that employs 15 family-practice physicians, 20 family practice nurse-practitioners, and 40 registered nurses, in addition to 40 support and management staff, that includes an internal information technology team. SFPA has been approached by a large HMO in the area to become a full-risk partner on their care team. Accepting the contract means that SFPA would assume a panel of 2500 adults and 500 children ages 1 to 8 years under a capitated payment plan. They would receive a capitated payment of $611 per adult member per month and a payment of $449 per month for each child between ages 1 year and 18 years. Children under age 1 year are reimbursed at the adult rate. The rate would include all care provided on an outpatient basis including all diagnostic work related to general care. Specialty care is reimbursed on a discounted fee-for-service basis, with a closed-panel approach so that only specialists within the HMO panel are reimbursed for care. Eighty percent (80%) of the capitated payment is made at the beginning of the benefit year and twenty percent (20%) of the capitated payment is withheld until the end of the payment year. The amount withheld is adjusted for plan migration as well as for any unanticipated large claims or other catastrophic costs on a negotiated basis.

The executive team at SFPA has been tasked by the practice owners to present a business risk analysis of the potential contract. If accepted, the panel will increase the practice volume by an estimated 35%, and this would require some additional staff. To expand the practice, a loan would need to be negotiated. The potential lenders have asked for a detailed analysis of the business risk that needs to be managed if the contract was accepted. The practice would assume all routine risks for the book-of-business represented by the proposed panel. The catastrophic cost reserve payment is not automatic, but would have to be the result of unanticipated injury of illness. For example, a diabetic in the panel who was admitted for hypoglycemic shock to the ICU care would not be eligible for the catastrophic payment because the practice should have been managing the diabetes to prevent such an occurrence.

You are the Chief Nursing Executive and have been asked to present the business risk analysis for your department. The family practice nurse practitioners are not your responsibility since they are allocated to the Chief Primary Care Officer who manages the nurse practitioners and physicians. You are, however, responsible for all nursing care, as well as all patient education, including preventive care and teaching for those who are chronically ill. Please do the following to prepare for the risk analysis:

1. Prepare a request to the HMO management team for all the information you require on the patient panel. Include all parameters that you will need to accurately assess the business risk inherent in the panel. Do not forget environmental health risks to the individuals in the panel as well as those posed by individual health history.
2. Outline the strategy you will consider for managing utilization and thus decreasing business risk in this panel. Although SFPA is not at risk for the cost of hospitalizations required by specialists, it is at risk for the cost of all other hospitalizations in the panel. This excludes maternity stays since all maternity care in the HMO is provided by OB/GYN specialists in the HMO panel. Routine pediatric care is the responsibility of SFPA. Hospitalizations are not expected in this population unless specialty procedures are needed or accidents occur. Large claims from catastrophic accidents can be assumed to be covered by the catastrophic adjustment at the end of the year.

You will be presenting your business risk case to the SFPA management team and Board of Directors. The total business risk analysis will be given to the Chief Financial Officer who will compile a recommendation on the amount of additional financial risk (usually in the form of loans) that will be assumed as a result of this contract. Since the SFPA management team's total salary reimbursement is based in part on an annual profit share, your annual salary depends in part on the accuracy of your work.

Strategic Financial Management Tools

This section summarizes the tools used by executives to manage the financial aspects of the health care enterprise, and their specific and general applications.

Revenue Management

Health care executives must define and manage revenue sources to assure achievement of the goals and objectives of the business. Common tools used to accomplish this task include revenue planning, revenue accounting and optimization, revenue matching, and account negotiation. Revenue planning tools focus on payer policies and procedures so that the payment terms and conditions for each health care contract are clearly understood. Management should be able to understand the beneficiary base of each health care contract and the mechanisms by which bills are presented and paid. If there are revenue withholds, per capita payments, or some incentive or penalty payments, the terms and conditions under which these payments are made should be clear.

Revenue accounting and optimization is an ongoing function of the financial staff. At the executive level, monthly revenue reports should be available that outline the revenue performance of each payer contract including timeliness of payment, number of payment appeals and settlement time of appeals, enrollee stability (also known as enrollee churning), and any legal or regulatory issues related to the payer. The financial department should be able to outline account optimization steps taken to assure accurate and timely payment as well as to minimize disputes of any type.

Cost Management

The tools of cost management include direct and indirect costing methods, such as the method used to allocate indirect costs to revenue producing departments, comparative costing systems that examine organizational cost performance against average peer group costs or other benchmarks, and the cost standardization tools in use, such as relative value units (RVU) or DRG costs.

All executives need to use these tools to understand the costs in their area of responsibility, as well as the overall cost behavior of the organization. This includes both the direct costs of care that can be traced to each revenue producing unit and the indirect costs allocated to revenue units. The basis for the allocation of indirect costs should be clear and consistently applied. If indirect costs are allocated and adjusted based on revenue performance, all levels of management should be aware of how these adjustments are made and the incentives such adjustments create. If a disproportionate level of indirect costs is allocated to one or two high performing revenue producers, the leaders of these departments will inevitably question this practice. Executives need to be aware of the rationale for any subsidies created and the effects on the productive members of the organization.

Comparative cost performance in the defined market is also a valuable part of executive information. Organizations that are not aware of their relative position in their market risk either delivering services below the accepted rate of payment and becoming overloaded, or pricing themselves out of the market and losing market share. Executives need to know how their costs compare to other organizations in their market peer group and analyze any significant differences. Comparative cost analysis is one area of executive management that requires boundary-spanning strategies, such as membership in local health care organizations that share information and risk management approaches, as well as local market and regulatory information. Boundary-spanning in organizations typically involves the creation of meaningful strategic alliances beyond organizational boundaries. Effective boundary-spanning requires analysis of the most time and cost-effective alliances that the executive can initiate as well as consistently manage (Williams, 2002).

Strategic Planning and Management Budgeting

Strategic planning and budgeting are two sides of the same management coin. Items in the strategic plan not represented in the budget will seldom be implemented. The saying that the organization budget represents the cost of the strategic plan is correct. The organization needs to carefully manage the relationship between these important documents to assure that an item in the strategic plan is also a budget item. One of the most important areas to examine carefully is the quality of care commitment most health care organizations make in their strategic plan. Few health care organizations would admit to devaluing quality of care, yet many organizations do not represent an explicit commitment to such quality in the budget. This is particularly true in decisions about the nursing workforce. The nurse executive needs to be aware of local and national developments in matters relevant to professional nursing and be able to communicate evidence-based information on the relationship between nurse staffing and quality patient management.

Budgeting tools that can help executives understand this cost/quality relationship include variance analysis that distinguishes between variance due to volume increases, or input prices, such as the cost of labor, supplies, or technology, and cost-benefit analysis that provides information on the sustainability of operational initiatives. If variances are due to input price increases, the cost/quality relationship of these increases must be clearly understood. For example, new patient care technology or trends in nursing education may be increasing the cost of a surgical procedure but may also be increasing the quality of care for the patient. Health care executives need very detailed variance information to understand the cost vs. budget performance of their organization, as well as the effect of the favorable or unfavorable variance not only on the cost, but on the quality of care.

Cost-benefit analysis is useful when deciding to initiate or continue projects and to expand or eliminate organizational services or departments. Project or department valuation methods are essential to conduct a credible cost-benefit analysis. The two most commonly used methods are net present value analysis and internal rate of return. Computerized systems that calculate these valuations are preferred over those that require less information and are easier to calculate. Two of the most common and fastest methods to determine value projects or services are payback and accounting rate-of-return. These methods are less data-intensive, although they do not provide accurate valuations when the time-value of money is a factor. Benefits of a given project or service can be limited to the direct financial benefits it provides to the organization in the profit margin, or the benefits analysis can be extended to non-tangible, indirect organizational and societal benefits. Executives should carefully consider both options when selecting a cost-benefit approach. Both approaches are often used when leaders must make decisions about terminating or expanding organizational operations.

Financial Performance Tools

In addition to essential financial reports delineated in Appendix A, the DNP nurse executive needs tools that calculate the cost and revenue related to the delivery of patient care. Internal performance measures, such as nurse-to-patient ratios, cost of each unit of care delivered, cost of each procedure, and direct costs per unit of care are important. Financial performance measurements or financial performance ratios are primarily used by finance and accounting personnel to monitor overall financial performance and financial risk. Table 8.2 summarizes the four common ratio categories.

Although the primary audience for these ratios is financial managers, all health care executives should understand the financial performance measures used by their organization, particularly those related to their area of operational responsibility. For example, asset turnover ratios are good measures of the overall efficiency of the organization. If these turnover ratios reflect inefficient performance, all executives should examine their operational area to identify any underlying issues that might influence performance. Profitability ratios are important to all health care organizations since the ability to earn a fair return on investment assures organizational survival. The often quoted saying—"no margin, no mission"—means that the inability to earn a return-on-investment leads to an organization without the funds for development. Merely recovering costs does not allow the organization to develop or improve, and this will eventually lead to a decrease in patient care quality and organizational demise.

The primary budget management tools that operational executives need to understand are variance analysis, longitudinal trend analysis in regard to relevant cost, revenue, and profitability categories, and the relationship between budgetary performance and organizational strategic goals. Budget performance is affected by all of these factors and is sub-

Table 8.2 Performance Ratios.

Ratio Group	Definition	Purpose	Ratio Definition
Profitability	Measures the organization's ability to generate enough net revenue to provide a return on investment and maintain and upgrade its healthcare.	Profit margin Return on assets	Net income/Total revenue Net income/Total assets
Liquidity	Measures the ability of the organization to convert its non-cash assets into cash.	Current ratio Quick ratio Accounts Receivable	Current ratio Current assets/Current liabilities Cash + marketable securities (if any) + net accounts receivable/Current liabilities Total accounts receivable/Gross fee-for-service charges × (1/12) or Medical Group Management Association (MGMA) Net accounts receivable/Sales revenue × 365
Long-term solvency ratios	Long-term (more than 1 year) financing of the practice, which indicates how it financed itself (use of debt or invested capital) and its ability to meet its loan obli- payments.	Debt/Equity Leverage Times interest earned	Total liabilities/Total equity Assets/Total equity or Debt/Total equity +1 Number of times earnings exceed interest payments: Earnings before interest and taxes/Required interest payments
Asset Management or Activity Ratios	The level of effectiveness in the practice's use of assets.	Asset turnover Fixed-asset turnover Inventory turnover	Operating revenues/Total assets Operating revenue/Net fixed assets Operating revenue/Inventory

ject to variations in internal and external environments. One of the most important factors that must be considered is the position of the organization in the health care market environment and the effect of various environmental changes on the organization. Adjustment in budgetary goals and objectives frequently lags behind the more dynamic changes in the external health care market and the adept strategic manager keeps abreast of these changes and understands their effect on cost and volume behavior within the organization.

Mini-Case #3: St Alban's Hospital Management Team

Immediately after securing your DNP degree, you have been appointed the Vice-President for Nursing at St. Alban's Hospital. Congratulations! After your orientation, you move into your new office and begin reviewing the monthly reports for the nursing department. You notice that the reports include nursing hours spent vs. those budgeted, and payroll and supply costs for nursing, compared to the budgeted costs. However, you do not find utilization statistics for each nursing unit, or any operational ratios. The information you have on quality of care is limited to summaries of the patient satisfaction survey administered to all discharged patients. The response rate for this survey is 20%.

You must now explain the unfavorable variances in nursing hours vs. the budgeted nursing hours, and present your analysis to the next meeting of the management team. Before you discuss this problem with your nurse managers, compile a list of the additional information you will request from the hospital information system, and the rationale for each request.

Chapter Takeaways

1. The fundamental social compact in the United States assumes that citizens consent to specific government roles in health care. The key relationship in health care is between the citizen and the provider. This relationship is complicated by third-party payers, as well as state and federal regulations that have developed over time.
2. The free market is the foundational approach that guides the consumption of goods and services in the United States. Health care deviates from free market principles in a number of important ways.
3. The management of business and financial risk in health care organizations is closely related. DNP organization executives and financial managers must coordinate their strategic initiatives to assure adequate risk management in health care organizations.

4. The risks imposed by regulation require boundary-spanning activities for all strategic executives. Information and interaction with professional groups, governmental advocacy groups, and lobbyists is essential for adequately managing regulatory risks.
5. Organizational financing and operational performance are reflected by four fundamental performance relationships: profitability, liquidity, long-term solvency, and asset management. Organizational executives need to understand the relationship between these performance indicators and their area of operations management.
6. Budget variance analysis and cost-benefit analysis are tools needed to shape decisions about operational performance and organizational services management. Budget variances may be due to factors that include input costs, service volume fluctuations, and environmental and regulatory effects. Organizational executives need to understand and use variance analytic tools to accurately manage and improve their department's performance.
7. Financial strategy at the corporate level is shaped by input from operational risk analysis, budget variance analysis, cost-benefit analysis, and external stakeholder mapping and management. Organizational executives need to understand these analytic tools and use the information to define and manage organizational financial strategy. Since all members of the executive team contribute to the discussion of financial strategy, management of organizational financial performance is an interdependent executive activity.

Chapter Summary

Financial management is a skill that has not been essential in professional nursing education. Advancement to executive positions in nursing or health care management requires that nurses expand their professional knowledge and skill to include financial management. While academic DNP programs provide healthcare finance curriculum content, this remains a challenging task since this knowledge has not been a foundational requirement for success as a clinical professional. This chapter introduces general principles familiar to financial professionals: free market characteristics, business and financial risk management, and financial management tools. The chapter provides insights into the social compact that makes financial tools and free market concepts essential for health care management. DNP prepared nurse executives must develop a working knowledge of the principles and skills introduced here. The three mini-cases provide the opportunity for practice in knowledge acquisition and use. Mastery of the information presented here is a map to guide development of financial knowledge and skills in health care. For professional success in a C-Suite role, the DNP nurse executive executives must move beyond these introductory concepts and develop a deeper understanding of these critical financial concepts.

Chapter Reflection Questions

1. How does the United States social compact influence the current health care system and affect your work as a professional nurse and a DNP prepared nursing executive?

2. The free market is a foundational principle of American markets and commerce. What is the effect of the variations from the free market on health care demand and supply in the United States?

3. The management of business and financial risk is a shared-responsibility of all C-Suite executives. In your position as a DNP prepared nursing executive, what macro- and micro-information would you need to be able contribute to managing these risks?

4. The organization's strategic plan is considered a roadmap for organization executives. As a DNP prepared nurse executive, what general financial information and strategies are needed to assure success in achieving the goals outlined in the strategic plan?

5. Discuss the primary uses and importance of two fundamental financial management tools: variance analysis and cost-benefit analysis. What is the general purpose of these tools and when should they be used?

References

Austin, D.A. & Hungerford, T.L. (2010). The market structure of the health insurance industry. *Congressional Research Service Report* R40834. Retrieved from www.fas.org/sgp/crs/misc/R40834.pdf.

Leonard, E.W. (2010, June). State constitutionalism and the right to health care. *University of Pennsylvania Journal of Constitutional Law, 12*(5), 1325-54. Retrieved from https://www.law.upenn.edu/journals/conlaw/articles/volume12/issue5/Leonard12U.Pa.J.Const.L.1325(2010).pdf

Paterson, M.A. (2014). *Healthcare finance and financial management: Essentials for advanced practice nurses and interdisciplinary care teams.* (1st ed.) Lancaster, PA: DEStech Publications Inc.

Pawlson, L. G. & O'Kane, M. (2002 May-June). Professionalism, regulation, and the market: Impact on accountability for quality of Care. *Health Affairs, 21*(3), 200–217. Retrieved from https://www.healthaffairs.org/doi/pdf/10.1377/hlthaff.21.3.20

Wood, G.S. (2009). *Empire of Liberty: A History of the Early Republic,* 1789–1815. New York: Oxford University Press, Inc.

U.S. Internal Revenue Service. (2017). Publication 969 (2017), Health savings accounts and other tax-favored health plans. (Internal Revenue Service Report 969.) Retrieved from https://www.irs.gov/publications/p969

Appendix A

Essential Financial Reports for the DNP Nurse Executive

The following list presents basic financial and operational reports that a nurse executive needs to effectively manage the nursing operations in health care organizations. This list can serve as a discussion tool during the orientation period upon entry to an executive-level position and should be updated and expanded as the nurse executive gains experience and knowledge.

It is very useful to request the current financial report, and at least three years of previous reports for comparative purposes.

1. Annual report of the organization including the annual financial report.
2. The most current strategic plan.
3. Monthly financial performance reports.
4. Annual and monthly departmental financial reports.
5. Organizational and departmental budget. (The organizational budget may be general in scope while the specific departmental budget may be much more in-depth.)
6. Budget monitoring reports (most current and at least the prior six months).
7. Financial and operational ratios that are routinely monitored. (If ratios are not monitored, request the current indicators that are monitored and at least a three- year trend analysis.)
8. Nurse staffing and recruitment reports for the previous 12 months.
9. Current list of third-party contracts and any available utilization data by payer. (After reviewing this list and the payer utilization data, you should request the specific contract for the three major utilizers of your facility.)
10. Department-specific current quality indicators and any available trend analysis of the indicators.
11. Organization-level quality indicators and available quality reports.
12. Current government compliance reports. The Medicare Cost report, if required from your organization, will be a large document that requires time to review. (Review of the current cost report is well worth the time, because it may suggest areas within your operational scope of responsibility that require additional information.)
13. Current large claims that are under management by any third-party payer and a summary of the large claims that have been subject to external management within the last 12 months.

Appendix B
Stakeholder Mapping

Stakeholder mapping is a powerful tool for the health care executive. It provides a way for the manager to analyze the environmental forces that require management attention, as well as a method to define essential strategic relationships and boundary spanning activities necessary to ensure organizational success. Strategic managers can also use stakeholder mapping as a delegation tool to ensure that the management team coordinates external contacts and gathers information essential to the smooth management of key external relationships. These relationships include but are not limited to regulatory agencies, major payers, and large employer groups. Depending on the size and scope of the organization, both state and federal regulatory stakeholders need to be managed, as well as professional organizations that directly impact on the organizational mission. Mapping the stakeholders active in a given area is a useful way to assure coverage of key areas important to the organization as well as a way to organize informa-

Example: Nursing Workforce Stakeholders for an Urban Non-Profit Hospital

Professional	Educational	State Government	Federal Government	Advocacy
State Nursing Association	Local two- and four-year nursing schools	State Nursing Association (note some states place nursing regulation under the state medical board)	Medicare (CMS) nursing staffing requirements. HRSA Nursing Workforce Group	AARP Center to Champion Nursing State Chapter
American Nursing Association	American Association of Colleges of Nursing	State Legislators that focus on nursing issues or are professional nurses.	Elected senators and representatives	Non-profit organizations focused on health such as the Red Cross.
Professional nursing collective bargaining organizations active in the area. These groups may or may not be affiliated with the state nursing association	Nursing school alumni and student groups.	State health consumer organizations active in state and local government	National Institute of Nursing Research (NINR)	Federal consumer groups interested in health such as Health Care for America Now or Families USA
Nursing Certification and Specialty Organizations	Campus recruitment and student placement offices	State professional certification and licensing groups with an interest in nursing		State consumer and payer groups interested in health.

tion that results from stakeholder contacts. Generally, a stakeholder map begins with a focus area and branches from main stakeholders to those that may be affiliated or peripheral influencers on the major stakeholders identified. There are a variety of stakeholder mapping tools available and many organizations designate a preferred template for this activity. The following example uses a simple table, but many templates employ a flowchart or force-field approach to indicate major and contributory stakeholders. The example following is a list of major organizations and organizational areas that a non-profit urban hospital would need to consider in regard to the nursing workforce. Depending on the issue, some of these groups would be major and some minor stakeholders, but all should be evaluated for their influence on the nursing workforce issue.

JOYCE E. JOHNSON

9

The C-Suite Business Case: The Critical Role of Business Planning

Chapter Objectives

- Describe the current business climate of the health care industry.
- Emphasize the critical importance of business skills for DNP nurse executives.
- Detail the essential components of a standard business plan.
- Identify the success factors for business planning.
- Develop business plans based on successful business plan exemplars authored by nurses.

KEY WORDS: Business acumen, business planning, core competency, doctorate in nursing practice, and entrepreneurship

Introduction

American health care today is a complex business challenged by the evolution of the Patient Protection and Affordable Care Act (ACA) and a myriad of other complex factors that require leaders in the C-Suite to have consummate business skills. This chapter reviews the complicated business climate of health care today, the critical need for nurse executives to possess consummate business skills and acumen, the role of entrepreneurship in business planning, the essential components of the classic business plan framework, and factors for success in business planning.

Business Acumen and the C-Suite DNP-Prepared Nurse Executive

The DNP prepared nurses who advance up the career ladder to top leadership positions in the C-Suites of today's health care institutions will be entering a new world, the world of big business. It is an increasingly complex business environment in which health care systems must adjust to the uncertain regulatory environment of highly politicized health care reform (ACA, 2010), exploding technology, significant personnel shortages (Carrier, Yee, & Stark, 2011), and mounting national pressures to improve health outcomes, patient satisfaction, and health care quality while also lowering costs and conserving resources. Such immense challenges have made financial viability a significant concern for today's healthcare leaders (Brown, 2017). Whether they serve as a chief nursing officer, chief operating officer, or the chief executive officer, greater numbers of nurses academically prepared at the doctoral level will be among these leaders of one of our country's largest and most complex industries–an industry that now equals 17.8% of the American gross domestic product (Amadeo, 2017).

Although executive leadership roles give nurses the opportunity to "practice to the full extent of their skills" and influence the American healthcare system (Wilson, Whitaker, & Whitford, 2012; Johnson *et al.* , 2012), the reality is that most aspiring nurse executives arrive in the C-suite with limited training in the regulatory, financial, and general operational business requirements of a complex health care organization. Like physicians, nurses' training has traditionally focused on professional practice, and not on learning business administration and developing business and finance acumen. According to Benner, Sutphen, Leonard, and Day (2009), nursing has been the most underserved group within healthcare in terms of general education and more specifically, business-related education. Rothausen and Bazarko (2015) suggest that nursing education has traditionally taught nurses to focus on each patient's experience of care, a focus that often did not consider resource consumption or outcomes. Yet, as Jain (2015) suggested, in the current health care environment, both physicians and nurses are "assuming a higher level of influence in the business of health care than ever before" (p. 1).

Gandolf (2014) reported that today's physicians are accepting the reality that health care is now a mega-business, and that to survive and thrive in the current business climate, physicians must have business training. Many universities have recognized this acute need and now offer dual MD-MBA degree options. According to Gandolf, in the past ten years, the number of dual programs in the US has grown to over 65, which include the University of Pennsylvania, Harvard, Dartmouth, and Cornell.

The reality that nursing leaders in executive roles need business training as well has not gone unnoticed by national nursing organizations. In 2006, the American Association of Colleges of Nursing (AACN) recognized this deficit of business skills, and defined core competencies for the doctorate in nursing practice (DNP) academic program accreditation in their *Essentials of Doctoral Education for Advanced Nursing Practice* (American Association of Colleges of Nursing, 2006). These core competencies include proficiency in using economic and financial principles "to redesign effective and realistic care delivery strategies" and the ability to "employ principles of business, finance, and economics" to develop effective plans for improving the quality of health care. This call to executive leadership in health care was accelerated by the Institute of Medicine's 2010 landmark report—*The Future of Nursing: Leading Change, Advancing Health*. This well-publicized national report emphasized the critical contribution of nursing leaders to ". . . building a health care system that will meet the demand for safe, quality, patient-centered, accessible, and affordable care" (p.1). The Institute of Medicine (IOM) report asserted that nurses were vital to making the health care of the future accessible, affordable, and acceptable. How nurses could specifically contribute to the future of health care was delineated five years later by the American Organization for Nursing Leadership (AONL) (formerly the American Organization of Nurse Executives) in AONL's updated nurse executive competencies (2015). This set of leadership competencies included business skills–categorized by AONL as financial management, human resource management, strategic management, and information management and technology—as one of the five critical skill domains needed by all nurses in executive roles.

The need for significant business savvy has driven the development of dual DNP/MBA programs, which like similar programs for physicians, now appear to be gaining ground in the U.S. (Carlson, 2015). As one nursing leader concluded, "Nursing leaders need to have the business acumen to analyze the way care is being delivered and apply clinical value analyses and the kind of 'lean' thinking that can reduce waste, inefficiency and costs" (O'Sullivan, 2016). Larson (2015) had reported that "such thinking involves understanding and adopting lean protocols, implementing best practice workforce strategies and tools that optimize labor and minimize time spent in management and administrative tasks, while creating economies of scale through reduced redundancies and standardization wherever possible" (p. 1). As Larson said, all are inherent in an enterprise approach to workforce management.

At the 2017 International Council of Nurses Congress in Barcelona, National Nursing Centers Consortium chief executive Tine Hansen-Turton reiterated the importance of including business skills in today's graduate nursing curriculum (Jones-Berry, 2017). As that change evolves over the long-term, some executive nurses are learning business skills through professional development partnerships with CFO's (Van Dyke, 2008) and continuing professional education in finance supported by hospitals, but driven by the nursing department (Douglas, 2010). However, Hansen-Turton argued that practically, executive nurses who plan to enter the C-suite and sit at the decision-making table can obtain the type of business skills they need without going to business school. "I think nurses are incredible entrepreneurs—we need to show them how to put a business plan together," Hansen-Turton said (p. 1).

Think Like an Entrepreneur

What does it mean for a nurse executive to be an "entrepreneur?" Around the beginning of the 19th century, Say coined the term entrepreneur from the French term entreprendre–to "undertake" (Stoy, 1999, p. 231). Say suggested that change agents seek opportunities for shifting economic resources away from areas of low productivity to those with the potential for higher productivity, higher yield, and greater value. Nurse entrepreneurs, according to Wilson *et al.* (2012), seek self-employment by developing diverse practices and businesses that give them the opportunity to "improve health outcomes with innovative approaches" (p. 1). These entrepreneurs recognize direct accountability to clients regardless of their status as an individual or a public/private organization that use their services (Liu & D'Aunno, 2011). According to Wilson *et al.* (2012), successful nurse entrepreneurs might have an independent clinical practice, own a business, such as a nursing home or pharmaceutical company, or operate a consultancy that offers research or educational services. Carlson (2016) added that these ambitious nurses also work as massage therapists, writers, coaches, filmmakers, bloggers, and product developers.

As agents of change, nurse entrepreneurs seek opportunities through which they can directly address gaps in direct patient care and the healthcare industry. These entrepreneurs must develop top-notch business skills, because they must convince decision makers and other stakeholders that their views of a new, improved way of doing business via an independent practice offer clear, data-driven advantages for patients and real value for the organization's bottom line as well. As Barberio (2010) concluded, an entrepreneurial spirit, a solid knowledge base, excellent clinical skills, and the desire to provide patients with quality healthcare are simply not enough to be successful in an independent practice. As Barberio (2010) said, business acumen and financial "know-how" are essential to the viability of nurse-managed practices.

These same attributes are needed by new DNP prepared executive nurses who begin working in the C-Suite of a health care institution. In contrast to nurses who lead independent nursing practices, executive nurses work as a member of an executive team that is responsible for assessing organizational productivity and performance, and, strategically and creatively shifting economic resources in a hospital away from areas of low productivity to those with the potential for higher productivity, higher yield, and greater value. In this environment, traditional bureaucratic thinking and maintaining the status quo simply cannot generate the new efficiencies, better speed, and transformational changes that create what is needed for success—greater efficiencies, greater value in health care, and ultimately, financial viability.

Nurse executives enter the C-Suite in a climate that requires entrepreneurial thinking. According to Jain and Tsang (2014), recent government incentives that support innovation have created a business case for performance improvement that did not exist in the past. There has been an influx of talent from other industries that all "recognize the enormous size of the opportunity to make a profit while improving care, lowering costs, and improving health" (p. 1). Access to higher quality data is also increasing the understanding of the weak links in health care and helping identify proactive approaches for anticipating illness and intervening at an earlier stage. Thus, DNP prepared executive nurses with an entrepreneurial mindset and the right toolkit of business planning skills, now have the opportunity to lead or join an executive team that can identify innovative approaches, products, and services that will define health care in the future.

Learn How to Write a Winning Business Plan

Deep in the large literature on business development lies a central truth—*business planning* is an essential business tool. Translating business planning efforts into a sophisticated, successful business plan remains an undisputed, effective necessity in any business endeavor (Sherman, 2016), but especially in the business environment of health care institutions today. In a *business plan*, nurse executives can make a data-based case for a proposed organizational change-identify specific goals and measurements to assess progress over time-establish the foundation for projected organizational performance with detailed financial analyses and where they can leverage critical industry intelligence and marketing data to demonstrate the value of a proposed organizational change before the institution's top decision makers agree to make a major change in a hospital program, policy, or procedure. In their role as champions of change and advocates for patients, savvy nurse executives depend on the traditional business plan as the vehicle for defining the what, why, who, and where of any proposed reform initiative.

The Business Plan Framework

Although business planning dates back to the 1960s (Taylor, 2016), the essence of business planning has changed very little over the years. A good business plan, with an average length between 10 and 35 pages, is a well-written, compelling document that explicitly defines the goals of a proposed business initiative and describes in detail the strategies to achieve those goals. The typical plan uses a single-spaced format, with tables and charts in the body of the plan, and references and appendices at the back.

As suggested by Sherman (2016), writing a business plan is similar to telling a story, one that flows logically through a traditional series of key elements, as shown in Table 9.1.

These elements are similar to those used in evidence-based projects,

Table 9.1 Key Elements of a Business Plan.

• Introduction
• Description of the Business
• Market & Competition Analysis
• Development Plan & Schedule
• Operational Plan
• Marketing Plan
• Organizational Plan
• Financial Plan
• Executive Summary

which according to Stephens (2013), build on the recommendations from the IOM (2001) and focus on "standardizing healthcare practices to science and best evidence and reducing illogical variation in care, which is known to produce unpredictable health outcomes" (p.1).

Introduction

The introduction sets the stage for the entire business plan. The introduction captures the readers' interest, introduces the author's area of specialization and envisioned future state of the organization, describes the need for and details of the proposed business initiative, and makes a convincing, compelling case that the plan has identified an important gap in patient care, or some other aspect of hospital administration. Most importantly, a business plan describes a practical plan for change that can close that gap and achieve important data-driven outcomes that affect patient care and a host of other variables that affect the organization's bottom line.

Description of the Business

According to Barberio (2016), this part of business plan defines the unique aspects of the proposed business or organizational change that distinguishes it from other competitors or concepts. Specialization, suggested Barberio, is a wise strategy because it reduces competition and drives reimbursement, both of which are essential for business ventures in the highly competitive, consumer-focused health care industry.

This section begins with a brief but detailed overview of the business or proposed organizational change, current service proficiency and offerings, existing customer base, and economic prospects. A complete description of the proposed business' essence, evolution, and market follows, as well as the current healthcare and practice trends that support the need for and sustainability of the new business concept. The section summary should include a broad and comprehensive perspective on industry, economic, regulatory, and competitive trends that affect the proposed new business.

Sample Business Description

The Lourdes Family Clinic provides primary medical care for family members of all ages. As a clinic seeking medical home certification, Lourdes Family Clinic utilizes nurse care-coordination to optimally manage chronic conditions such as asthma and diabetes. The clinicians use the Creighton Model Fertility Care System as a method to monitor and maintain women's gynecological health. The clinic follows the medical and surgical methods of NaPro Technology to treat a variety of women's health problems (see Appendix A for more information on NaPro Technology). For obstetric deliveries and minimum invasive NaPro Technology surgeries for women, the clinic plans to obtain OB/Gyn physician privileges at Fairview Southdale Hospital in Edina, Fairview Ridges in Burnsville, and St. Francis Hospital in Shakopee. The founding clinicians seek to find office space in the northeastern area of Eden Prairie. The location offers convenient access to 169 and 494, a central location for the four targeted counties, and an office space price ranging from $10–$22 per square feet (see Appendix C for map of location). The clinic anticipates the need for office space with at least 7,000 square feet and preferably 8,000 to 10,000 square feet.

Mission: To spread God's Kingdom of Life by providing exceptional Catholic medical care that respects the inherent dignity of the human person at all stages of life.

Vision: To become a leading center for advanced Catholic healthcare in the Midwest.

Values: Respect for human life, integrity, joy in serving.

Goals: Short-term goals include opening the Lourdes Family Clinic and attaining a patient volume of 13,875 in the first year. Long terms goals include expanding the clinic's operational hours to evening business hours and Saturday day hours. The clinic intends to obtain certification as a Health Care Home (HCH) within the first four years of operation. Beyond five years, the founders aim to eventually build a clinic to fit specific needs and preferences of Lourdes Family Clinic and highlight the Catholic identity of the practice.

Courtesy of P.J. Mantel, MSN, RN AGNP-BC, FNP-BC, 2017.

Market and Competition Analysis

This analysis must present sufficient data to convince the top leaders of the institution or potential investors that the proposed venture has a

Table 9.2 Sample SWOT Analysis.

Strengths	Weaknesses
• Clinically-expert APNs • Location adjacent to target community • Clinical specialty has few competitors	• Aging population limits family practice opportunities • Growing hospital system employs physician practices • Lack of practice owner experience
Opportunities	**Threats**
• Potential to link with practices interested in specialty referrals • Reconfiguration of practice patterns may enable significant market penetration • Growth potential significant based on absence of alternative options	• Aggressive hospital system entry into marketplace • Insufficient funding support may limit immediate practice expansion • Practice marketing efforts overshadowed by hospital system market penetration strategy.

substantial market in the healthcare industry. This analysis identifies the *target population*, describes the *size* of the current and potential market, and details the *competition* that exists in the market place. The "SWOT assessment" with the classic four-square matrix format (Taylor, 2016) is the framework for this analysis, as shown in Table 9.2.

Fallon (2016) said that a SWOT analysis can "help your company face its greatest challenges and find its most promising new markets" (p. 1). Berry (2016) suggested viewing strengths and weaknesses as those factors that are internal to the proposed business and that you can change over time. According to Fallon (2016), strengths and weakness include a variety of resources—financial, physical, and human—as well as current processes such as employee programs, department hierarchies, and software systems. In contrast, opportunities and threats are external to the business, exist in the market, and are beyond your control. Fallon (2016) cited market and economic trends, funding sources, demographics, relationships with suppliers and partners, and political, environmental, and economic regulations as external factors.

Each part of the SWOT analysis forces the author to answer some critical questions (Johnson & Garvin, 2017). When considering *strengths*, it is helpful to answer the following questions:

- What is your *real* strength?
- Are you associated with specialty physicians for referrals?
- Do you have competent administrative and management personnel?
- Are your personnel specialty trained and educated in ways that differentiate their expertise from others offering similar services?
- Is your patient flow paradigm preferential?

The analysis of *weaknesses* might include answers to the following questions:

- What are the weaknesses in your skills and experience?
- Are there problems in your facility?
- Do you lack business expertise?
- Does your business have limited resources?
- Do you lack necessary clinical expertise to expand your practice?
- Is the management of your patient flow a problem?
- Do you have an unacceptable patient wait time?
- Do you have inadequate supplies to meet patient needs?
- Is your business in a poor location?

Identification of the *opportunities* can include answering some different types of questions such as:

- Are market trends favorable to your volume projections?
- Are demographics, such as age or gender, favorable to your practice?
- Is the payer mix in your location favorable?
- Can you envision vendor or supplier collaborations and associated cost reduction?
- Can you maximize benefit from economic and financial trends?

In contrast, threats require answers to a different set of questions:

- Are other nearby practices expanding?
- Have new practices open in your area?
- Are accountable care organizations affecting your practice's potential development and growth?
- Are hospital systems aligning market flow to their practices and acute care facilities?
- Are there government regulations (such as those focused on the implementation of electronic health records) that are challenges for your proposed practice?
- Are there economic projections that could negatively the practice you envision?
- Does a new product or technology make your services obsolete?

Describing threats from government regulations is an especially critical part of the threat assessment. In a 2012 national survey conducted by KPMG, 60% of healthcare executives said that regulatory and legislative pressures were the most significant barriers to their company's growth projections for the next year (PR Newswire, 2012).

Patrishkoff (2015) suggested that the SWOT assessment is only the foundation of a good strategic plan and is not the final analysis. As Berry

(2016) concluded, the "the true value of this exercise is in using the results to maximize the positive influences on your business and minimize the negative ones," (p. 3).

Development Plan and Schedule

This section includes the details of the what, how, and when of developing the new product or service. The proposed services are defined and described in detail. This should leave no questions about what the product is and what it is not. Using the development cycle, all the resources must be described such as equipment, staff, facilities, supplies, technology, and finances. Also described are the planning, program, and policy development required for the new enterprise or initiative; all construction equipment that must be purchased; and the plans for marketing, staffing, training, and hospital operations.

The development plan typically includes a step-by-step timeline that details the evolution of the initiative from planning to completion, as well as a comprehensive, multistage evaluation plan that will document the quantitative and qualitative impact and also assure potential funding sources in the future. Such sources require data-driven metrics and system-wide mechanisms for quality control, continuous improvement, and risk abatement. According to Wolters Kluwer (2012), new businesses typically face two primary risks—introducing a product that customers will not buy, or not introducing new products often enough (p. 1). The first risk can be reduced by being clear about the target population and doing sufficient market research at each step of the development process, and the second risk by being knowledgeable about shifting market conditions and making a strong commitment to the proposed business' development strategy.

Organizational Plan

This section of a business plan provides a thorough view of the staff and

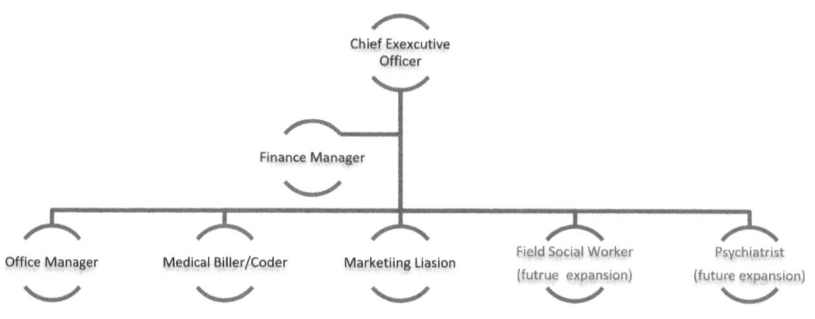

Figure 9.2. Sample Organization Chart.

the organizational relationships within the proposed business. This section includes an organization chart, shown in Figure 9.2. The chart must clearly depict the hierarchical structure of the initiative; defines the chain-of-command, and lines of direct authority and reporting; and the direct and indirect linkages with a larger health care system.

The organizational plan also includes detailed descriptions of the key members of the team that will assume responsibility for the business' success. These should include qualification profiles that detail key skills, competencies, and prior experience. Traditionally, a business plan includes complete job descriptions for all key personnel, along with expected salaries, in an appendix to the plan. Fontinelle (2016) believes that all business plans should identify any external consultants or other independent contractors to be hired, and describe their unique function and contribution.

Sample Marketing Plan—Lourdes Family Clinic

The clinic plans to print a brochure about Lourdes Family Clinic prior to opening day and distributing the brochure at Catholic parishes and schools in the three targeted counties. Along with the brochure, the clinic intends to advertise the open house three months in advance in parish bulletins and on the local Catholic radio station Relevant Radio starting at the beginning of October 2017. The clinic will encourage word-of-mouth patient recommendations by giving patients who come to our clinic an extra brochure along with an invitation for them to distribute to one person they know. The clinic also plans to place weekly regular advertisements in Catholic church bulletins. The founders and spouses/children of the founders plan to advertise the clinic at various Catholic conferences and events in the Twin Cities throughout the year. Many Catholic events take place in the Twin Cities, providing an opportunity to obtain a booth to promote Lourdes Family Clinic by distributing brochures and speak to persons about the Lourdes Family Clinic. The clinic will advertise on the local Catholic radio station Relevant Radio as well. The budget for marketing consists of $10,000 for initial advertising with the printing of a brochure and relevant radio advertisement, and $10,000 for each year.

Courtesy of P.J. Mantel, MSN, RN AGNP-BC, FNP-BC, 2017.

Marketing Plan

According to the U.S. Small Business Administration (SBA) (2016), the marketing plan ensures that "you're not only sticking to your schedule, but that you're spending your marketing funds wisely and appropriately,"

(p. 1). The plan, suggests the SBA, details "everything from understanding your target market and your competitive position in that market, to how you intend to reach that market (your tactics) and differentiate yourself from your competition in order to make a sale," (p. 1).

Abrams (2015) suggests that the marketing plan must address four factors: (1) *fit*—this means that the marketing vehicles you have chosen match the professional image of your institution and can actually reach the target customers, whether internal or external, (2) *media mix*—in today's uber media market, a marketing plan must incorporate multiple media channels to obtain maximum exposure; these might include traditional media (brochures, on-line advertising, direct or email mailings, and print or broadcast media) and new media such as Facebook, other websites, and social networking platforms such as Twitter, (3) *extent of repetition*—this means that an organization must plan and pay for many exposures to achieve the maximum media saturation that is needed, and (4) *affordability*—marketing requires a substantial budget, as well as a significant commitment of human resources.

Beyond these general guidelines, a marketing plan should reflect the tried-and-true principles of diffusion of innovation derived from the seminal work of Rogers (2003). Rogers said that five attributes influence the rate of adoption of any innovation: (1) *relative advantage* –the degree to which an innovation is seen as being better that the idea it supersedes; the greater the relative advantage of an innovation, the greater the rate of its adoption. Rogers said that relative advantage (such as economic profitability, low initial cost, a decrease in discomfort, social prestige, savings of time and effort, or an immediate reward) is one of the strongest predictors of an innovation's rate of adoption (p. 233), (2) *compatibility*—the degree to which an innovation is perceived as consistent with the existing values, past experiences, and needs of potential adopters (p. 240); thus, a nursing innovation might revolve around a core of caring, healing and holism, dedication to the well-being of patients and nurses, appreciation of the opportunity to serve others, focus on comfort, and honor for the human spirit, (3) *complexity*—Rogers suggested that a high degree of complexity is a barrier to adoption; thus a new innovation in a hospital setting should be straightforward, simple, and easy to understand, (4) *trialability*—this is "the degree to which an innovation may be experimented with on a limited basis" (p. 258). Since trialability is positively related to the rate of adoption, conducting an initial trial or pilot study is often preferable to a longer, more permanent intervention; (5) *observability*—this was defined by Rogers (2005) as "the degree to which the results of the innovation are visible to others" (p. 258); the more easily the results of an innovation can be seen by others, the greater the rate of adoption. This reaffirms the important role of communication in any change or entrepreneurial initiative.

Another critical feature of the marketing plan is the proposed plan for evaluating the success of a new organizational initiative. The SBA refers to this as "measuring your spend" (2016, p. 1), i.e., monitoring the effect of specific marketing strategies on revenues and other factors during a fixed period of time as compared to another fixed time period. To assure the most accurate assessment of impact, the evaluation plan should ideally include multiple methods of data collection that will generate both quantitative and qualitative data [U.S. Agency for International Development (USAID), 2013]. Use of multiple methods helps to balance the limitations of one data collection method with the strength of another. This might include quantitative outcome measures from existing databases and new surveys, as well as qualitative data from structured observations, key informant interviews, and focus groups. Qualitative data are important in the evaluation process because qualitative analysis increases understanding of ". . . how people involved with the program being studied understand, think about, make sense of, and manage situations in their lives and environment and/or to describe the social or environmental contexts within which a program is implemented," [U.S. Agency for International Development (USDHHS, 2016)].

The SBA left no doubt about the critical importance of the marketing strategy in a business plan. "The time spent developing your marketing plan is time well spent because it defines how you connect with your customers, and that's an investment worth making" (SBA, 2016, p. 1).

Financial Plan

This section of a business plan defines the business strategy and goals of the new initiative, identifies the payer priorities, and specifies what the potential customers value and need. Wasserman (2016) emphasized that the financial section of a business plan *does not equate to traditional accounting*. According to Wasserman (2016), although the financial projections (profit and loss, balance sheet, and cash flow) look similar to accounting statements, accounting looks back in time, while business planning looks forward into the future.

Writing a financial plan requires a clear understanding of the health care industry and the proposed organizational initiative, basic knowledge of financial planning, and knowledge of financial tools that measure the performance and success of a business enterprise. Nurse executives who have limited experience with financial planning may require additional assistance when writing this part of a business plan. There are certainly some good reference texts available (Abrams, 2015; Baker & Baker, 2014; Paterson, 2014) and many on-line resources as well (Fontinelle, 2016b; U.S. Small Business Administration, 2016). However, many new nurse executives may elect to either partner with the Chief Financial Officer (CFO) from their institution (Van Dyke, 2008), or opt for hiring an external financial consultant who can assist them in creating a very complete, concise, and *realistic* overview of the proposed new business' financial future. Fontinelle (2016) recommends hiring an expert, unbiased professional who can assure that your financial projections are well done and realistic. These projections typically include an income statement, balance sheet, and the cash flow statement with a number of different analyses.

Income Statement

This statement summarizes the revenue and expenses associated with the new initiative or business. According to Patterson (2014), the income statement must list all sources of income, estimate the volume of patients that might be affected and the payer mix, determine the expected revenue per unit, and calculate the expected total revenue per year (p. 104). Some factors that should be considered in these calculations include ambulatory payment classifications (which may apply to free-standing practices such as an ambulatory surgery center not associated with a hospital); Healthcare Common Procedure Coding System (HCPCS) codes; payer fee schedules; percent of charges; relative value units (RVUs), the basis of reimbursement in ambulatory care; and an allowance for bad debt.

For a new start-up endeavor, the financial plan must include total project expenses that include payer mix information, labor projections for all staff by category and with benefits and overtime, the expected capital costs, and the indirect costs or overhead. Indirect costs, which are determined by allocation methods set by the health care organization, recognize the reality that all new services require general organizational resources, such as leasing costs for additional space, furnishings, technology support, heat and other utilities, as well as all administrative or supervisory staff. While the income and expense statement provide an estimated organization-wide pool of indirect expenses, new practices or businesses demand the estimation of detailed indirect expenses as well as direct expenses. The total of direct and indirect expenses is then divided by direct expenses to produce the *loading factor* that shows the excess of total costs over direct costs for the new business.

Balance Sheet

Fontinelle (2016a) suggests that the balance sheet simply shows potential funders that the expected assets of the proposed initiative balance with the projected liabilities. These figures are speculative for a brand new enterprise, although it is helpful to benchmark the figures with financial figures from another similar type of business. Assets might include accounts receivable, cash, inventory, and equipment. Liabilities include accounts pay-

Break-Even Analysis Chart

— Projected Revenue   — Projected Expenses

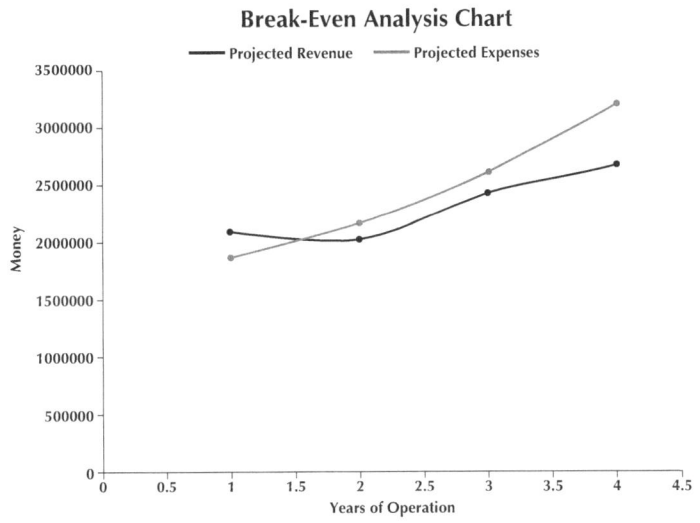

Figure 9.3. Sample—Break Even Analysis. Courtesy of P.J. Mantel, MSN, RN AGNP-BC, FNP-BC, 2017.

able and loan balances. An easy way to remember the balance sheet is that it describes "what you own vs. what you owe," (Fontinelle, 2016a, p. 1).

Cash Flow Statement

This statement includes a number of interesting analyses that demonstrate cash flow in a given timeframe. The general requirement is that a business plan should include a cash flow estimate by month for at least one year, and a longer-term, "pro-forma" projection of at least three years of business performance. These estimates might include sales forecasts, cash vs. credit receipts, the predicted time frame for collecting accounts receivable (Fontinelle, 2016b), and any projected variance in the budget. It is critical to perform a strategic analysis of budget variances that might be due to factors such as lower service volume and higher resource use than expected, and to identify all potential management strategies that could minimize the budget variances.

Another critical part of the financial plan is the breakeven analysis. This is the critical calculation that demonstrates the point at which income exceeds costs and the new initiative begins making a profit. The operative question to be answered by this analysis is ". . . at what operational point has a new business earned enough revenue to recoup its costs"? At the breakeven point, a new business makes no profit but also does not lose money. At this point, a new business venture has covered the cost of staying in business and has begun building the kind of volume that will lead to profitable returns for the institution.

The breakeven analysis involves calculating the total costs (all fixed, variable/semi-variable, and opportunity costs), the payer mix and the actual revenue per customer, and the actual and projected patient volumes over a three-year period. The figure for actual revenue per patient is multiplied by patient volume to obtain the total revenue. Along with total expenses and current and projected volume for the next three years, there should be sufficient information to construct a simple breakeven analysis that can demonstrate a profitable enterprise over the next three years. This analysis represents a major step in defining the financial and investment strategy of a new business venture and convincing the top leadership of your institution and other stakeholders of the new business' potential profitability.

The Executive Summary

Written last but placed at the beginning of the business plan is the all-important executive summary. The U.S. Small Business Administration says "... The executive summary is often considered the most important section of a business plan. This section briefly tells the reader where the company is, where the executive wants to take it, and why the business idea will be successful. If the executive is seeking financing, the executive summary is also the first opportunity to grab a potential investor's interest," (p.1). It is important to create an outstanding executive summary because many business proposals are rejected on the basis on the executive summary alone.

In *no more than one page of concise and compelling writing*, the executive summary has two goals—convince top leadership and all potential funders that the entire business plan is worth reading and that the proposed business venture is worth funding. Some experts warn that professionals who are new to the business environment should use the upfront executive summary to tell potential funders exactly what they want and to avoid the common mistake of burying their needs deep inside the business plan (Entrepreneur, 2016).

Choosing what to include in this critical one-page document is a challenge because every word counts. In total, the executive summary should include:

- A brief description of the proposed business, including a historical overview that includes date of formation, company founders, and projected number of employees
- A summary of the business' mission, goals, and objectives
- Solid description of the target market and the need for the business
- High-level justification for the viability of the proposed business along with a quick look at the competition
- Growth and service projections

- Marketing strategies—how the business will attract customers
- Financial projections, including bank references and investors
- Future plans that detail the direction of the business development (DiscoverBusiness.us, 2016)

Sample Business Plan—Lourdes Family Clinic

Executive Summary

As a new independent medical clinic located in the southwestern Twin Cities region, the Lourdes Family Clinic will offer family primary care, women's obstetrical care, and innovative NaPro Technology gynecological services for women in accordance with Catholic bioethical principles. The experienced team of Lourdes clinicians consists of three physicians and one Family Nurse Practitioner who will practice medicine with integrity, joy, and respect for the inherent dignity of all human life. The Lourdes Family Clinic targets male and female Catholics of all ages and ethnic backgrounds in Hennepin, Scott, and Carver counties and parts of Dakota county. Although large managed systems dominate the healthcare landscape in Minnesota and the Aalfa Family Clinic affords Catholic competition, the clinic's competitive edge consists in providing medical care according to Catholic values at a new and convenient location for Catholic healthcare in the southwest metro, offering convenient evening and Saturday hours, and delivering healthcare with the technologically advanced EMR system eClinicalWorks to improve the efficiency and quality of Catholic medical care in the Twin Cities. The clinic will begin medical services on January 22, 2018, with regular Monday through Friday business hours, expand to offer two evenings of clinic hours in the second year, four evenings of clinic hours in the third year, and Saturday hours in the fourth year. Marketing strategies include colorful advertising in Church bulletins, a printed brochure distributed at local parishes and Catholic schools, encouraging word-of-mouth patient promotion of the clinic, maintaining advertisement booths at local Catholic conferences and events, and local Catholic radio advertisement. The structure of the clinic management consists of CEO Dr. Harold Jones as the overall director of the clinic, Vice President Dr. Nancy Smith in charge of clinicians and marketing, a Clinic Manager responsible for clinical operations, and a RN care coordinator as supervisor of the medical assistants and ultrasound technologist. By reaching 13,875 patient appointments in the first year and increasing the patient volume by 15% each year, projections indicate the clinic reaches a break-even point at the 19th month of operation and achieves a yearly profit of $527,000 at the end of the fourth business year.

Introduction

In January of 2018 the Lourdes Family Clinic will open as a new independent family medical clinic in the southwestern Twin Cities metro area. The clinic offers family primary care and women's obstetrical/gynecological health care in harmony with Catholic bioethical norms.

Goals:
- To provide exceptionally high quality primary and OB/Gyn medical care to families we serve.
- To provide advanced women's healthcare through NaPro Technology, including minimally invasive surgical services to treat a variety of women's health problems.
- To practice medicine following Catholic bioethical principles as described by the Ethical and Religious Directives for Catholic Health Care Services of the U.S. Catholic Bishops Conference and the National Catholic Bioethics Center.
- To use advanced electronic medical records (EMR) in order to provide efficient and the highest possible quality of healthcare.
- To obtain recognition as a Health Care Home (HCH) by the Minnesota Department of Health within the first four years of operations.
- To create a practice which reaches financial self-sufficiency by the end of the second business year.

Objectives:
- Acquire a business loan and a lease for office space with at least 8 exam rooms in a strategic location.
- Hire staff and purchase required furniture and equipment to meet clinical and operational needs, including the purchase and installation of a highly advanced EMR system.
- Attain average visits per month of 1,156 in the first year and increase patient volume by 15% each year.
- Limit financial losses due to bad debt to less than 5% each year.

Problems the clinic addresses:
- Currently no Catholic healthcare clinic exists in Minneapolis or the southwestern metro suburbs. To obtain Catholic healthcare many families in the area travel a long distance to a northeastern suburb of St. Paul.
- A growing demand exists in the Catholic population for NaPro Technology services to treat a number of women's health issues.
- No Catholic healthcare clinic in the Twin Cities metro region receives above average ratings by MN Community Measurement.
- No Catholic healthcare clinic in the area uses advanced technology found in EMR.

General description: The Lourdes Family Clinic seeks to meet the health care needs of Catholic families residing in the Hennepin County and surrounding region. Two board-certified, family practice medical doctors and one certified family nurse practitioner (FNP) will provide primary care to patients of all ages according to Catholic values at the proposed Lourdes Family Clinic. One OB/Gyn physicians trained in NaPro Technology will provide OB/Gyn services for women including hospital deliveries and outpatient minimal invasive NaPro Technology surgeries at a local hospital. One of the family practice physicians also possesses board certification as a OB/Gyn and will perform a limited number of deliveries at a local hospital as demand dictates. The clinic will use eClinicalWorks EMR to provide top quality Catholic healthcare for patients of all ages. The founders determined Eden Prairie affords a strategic location for the clinic.

Outcome: Outcomes sought include the establishment of a profitable and reputable Catholic family practice in a southwestern suburb of Minneapolis. The clinic intends to achieve above average state quality ratings and exceed patient expectations by providing exceptional patient-centered medical care according to Catholic bioethical principles.

Description of the Business

History: The two physician Dr. Harold Jones and Dr. Nancy Smith envisioned The Lourdes Family Clinic and lead the effort to transform their vision into reality. Dr. Jones carries the title of CEO of the Lourdes Family Clinic. Dr. Jones possesses board-certification as a family medicine physician and OB/Gyn with 10 years of experience working in a family medicine practice in Houston and an Allina Health clinic Minneapolis. Dr. Nancy Smith assumes the title of vice president of the Lourdes Clinic. Dr. Smith practiced for 5 years as a board certified family medicine physician at a HealthEast clinic in St. Paul. Both Dr. Jones and Dr. Smith hold certification as a Creighton Model Medical Consultant as well. The Lourdes Family Clinic team also includes Dr. Diane Fredrickson. As an OB/Gyn physician, Dr. Fredrickson possesses 15 years of experience at the Mayo Clinic in Rochester in both clinical, hospital, and surgical gynecology. She completed medical and surgical NaPro Technology training at the Pope Paul VI Institute. An advanced practice registered nurse (APRN) joins the medical team as well. Although newly certified as a family nurse practitioner (FNP), Patty-Jo Mantel possesses 8 years of hospital experience as a medical-surgical registered nurse and also works as a volunteer Creighton Fertility Care Practitioner teaching and promoting the Creighton method of natural family planning which serves as the foundation for NaPro Technology.

The Lourdes Family Clinic provides primary medical care for family members of all ages. As a clinic seeking medical home certification,

Lourdes Family Clinic utilizes nurse care-coordination to optimally manage chronic conditions such as asthma and diabetes. The clinicians use the Creighton Model Fertility Care System as a method to monitor and maintain women's gynecological health. The clinic follows the medical and surgical methods of NaPro Technology to treat a variety of women's health problems (see Appendix A for more information on NaPro Technology). For obstetric deliveries and minimum invasive NaPro Technology surgeries for women, the clinic plans to obtain OB/Gyn physician privileges at Fairview Southdale Hospital in Edina, Fairview Ridges in Burnsville, and St. Francis Hospital in Shakopee. The founding clinicians seek to find office space in the northeastern area of Eden Prairie. The location offers convenient access to 169 and 494, a central location for the four targeted counties, and an office space price ranging from $10-22 per square feet (see Appendix C for map of location). The clinic anticipates the need for office space with at least 7,000 square feet and preferably 8,000 to 10,000 square feet.

Mission: To spread God's Kingdom of Life by providing exceptional Catholic medical care that respects the inherent dignity of the human person at all stages of life.
Vision: To become a leading center for advanced Catholic healthcare in the Midwest.
Values: Respect for human life, integrity, joy in serving.

Current practice trends:

Broad industry trends in Minnesota since the 1990s include rapid consolidation of health care clinics and systems. Large integrated delivery systems (IDSs) and health maintenance organizations (HMOs) dominate most of the medical market in Minnesota. Five years ago Park Nicollet merged with the larger HealthPartners system. Last month Fairview and HealthEast announced a new merge. Since Mayo Clinic largely operates southeast of the Twin Cities, the main three entities in the metro area include HealthPartners/Park Nicollet, Fairview/HealthEast, and Allina Health. North Memorial holds a smaller share of the market in mainly the northwestern metro region. Few independent clinics exist in Minnesota due to the difficulty of competing with these large IDSs/HMOs.

Economic trends in Minnesota mirror national and international trends towards increasing spending on healthcare. The Minnesota Health Department reports total healthcare spending in Minnesota in 2013 as $40.9 billion. Private insurance accounted for 38.3%, Medicare 19.3%, Medical Assistance 21.2%, out-of-pocket 12.4%, public spending 6.2% (MNcare, Veterans Healthcare, government worker compensation), and private 2.5% (private workers' compensation, auto medical insurance). Healthcare spending in Minnesota increased 35% from 2005 through 2015 though the Minnesota economy grew only 22%. This aligns with global trends of increased healthcare spending. The UK financial advisory firm Deloitte projects healthcare spending to increase 4.3% in North America and globally by the year 2020.

Regulatory trends in Minnesota reflect efforts made in the Affordable Care Act to improve healthcare access. Minnesota ranks as one of the states with the lowest number of uninsured persons. In the Twin-Cities metro region 63% of residents carry commercial insurance with only 9% uninsured. Minnesota passed several pieces of legislature to provide insurance coverage and medical assistance to low-income and high-risk persons. MinnesotaCare (1992) provides a state-subsidized insurance plan for persons with low to moderate incomes who fail to qualify for Medicaid but remain unable to pay for insurance. After the passage of the Affordable Care Act, Minnesota passed legislation to expand Medicaid in 2010 for adults with incomes up to 75% of Federal Poverty Level. In 2013 the state-based exchange MNsure began.

Although Minnesota consistently ranks as one of the top states in population health outcomes, the state faces similar health trends and challenges as the rest of the country such as an increase in expensive chronic conditions. The Minnesota Department of Health reports the obesity rate in 2015 as 26.1% of the population, while twenty years prior in 1995 the rate stood at 14.6% of the population. The number of persons in Minnesota with diabetes almost doubled during this twenty-year timespan. Minnesota faces a quickly aging population, with a state projection of the older adult population doubling between 2010 and 2013. A higher immigrant population reside in Minnesota with the fastest growing groups from Africa. The non-white population in the 2015 rose to 19% of the total population.

As one of the core initiatives of the 2008 Minnesota legislation Health Care Reform Act, the Health Care Home (HCH) improves health outcomes in patients with chronic or complex health conditions by promoting patient-centered care and prevention strategies. The HCH approach relies highly on care coordination to improve patient self-management. In order to receive certification as a Health Care Home, primary care clinics must meet certain HCH standards and regularly report data for evaluation and benchmarking purposes. The state compensates HCHs for care coordination if they reach the set standards goals. The Minnesota Department of Health collects data from HCHs on colorectal screening, diabetes, asthma, depression, and pediatric mental health.

Goals: Short-term goals include opening the Lourdes Family Clinic and attaining a patient volume of 13,875 in the first year. Long terms goals include expanding the clinic's operational hours to evening business hours and Saturday day hours. The clinic intends to obtain certification as a HCH within the first four years of operation. Beyond five years, the founders aim to eventually build a clinic to fit specific needs and preferences of Lourdes Family Clinic and highlight the Catholic identity of the practice.

Market and Competition Analysis

Target population: The Lourdes Family Clinic primarily targets Catholics (men, women, children, older persons) of any ethnic background in Hennepin, Scott, and Carver Counties and parts of Dakota County such as Burnsville and Lakeville (see Appendix B for map). The Catholic population in Minnesota continues to grow as more pro-life Catholic married couples give birth to a large amount of children. In the Twin Cities, an increasing number of conservative/traditional Catholic families include 7 to 10 children in their household. Along with younger growing Catholic families, Lourdes also seeks to attract older Catholic adults in the area who desire healthcare that harmonizes with their faith. The population of the sixteen-county Twin Cities region (federal government defined) consists of 3.5 million residents. Fourteen Minnesota counties and two Wisconsin counties make up the Twin Cities metro area. The population of the metro region grew by 5% from 2010 to 2015. Hennepin County contains the city of Minneapolis and surrounding suburbs, while Ramsey County contains St. Paul and surrounding suburbs. The U.S. Census Bureau estimates the 2016 Hennepin County population as 1.23 million persons. Approximately 825,000 Catholics in 187 parishes live in the 12-county area of the Archdiocese of Saint Paul and Minneapolis (2017). Approximately 215,205 Catholics (18.7% of the population) live in the target market area of Hennepin County. About 39,912 Catholics (30.7% of the population) live in Scott County and 14,887 Catholics (16.4% of the population) reside in Carver county. Potential market includes Catholics living in the northwestern metro Wright County (18,699 Catholics or 15% of population) as well as the counties to the south and west of the metro area such as Mcleod, Sibley, Nicollet, and LeSuer. Although most likely families in these more distant counties choose not to come to the clinic for primary care, perhaps Catholic women with specific women's health issues or infertile couples consider the Lourdes Family Clinic for NaPro Technology. Potential additional market includes persons belonging to other religions or no religion who desire to receive the high-quality person-centered services provided. A potential market includes particularly pro-life Protestant Christians who desire a medical clinic which practices exclusively according to pro-life values. Approximately 193,498 (16.8%) persons in Hennepin County identify as Mainline Protestants and 162,094 (14.1%) identify as Evangelical Protestants.

Competition: The competitors of the Lourdes Family Clinic in the southwestern Twin Cities area include HealthPartners/Park Nicollet, Fairview Health Systems, and Allina Health (see Appendix C). Compared to these large healthcare corporations, the Lourdes Family Clinic's advantage lies in the practice of Catholic values and the person-centered approach of a medical home. A 2011 research study funded by the Robert Wood Foundation reported clinics independently owned by physicians fared the same as large managed care system with regard to patient outcomes. Within the Catholic population in particular, the Aalfa Family Clinic in White Bear Lake comprises the main business competition. The clinic provides primary care and OB/Gyn and practices NaPro Technology. Aalfa refuses to use Electronic Medical Records (EMR) and operates with a paper charting system. Patients report long wait at the clinic for appointments. While in 2014 and 2015 reports by the nonprofit healthcare data organization MN Community Measurement ranked the Aalfa clinic's quality as average, in the latest report for 2016 the clinic dropped to below average for adult health care. Aalfa offers clinic visits Monday through Friday during day time hours.

SWOT analysis: Strengths of the Lourdes Family Clinic include the new location for a Catholic family clinic in the south-western region of the Twin Cities and a technologically up-to-date delivery of Catholic health care in the area with the use of EMR. The Lourdes Family Clinic brings a distinctive Catholic approach which respects the sacredness of human life from the moment of conception. The clinic features experienced clinicians and utilizes evidenced-based advances in women's healthcare with NaPro Technology. A weakness of Lourdes Family Clinic includes a need for funding. The clinic plans to explore options for obtaining funding for the first year of operation. Lourdes lacks the advantages that comes from a clinic with established reputation, but the clinic plans to strive for an excellent reputation. Lourdes offers similar family care services compared to the Aalfa Family Clinic and many managed care operations in the Twin Cities. Lourdes offers a limited amount of services and specialties compared to managed care competition. Opportunities exist for increased demand as young, Catholic families continue to grow and thrive in the Twin Cities. Opportunities exist for expansion in the future of hours when the clinic operates, hiring additional clinicians, and providing services for home births. Threats to Lourdes Family Clinic include robust competition with managed care healthcare groups and the Aalfa Family Clinic. Many employee insurance plans contain a preferred provider network which excludes the Lourdes Family Clinic. Several Catholic churches in the area include a large number of undocumented immigrants who lack health care insurance. Providing care for too many persons without insurance leads to an unsustainable level of financial loss (see Appendix D for SWOT chart).

Development Plan and Schedule

Services Offered

Family primary care. The Lourdes Family Clinic predominantly provides family primary care and offers same-day appointments to fill empty schedule spots. To perform these services, the clinic requires an office space with at least 8 exam rooms and preferably 10 to 12. The clinic needs basic clinic equipment such as electronic blood pressure machines, thermometers, and exam tables for each exam room. The clinic requires disposable clinic supplies such as gauze and sutures. The clinic plans to purchase an x-ray machine to perform on-site basic x-rays. The clinic will send patients to Center for Diagnostic Imaging (CDI) in nearby Eden Prairie for specialized x-rays, CT scans, MRIs, Bone Density screening, and medical ultrasounds. The clinic will contract an off-site medical laboratory to process specimens. On the technological side, the clinic requires computers and an EMR system as well office equipment such as a printer/fax machine (see Appendix E for list of direct care equipment/supply needs and training required).

Obstetric services. The clinic provides pre-natal appointments as well as vaginal and C-section deliveries at certain hospitals where our physicians hold privileges. Whether or not our physicians deliver the baby for a woman seen for pre-natal care depends on patient preference and specific circumstances at the time of labor. In addition to basic clinic equipment, the OB/Gyn physicians require handheld fetal Doppler machines for pre-natal visits. The clinic will provide OB/Gyn ultrasounds in the clinic on certain days of the week for the first three year of operation and plans to increase ultrasound hours as volume increases. On days without OB/Gyn ultrasound, the clinic will send women to CDI for ultrasonography. The Knights of Columbus graciously offered to donate an OB/Gyn ultrasound machine to the clinic.

Minimally Invasive NaPro Technology Surgeries. Dr. Fredrickson will perform outpatient NaPro Technology surgeries for women's gynecological health problems (such as endometriosis) at certain local hospitals. The hospitals possess DaVinci laser for the laparoscopic procedures. The equipment and supplies belong to the hospitals. The hospitals will also provide nursing staff and an anesthesiologist for procedures.

Development Plan

The Lourdes Family Clinic's development plan consists of strategic initiatives designed to keep the clinic on the path to achieving our goals (see Appendix F for Achievement Timeline).

Preparation: The founders intend to secure a loan for the amount needed to operate in the first two years of operation and obtain a lease for office space in the Eden Prairie suburban area. The space most likely requires some construction to transform it into a functional medical clinic site. Additionally, furnishing and decorating the space will transform it into a welcome environment. The clinic will register and comply with all regulations to obtain clinic licensure in the state of Minnesota. The CEO and Vice President plan to complete a comprehensive policy and procedure handbook to guide clinical practice by October.

Year One of Operations: The clinic intends to open on January 22, 2018, the 45th anniversary of the legalization of abortion in the United States. The founders chose this symbolic date to signify the triumph of life over death . . . the respect for life as practiced by the clinic over the tragedy of abortion. The clinic plans to open with a regular business hour schedule of Monday through Friday, 8:00 A.M. to 4:00 P.M.

Year Two of Operations: At the beginning of the second year the clinic will open evening hours two days per week, expanding the normal business hours to 8:00 P.M. on Tuesday and Wednesday. Dr. Jones agrees to change his hours to 12:00 P.M. to 8:00 P.M. for two business evening hours in the second year. This move enables the clinic to softly test patient response to evening hours. The clinic plans to hire a part-time receptionist to cover these additional hours.

Year Three of Operations: If evening hours proves successful in year two, the clinic intends to expand to Monday through Thursday evening hours at the beginning of year three. Dr. Jones will continue to work the two evenings per week and Patty-Jo Mantel, FNP, will work the other two evenings. The clinic will consider hiring an additional FNP/PA for day/evening hours depending on the demand and a part-time or full time medical assistant.

Year Four of Operations: In the fourth year, the clinic plans to open Saturday clinic hours 8:00 A.M. to 2:00 P.M. and hire staff as needed for this new work day. If not accomplished in the third year, the clinic will hire a FNP/PA to cover Saturday and evening hours. Doctors Jones and Smith agree to alternate working on Saturdays instead of a weekday in the beginning of the fourth year. Depending on demand trends, the clinic will consider hiring an additional physician or mid-wife. Utilizing a mid-wife to assume more of the normal vaginal births frees Dr. Fredrickson to concentrate on high-risk pregnancies and NaPro Technology surgeries. The clinic aims to attain HCH certification by the end of year four.

Marketing Plan

The clinic plans to print a brochure about Lourdes Family Clinic prior to opening day and distributing the brochure at Catholic parishes and schools in the three targeted counties. Along with the brochure, the clinic intends to advertise the open house three months in advance in parish bulletins and on the local Catholic radio station Relevant Radio starting at the beginning of October 2017. The clinic will encourage word-of-mouth patient recommendations by giving patients who come to our clinic an extra brochure along with an invitation for them to distribute to one person they know. The clinic also plans to place weekly regular advertisements in Catholic church bulletins. The founders and spouses/children of the founders plan to advertise the clinic at various Catholic conferences and events in the Twin Cities throughout the year. Many Catholic events take place in the Twin Cities, providing an opportunity to obtain a booth to promote Lourdes Family Clinic by distributing brochures and speak to persons about the Lourdes Family Clinic. The clinic will advertise on the local Catholic radio station Relevant Radio as well. The budget for marketing consists of $10,000 for initial advertising with the printing of a brochure and Relevant Radio advertisement, and $10,000 for each year.

Organizational Plan

Organizational Chart (See Appendix G)
Staff Analysis

The Chief Executive Officer (CEO) exercises responsibility for the overall viability of the clinic with the assistance of the Vice President (VP). The CEO provides general management of employees, oversees the lease and loan contracts, and clinic policies. The VP assumes responsibility for marketing and also heads the physicians and mid-level providers, assuring quality of clinician care. As the founders of The Lourdes Family Clinic, Dr. Jones and Dr. Smith agree to forego any compensation for the CEO or Vice President position in order to decrease spending costs. The clinic manager heads the daily activities of the clinic by budgeting, scheduling, hiring, managing service contracts, and ordering equipment and supplies. The manager monitors appointment volume, revenue, and patient satisfaction, working to ensure the clinic meets financial and quality goals. Physicians and mid-level practitioners provide comprehensive direct patient care by examining, diagnosing, and treating patients with a variety of diseases and conditions. The RN coordinates care for patients with chronic conditions and works to assure the clinic reaches outcome goals in compliance with the Minnesota Health Department in order to attain certification as a Medical Care Home. The RN Care Coordinator also oversees work of the medical assistants and ultrasound technician. The receptionist schedules patient appointments, obtains the necessary insurance information for billing purposes. The Billing specialist covers the financial workings of the clinic, assuring that the clinic receives the agreed payment for services and negotiates with third-party insurances. The billing specialist also handles medical records requests. A coding specialist assures accurate coding for billing integrity and in order that the clinic obtains the maximum amount of revenue for services provided. The medical assistant performs a variety of clinic tasks such as guiding the patient to the exam room, taking weight/height and vital signs, giving immunizations, drawing blood, cleaning exam rooms after use. The ultrasound technician obtains ultrasound images of women's pelvic area for perinatal and gynecological purposes.

Qualifications for key personnel

CEO: Qualifications include physician licensure in good standing, at least five years of clinical experience, excellent communication skills, passion for Catholic bioethics. Ability to lead and work effectively as a team to reach clinic goals.

Vice President: Qualifications or a Vice President include clinician (physician/APRN/PA) licensure in good standing, at least five years of clinical experience, excellent communication skills, passion for Catholic bioethics.

Clinic manager/scheduler: Bachelor's degree in business or healthcare administration. Previous management experience and at least five years of experience working in the healthcare industry. Familiarity with medical terminology, practices, and procedures. Excellent judgement to plan and achieve goals. Computer proficiency.

Physician:
Family Practice: Successful completion of an accredited Family Medicine Residency with 2 years or more of experience. Current board certification by the American Board of Family Medicine (ABFM) or the American Osteopathic Board of Family Medicine (AOBFM). Unencumbered license to practice medicine as a MD/DO in the state of Minnesota. DEA certificate. Insurability (malpractice). BLS/ACLS. Experience with EMR.

OB/Gyn: Successful completion of an OB/Gyn Residency Program with 2 years or more of experience. Current board certification by the American Board of Family Medicine (ABFM) or the American Osteopathic Board of Family Medicine (AOBFM). Board certified or eligible in Obstetrics and Gynecology. Unencumbered license to practice medicine as a MD/DO in the state of Minnesota. DEA certificate. Insurability (malpractice). BLS/ACLS certified. Experience with EMR.

APRN/PA: Completion of an accredited master's program in nursing or physician assistant program. AANP, ANCC, or NCCPA certified. Minnesota APRN or PA license and DEA. BLS/ACLS certified. Experience with EMR.

RN Care Coordinator: BSN in nursing from an accredited college or university. Current RN license in the state of Minnesota. At least three years of clinical nursing experience. EMR experience. BLS certified. Patient advocacy and case management experience. Critical thinking and patient motivational/coaching skills.

Receptionist: High school graduate of GED. Prior experience in a medical clinic preferred. Experience with medical terminology preferred. Interpersonal and communication skills. Strong customer service and phone skills. Exceptional organizational skills and attention to detail.

Billing specialist: Minimum of two-year degree in accounting/finance, four-year degree preferred. CPC certified. Minimum two years of billing experience in a health care setting. Excellent computer skills including

Microsoft Office suite. Excellent organizational skills and ability to meet deadlines.

Coding specialist: Credentialed by RHIA, RHIT, or CCS-P. Possess expertise in the ICD-10 and CPT coding systems. Minimum of two years related coding experience directly applying codes.

Medical Assistant: Medical Assistant diploma from an accredited vocational institution or community college. National certification as a registered medical assistant preferred. Previous experience in family medicine preferred. BLS certified.

Ultrasound technician: Vocational/Technical training or college degree. Registered by American Registry for the Diagnostic Medical Sonography (ARDMS). OB/Gyn credentials required. NT certification preferred. Minimum of two years' experience as an OB Ultrasonographer. BLS certified.

Financial Plan

Volume:

The founders project a patient volume of 13,875 the first year and predict an increase volume rate of approximately 15% for the first four years. The number of women who come for pre-natal visits remains difficult to foresee, as with the number of women choosing our physicians for delivery or laparoscopic gynecological surgery. The Lourdes Family Clinic remains ready to respond to decreased or increased service demand. For the first several months, Dr. Fredrickson agrees to work three days per week and increase hours according to demand. The clinic budgeted Dr. Fredrickson for full-time the first year in order to account for expense. Likewise, the FNP agrees to work part-time three days per week the first several months and increase hours to full-time according to patient volume.

Type of patient	Volume per day yr 1	Volume per day yr 2	Volume per day yr 3	Volume per day yr 4	Total volume yr 1	Total volume yr 2	Total volume yr 3	Total volume yr 4
Medical	49.0	56.0	68.0	75.0	12348	14112	17136	21000
Pre-natal visits	6	7	8	9	1512	1764	2016	2250
Outpatient surgeries	0.04	0.07	0.13	0.25	10.20	17.85	33.15	63.75
Vaginal births	0.02	0.14	0.2	0.3	5.10	35.70	51.00	76.50
C-sections	0	0.011	0.019	0.025	0.00	2.81	4.85	6.38
Total medical & prenatal visits, births, and surgeries					13875	15932	19241	23397
Patient volume per month					1156	1327	1603	1949

Clinical service mix: Family medicine primary care 90%, OB/Gyn 10%.

Market and payer mix: 80% private insurance, 12% Medicare, 5% bad debt/charity, 2% cash payment, 1% Medicaid/MNSure.

Information Technology requirements: The Lourdes Family Clinic plans to use the eClinicalWorks EMR system and considers this a vital investment for the success of the clinic. eClinicalWorks ranks as the second most widely used EMR system in Minnesota (after the hospital system Epic) and accounts for 9% of the market share. eClinicalWorks includes EMR, eprescribing and formula checking, practice management that includes a scheduling system, billing services, and a Patient Portal for patient online access of health records and self-scheduling. The system costs $599 per month for each provider with no start-up costs. If the clinic decides in the future for more advanced Revenue Cycle Management (RCM), eClinicalWorks offers a RCM total service for 2.9% of practice collections. This price falls well below many other companies offering similar services.

	Year 1	Year 2	Year 3	Year 4
EMR cost per year	$28,752	$28,752	$35,940	$43,128

Profit margin requirement:

With our advanced EMR and billing system, the Lourdes Family Clinic aims at a high net profit margin of 0.95.

	Year 1	Year 2	Year 3	Year 4
Net Revenue	$1,876,681	$2,162,625	$2,600,345	$3,186,775
Total (gross) Revenue	$1,965,980	$2,221,141	$2,674,619	$3,283,575
Net Profit Margin	0.95	0.97	0.97	0.97

In the first year, the gross profit margin calculates to as negative at (−5.87%). In the second year, the gross profit margin crosses to the positive side at 11.22% and continues rising through the fourth year.

	Year 1	Year 2	Year 3	Year 4
Total costs	$2,081,405	$1,972,015	$2,299,727	$2,541,112
Total (gross) Revenue	$1,965,980	$2,221,141	$2,674,619	$3,283,575
Gross profit	(−115,425)	$249,126	$374,892	$742,463
Gross Profit Margin	(−5.87%)	11.22%	14.02%	22.61%

Total revenues:

Projected net revenue in year one equals $1.7 million dollars, which increases in year two by $300,000. In year three revenue increases by $438,000 compared to the second year, and in year four increases by $586,000 compared to the third year. This demonstrates a steady increase in net revenue for the clinic as total volume increases (See Appendix H for complete gross revenue chart).

Year	Average patients per day	Total Volume	Projected Gross Revenue (GR)	Projected inflation	Inflation Amount	GR with inflation	Minus 5% bad debt	Projected Net Revenue
1	55.0	13875	$1,965,980	N/A	N/A	$1,965,980	$98,299	$1,867,681
2	63.0	15932	$2,221,141	2.49%*	$55,306	$2,276,447	$113,822	$2,162,625
3	76.0	19241	$2,674,619	2.34%	$62,586	$2,737,205	$136,860	$2,600,345
4	84.0	23397	$3,283,575	2.16%	$70,925	$3,354,500	$167,725	$3,186,775

*(Statista, 2017)

Direct and indirect expenses:

Direct Costs	Year 1	Year 2	Year 3	Year 4
Direct medical care salaries	$1,362,306	$1,362,306	$1,540,003	$1,717,700
Medical supplies/stock drugs	$75,000	$100,000	$150,000	$175,000
Equipment depreciation		$40,000	$40,000	$40,000
Medical waste	$3,000	$4,000	$5,000	$6,000
Hospital privileges	$3,000	$3,000	$3,000	$3,000
Direct care equipment (see Appendix E)	$86,570			
Telephones for medical purposes	$2,500			
Continuing medical education/staff training	$20,000	$20,000	$20,000	$20,000
Malpractice insurance	$55,000	$55,000	$60,000	$65,000
Total direct costs	$1,532,376	$1,509,306	$1,738,003	$1,941,700

Indirect Costs	Year 1	Year 2	Year 3	Year 4
Building lease	$120,000	$120,000	$120,000	$120,000
Business liability insurance	$15,000	$15,000	$15,000	$15,000
Utilities	30,000	$30,000	$30,000	$30,000
Administrative salaries	$107,957	$115,957	$123,957	$132,957
Admin. contract labor	$35,000	$43,000	$51,000	$60,000
Janitorial services	$1,500	$1,500	$1,500	$1,500
Interest on loan	$0	$0	$62,172	$62,172
Security system	$500	$500	$500	$500
Office supplies	$12,000	$15,000	$18,000	$21,000
Printing/mailing	$12,000	$15,000	$18,000	$21,000
Answering service	$4,000	$4,500	$5,000	$5,500
Marketing	$10,000	$10,000	$10,000	$10,000
Legal services	$5,000	$5,000	$5,000	$5,000
Indirect care equipment (see Appendix E)	$11,200			
Total indirect costs	$364,157	$375,457	$460,129	$484,629
Total direct & indirect costs	$1,896,533	$1,884,763	$2,198,132	$2,426,329

Fixed & variable expenses:

	Costs	Year 1	Year 2	Year 3	Year 4
FIXED COSTS	Lease	$120,000	$120,000	$120,000	$120,000
	Salaries (see Appendix J)	$1,435,263	$1,435,263	$1,612,960	$1,790,657
	Licenses and permits	$7,000	$7,000	$7,000	$7,000
	Business liability insurance	$15,000	$15,000	$15,000	$15,000
	Malpractice insurance	$55,000	$55,000	$60,000	$65,000
	Loan interest	$11,102	$11,102	$11,102	$11,102
	Hospital privileges	$3,000	$3,000	$3,000	$3,000
	Legal services	$5,000	$5,000	$5,000	$5,000
	Credentialing service			$155	$155
	Continuing medical education	$20,000	$20,000	$20,000	$25,000
	Internet	$3,000	$3,000	$3,000	$3,000
	EMR	$28,752	$28,752	$35,940	$43,128
	Janitorial services	$2,000	$2,000	$2,000	$2,000
	Website	$5,000	$5,000	$5,000	$5,000
	Maintenance and repairs	$5,000	$5,000	$5,000	$5,000
	Security system	$500	$500	$500	$500
	Magazine subscriptions	$500	$500	$500	$500
	Marketing	$10,000	$10,000	$10,000	$10,000
	Staff education/training	$10,000	$10,000	$10,000	$10,000
	Furniture/equipment depreciation		$40,000	$40,000	$40,000
	Start-up costs (see Appendix I)	$199,890			
	Total fixed costs	$1,910,405	$1,750,515	$2,002,727	$2,192,612
VARIABLE COSTS and SEMI-VARIABLE COSTS	Variable costs				
	Medical supplies/stock drugs	$75,000	$100,000	$150,000	$175,000
	Office supplies	$12,000	$15,000	$18,000	$21,000
	Printing/mailing	$12,000	$15,000	$18,000	$21,000
	Medical waste	$3,000	$4,000	$5,000	$6,000
	Semi-variable costs				
	Utilities	$30,000	$40,000	$50,000	$60,000
	Answering service	$4,000	$4,500	$5,000	$5,500
	Contract labor	$35,000	$43,000	$51,000	$60,000
	Total variable/semi-variable costs	$171,000	$221,500	$297,000	$348,500
	TOTAL COSTS	$2,081,405	$1,972,015	$2,299,727	$2,541,112

Total expenses:

Year (A)	Inflation (B)	Fixed Expenses (C)	Variable Expenses (D)	Loan Payoff (E)	Total of C - E	Inflation Amount	Total Expenses with inflation
1	N/A	$1,910,405	$171,000		$2,081,405	N/A	$2,081,405
2	2.49%*	$1,750,515	$221,500		$1,972,015	$49,103	$2,021,118
3	2.34%	$2,002,727	$297,000	$62,172	$2,361,899	$55,268	$2,417,167
4	2.16%	$2,192,612	$348,500	$62,172	$2,603,284	$56,231	$2,659,515

*(Statista, 2017)

Break-even analysis chart:

Year	1	2	3	4
Projected Volume	13875	15932	19241	23397
Projected Net Revenue	$1,867,681	$2,162,625	$2,600,345	$3,186,775
Projected Expenses	$2,081,405	$2,021,118	$2,417,167	$2,659,515

The projected break-even point occurs at approximately 19 months of operation, which corresponds to an accumulated patient volume of 23,000 patient visits/encounters. After this time the projected net revenue surpasses the expenses. By the end of the fourth year with an accumulated patient volume of 49,000 the net revenue surpasses the expenses by approximately $527,000.

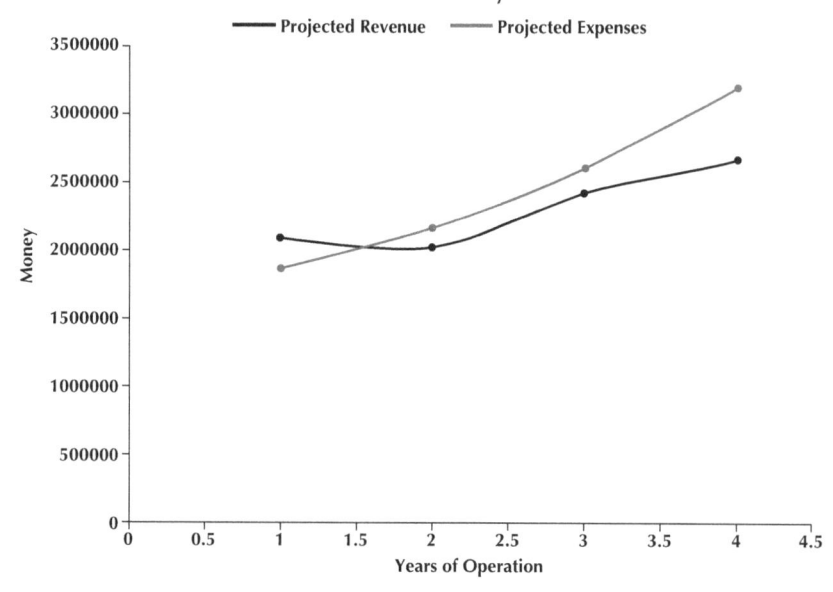

Break-Even Analysis Chart

Financing the Lourdes Family Clinic:

In order to achieve the goals of the new clinic, the Lourdes Family Clinic will secure a small business loan for the capital needed to start the clinic and sustain it until the clinic subsists on its own revenue at 19 months. The founders plan to acquire a new business loan of $500,000. This covers the initial start-up costs of $199,890 as well as expenses for the first four months and provides a comfortable level of capital for expenses beyond the net revenue for the first 19 months. The payment for the loan begins in the third year of operation. Estimates for the cost of a 10-year term loan of $500,000 at an interest rate of 4.50% equals $5,182 per month or $62,184 per year (Calculator.net, 2017).

References

Archdiocese of Saint Paul and Minneapolis. (2017). About the archdiocese. Retrieved from www.archspm.org/about-us/

Association of Statisticians of American Religious Bodies. (2010). 2010 U.S. religion census: religious congregations & membership study. Retrieved from www.city-data.com

Calculator.net (2017). Loan Calculator. Retrieved from http://www.calculator.net/loan-calculator.html?cloanamount=500000&cloanterm=10&cloantermmonth=0&cinterestrate=4.50&ccompound=monthly&cpayback=month&x=93&y=9

Deloitte. (2017). 2017 global health care outlook. Retrieved from https://www2.deloitte.com/global/en/pages/life-sciences-and-healthcare/articles/global-health-care-sector-outlook.html

Kralewsit, J.E., Dowd, B.E., & Xu, Y. (2011). Differences in the cost of health care provided by group practices in Minnesota. *Minnesota Medicine, 2*, 41-44.

Minnesota Business Partnership. (2015, January). Minnesota's health care performance scorecard. Retrieved from mnbp.com/wp-content/uploads/2015/02/MBP_Health-Scorecard.pdf

Minnesota Department of Health. (2016). Minnesota health care markets chartbook. Retrieved from http://www.health.state.mn.us/divs/hpsc/hep/chartbook/

Minnesota State Demographic Center. (2017). Aging. Retrieved from https://mn.gov/admin/demography/data-by-topic/aging/

MN Community Measurement. (2017). 2016 cost & utilization report. Retrieved from http://mncm.org/wp-content/uploads/2016/12/16CostUtilityReport.pdf

The Pew Research Center. (2016, September 28). Where the public stands on religious liberty vs. nondiscrimination. Retrieved from http://www.pewforum.org/2016/09/28/4-very-few-americans-see-contraception-as-morally-wrong/

Beal, D. (2013, March 22). MN's independent doctors are in critical condition. Retrieved from http://tcbmag.com/Industries/Health-Care/Minnesota-s-Independent-Doctors-Are-in-Critical-Co

Statista (2017). Projected annual inflation rate in the United States from 2008 to 2021. Retrieved from https://www.statista.com/statistics/244983/projected-inflation-rate-in-the-united-states/

United Status Census Bureau. (2017). American Fact Finder. Retrieved from https://factfinder.census.gov/faces/nav/jsf/pages/index.xhtml

Appendix A—Explanation of the Creighton Model Fertility Care and NaPro Technology

Nationally known as a researched and method of natural fertility-awareness, the Creighton Model Fertility Care assists women to either obtain or delay pregnancy. The Creighton Model also serves as a valuable tool to gauge women's gynecological health through the objective evaluation of the appearance of biomarkers during a women's menstrual and fertility cycles. Dr. Thomas Hilgers created the Creighton Model and Natural Procreative Technology (NaPro Technology) as the fruit of thirty years of research and practice at the Pope Paul VI Institute in Omaha, Nebraska. The Creighton Model serves as a foundation for the new women's health science of NaPro Technology. NaPro Technology uses medical and surgical treatments that work in harmony with the female reproductive system rather suppress it. NaPro Technology possesses a high rate of success in treating women's health problems such as menstrual cramps, post-partum depression, irregular cycles, irregular bleeding, recurrent ovarian cysts, endometriosis, and infertility. While modern women's health and reproductive medicine treat symptoms and neglect to find the causes, NaPro Technology successfully analyzes the underlying pathophysiology to discover the root causes and target them with evidenced-based treatments. For more information, see http://www.naprotechnology.com.

Appendix B—Strategic location for Lourdes Family Clinic

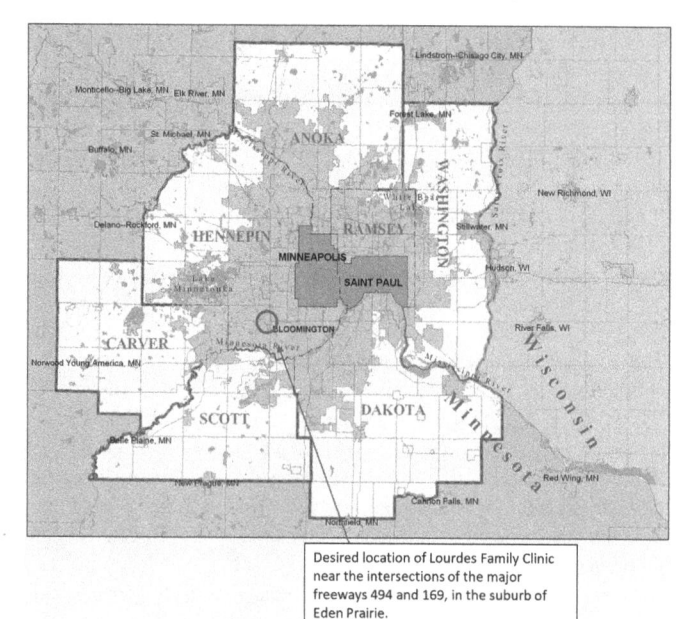

Desired location of Lourdes Family Clinic near the intersections of the major freeways 494 and 169, in the suburb of Eden Prairie.

Appendix C—List of Services Provided by the Competition

Health System/Clinic	Services and Location
Health Partners (HP) & Park Nicollet (PN)	• PN family practice clinic in Eden Prairie • HP family practice clinic in east Bloomington • PN family practice clinic in west Bloomington • PN family clinic, urgent care, multiple specialties near Methodist Hospital in St. Louis Park • PN family clinic, urgent care, multiple specialties in Burnsville and Chanhassen • PN women's center in St. Louis Park
Fairview Health System	• Fairview clinic in Eden Prairie with family practice, gynecology, pediatrics • Urgent care in downtown Bloomington • Fairview Southdale Hospital in Edina with many clinics and specialties surrounding the hospital • Fairview women's center in Edina
North Memorial	• Family practice clinic in Eden Prairie
Allina Health	• Family practice clinics in Bloomington, Edina, Chanhassen, Shakopee, Burnsville, Hopkins.
Aalfa Family Clinic	• Primary care, urgent care, OB/Gyn in White Bear Lake

Appendix D—SWOT Chart for Lourdes Family Clinic

Strengths	Weaknesses
• *Location*: Lourdes Family Clinic offers pro-life, Catholic family and OB/Gyn care primary care in the southern Hennepin County area. • *Technology*: Lourdes Family Clinic practices as the first Catholic healthcare clinic in the Twin Cities with convenient, efficient EMR. • *Values*: Lourdes Family Clinic practices medicine according to pro-life, Catholic values. • Experience: Educated, experienced clinicians work at Lourdes Family Clinic. • *Advanced services*: Lourdes Family Clinic offers gynecology with an advanced NaPro Technology approach.	• *Lack of capital*: Lourdes Family Clinic requires investments to fund the first year of operation. • *Similarity*: Lourdes Family Clinic provides similar services as Aalfa Family Clinic including NaPro Technology, and similar family—OB/Gyn services to many non-Catholic clinics in the Minneapolis area. • *Lack of service depth*: Lourdes Family Clinic practices limited services/specialties. • *Lack of reputation*: As a new clinic, Lourdes Family Clinic lacks an established reputation.
Opportunities	**Threats**
• *Area growth*: Growing population of young conservative/traditional Catholic families. • *Congestion in competition*: Crowded normal business hour clinic visits at Aalfa Family Clinic. • *Lack of technology use in competition*: Use of paper charting rather than EMR at Aalfa Family Clinic. • *Quality rating of competition*: Aalfa Family Clinic rates below average in adult care. • *Expansion*: Possibility for evening and Saturday hour appointments and the hiring of additional clinicians.	• *Competition*: Aalfa Family Clinic and many large, managed care healthcare groups in the area. • *Insurance companies*: Employee insurance which excludes Lourdes Family Clinic from their network of preferred providers. • *Charity services*: Many undocumented Catholic immigrants in the Twin Cities possibly leads to an amount of fiscally unsustainable charity care given. • *Medicare, Medicaid, MNsure*: A possibly unexpected higher patient mix of Medicaid and MNsure patients. Unknown number of Medicare patients, and amount of Medicare patients with supplemental 3rd party insurance.

Appendix E—Offered Services with Required Equipment

	Service	Equipment Needed	Cost	Initial Staff Requirements	Staff Training
Direct Care Equipment and Costs	Family Practice	Digital x-ray	$30,000	2 Physicians (one OB/Gyn certified) 1 FNP 1 RN 3 MA's	MA's training on the x-ray, EKG machine, spirometry machine, scales, BP machine, thermometer. MA's trained in supplies for blood draws, laboratory collection. MA training in rooming patients and cleaning rooms. All staff training on computers and EMR according to role. MD/FNP trained in viewing x-ray, EKG, spirometry results. RN training on requirements for Minnesota Health Care Home certification, including the clinical outcomes measured and the necessary results to obtain certification.
		Lead walls for x-ray	$3000		
		Radiology supplies	$500		
		Blood pressure machine(10)	$5500		
		EKG machine	$2000		
		Spirometry machine	$2241		
		Pulse oximeter (3)	$1359		
		Ophthalmoscope/ Otoscope (10)	$8400		
		Baby scale	$1280		
		Thermometer (10)	$3000		
		Standing scale	$1200		
		Medication/vaccine refrigerator	$1500		
		Miscellaneous equipment	$3000		
		18 computers for exam rooms, providers, RN, Mas	$18,000		
		Telephones for medical purposes	$2500		
	Obstetric services	OB doppler (2)	$1268	1 OB/GYN physician 1 Medical Assistant 1 Ultrasound tech RNs/anesthesiologist at hospital	MD training in Doppler use, birthing equipment at hospital. Medical Assistant training (in addition to duties above), specific training in rooming OB patients. Certified ultrasound technician training on ultrasound machine.
		Ultrasound	Donation		
		Basic office supplies	Listed under family practice		
		Birthing equipment	Provided by hospital		
	Minimally Invasive NaPro Technology Surgeries		$40,000	$40,000	The receptionist requires training in the computers and EMR, including entering patient insurance information and scheduling patient appointments. The receptionist also needs training in using the credit card processor to obtain co-pays and private pay revenue, and how to use the phone and copier/fax machine. The billing specialist and coder require training in the computer, obtaining insurance/code information in the EMR.
Indirect Care Equipment and Costs	Family Practice and OB/Gyn services	HP LaserJet all-in-one printer	$2,000	1 Clinic Manager 1 Receptionist 1 Billing Specialist 1 contracted coder	
		Office computers	$7000		
		Credit card scanners (2)	$700		
		Administrative telephones	$1500		

Appendix F—Achievement Timeline

	Milestone	Start Date	End Date	Person/s Responsible
Preparation	Obtain initial investors	5/1/2017	12/31/2017	CEO
	Obtain Small Business Loan	8/1/2017	10/1/2017	CEO
	Decide on Practice Site	5/1/2017	8/1/2017	CEO/VP
	Secure Lease	8/2/2017	10/1/17	CEO
	Legal entity established	5/1/2017	11/1/2017	Vice President
	Clinic Construction	10/2/2017	11/15/2017	Vice President
	Redecorate and furnish clinic	11/15/2017	11/30/2017	Vice President
	Obtain medical equipment and supplies	6/1/2017	11/30/2017	Clinic manager
	Obtain office equipment and supplies	6/1/2017	11/30/2017	Clinic manager
	Secure Staff	5/1/2017	12/1/2017	CEO
	Launch website	10/1/2017	12/1/2017	Vice President
	Install and test EMR system	12/1/2017	1/5/2017	CEO
	Obtain hospital privileges	9/1/2017	10/1/2017	Vice President
	Complete policy and procedure handbook	6/1/2017	10/1/2017	CEO/VP
	Employee training	1/8/2018	1/19/2018	CEO/VP
	Finish printed material	6/1/2017	10/1/2017	Vice President
	Develop radio advertisement	6/1/2017	10/1/207	Vice President
	Start pre-opening marketing with distributing brochures and radio advertisement	10/1/2017	1/21/2018	Vice President
	Hold open house	1/16/2018	1/16/2018	CEO
Year One	Begin first appointments	1/22/2018	1/22/2018	CEO
	Reach 1,156 appointments per month	2/22/2019	1/20/2019	Clinic manager
Year Two	Begin two days of evening appointments	1/21/2019	1/21/2019	CEO
	Hire part-time Medical Assistant and receptionist as needed	1/21/2019	1/21/2019	Clinic manager
	Reach 1,327 appointments per month	9/30/2019	9/30/2019	Clinic manager
Year Three	Begin Mon-Thurs evening appointments	10/1/2019	10/1/2019	CEO
	Hire NP or Mid-wife according to demand	10/1/2019	9/30/2020	Clinic manager/CEO
	Hire part-time Medical Assistant and receptionist if needed	10/1/2019	9/30/2020	Clinic manager
	Reach 1,603 appointments per month	9/30/2020	9/30/2020	Clinic manager
Year Four	Begin Saturday appointments	10/1/2020	10/1/2020	CEO
	Obtain HCH certification	10/1/2020	10/1/2020	RN
	Hire NP or Mid-wife or physician according to needs	10/1/2020	9/30/2021	Clinic manager/CEO
	Reach 1,950 appointments per month	9/30/2021	9/30/2021	Clinic manager

Appendix G—Organizational Chart

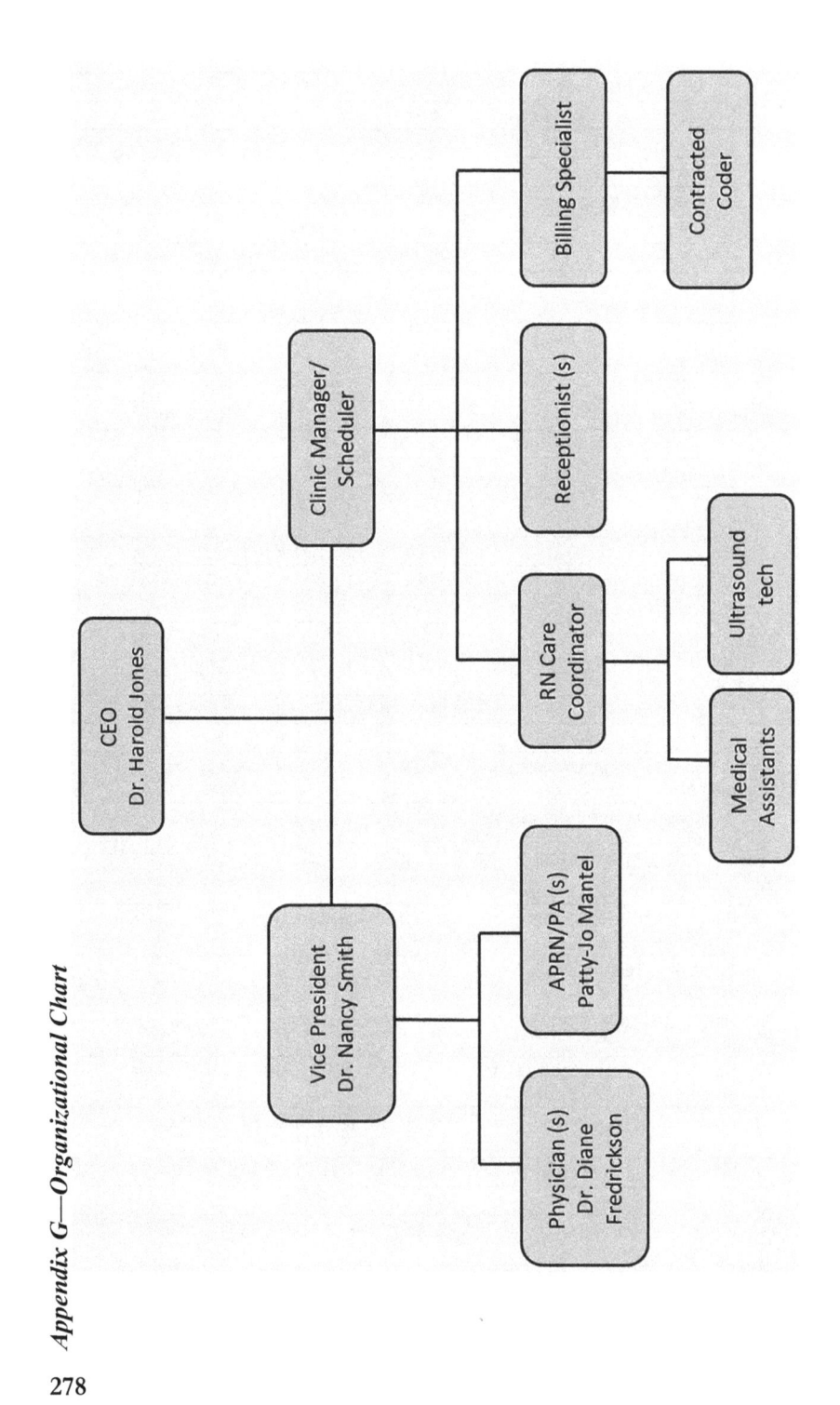

```
                          CEO
                     Dr. Harold Jones
                            |
          ┌─────────────────┴─────────────────┐
   Vice President                    Clinic Manager/
   Dr. Nancy Smith                      Scheduler
          |                                 |
   ┌──────┴──────┐              ┌───────────┼───────────┐
Physician(s)  APRN/PA(s)   RN Care      Receptionist(s)  Billing
Dr. Diane     Patty-Jo     Coordinator                   Specialist
Fredrickson   Mantel           |                             |
                        ┌──────┴──────┐                 Contracted
                     Medical      Ultrasound              Coder
                     Assistants      tech
```

278

Appendix H—Complete Gross Revenue Chart

Procedure	Volume Year 1	Volume Year 2	Volume Year 3	Volume Year 4	Average Revenue per procedure	Revenue Year 1	Revenue Year 2	Revenue Year 3	Revenue Year 4
New patient 20 min	2100	800	800	800	$140	$294,000	$112,000	$112,000	$112,000
New patient 30 min	900	500	500	500	$175	$157,500	$87,500	$87,500	$87,500
New patient 45 min	10	10	10	10	$250	$2,500	$2,500	$2,500	$2,500
Established pt 10 min	500	800	900	1000	$75	$37,500	$60,000	$67,500	$75,000
Established pt 15 min	3228	5482	7606	10370	$110	$355,080	$603,020	$836,660	$1,140,700
Established pt 25 min	800	1200	1500	1600	$135	$108,000	$162,000	$202,500	$216,000
Established pt 40 min	10	20	20	20	$155	$1,550	$3,100	$3,100	$3,100
Preventative < 1 yr	1,000	1100	1200	1400	$130	$130,000	$143,000	$156,000	$182,000
Preventative 1 to 4 yr	800	900	1000	1100	$135	$104,000	$117,000	$130,000	$143,000
Preventative 5 to 11 yr	600	700	800	900	$140	$84,000	$98,000	$112,000	$126,000
Preventative 12 to 17 yr	600	700	800	900	$150	$90,000	$105,000	$120,000	$135,000
Preventative 18 to 39 yr	500	500	500	600	$160	$80,000	$80,000	$80,000	$96,000
Preventative 40 to 64 yr	600	600	600	700	$200	$120,000	$120,000	$120,000	$140,000
Preventative > 65	700	800	900	1100	$210	$147,000	$168,000	$189,000	$231,000
Pre-natal visits	1512	1764	2016	2250	$150	$226,800	$264,600	$302,400	$337,500
Outpatient Gyn surgery	10.2	17.85	33.15	63.75	$2,000	$20,400	$35,700	$66,300	$127,500
Vaginal birth	5.10	35.70	51.00	76.50	$1,500	$7,650	$53,550	$76,500	$114,750
C-sections	0	2.81	4.85	6.38	$2,200	$0	$6,171	$10,659	$14,025
					TOTAL GROSS REVENUE	$1,965,980	$2,221,141	$2,674,619	$3,283,575

279

Appendix I—Start-up Costs

	Start-up Costs
Initial lease	$12,000
Renovation	$30,000
License/permit	$5,000
Credentialing	$1,120
Website	$500
Frontpoint security	$500
Opening celebration	$500
Brochure/initial marketing	$10,000
Staff training	$20,000
Digital x-ray	$30,000
Room build out for x-ray (lead walls)	$3,000
Radiology supplies	$500
Blood pressure machines (10)	$5,500
EKG machine	$2,000
Spirometry machine	$2,241
OB doppler (2)	$1,268
Pulse oximeter (3)	$1,359
Ophthalmoscope/Otoscope (10)	$8,400
Baby scale	$1,280
Thermometers (10)	$3,000
Standing scale	$1,022
HP LaserJet Enterprise all-in-one printer	$2,000
Office/Exam room furniture	$25,000
Telephones	$2,500
Computers	$25,000
Employee refrigerator	$1,500
Medication/vaccine refrigerator	$1,500
Electronic time clock	$500
Credit card scanner (2)	$700
Miscellaneous equipment	$2,000
TOTAL START-UP COSTS	**$199,890**

Appendix J—Projected Payroll

Staff	Base Salary	24%	MN Tax	Total to Hire	Year 1 Total	Year 2 Total	Year 3 Total	Year 4 Total
OB/Gyn surgeon	$230,000	$55,200	$11,377	$296,577	$296,577	$296,577	$296,577	$296,577
Physicians	$190,000	$45,600	$10,652	$246,252	$492,504	$492,504	$492,504	$492,504
APRN	$95,000	$22,800	$7,817	$125,617	$125,617	$125,617	$251,234	$376,851
Clinic Manager	$65,000	$15,600	$5,522	$86,122	$86,122	$86,122	$86,122	$86,122
RN	$65,000	$15,600	$5,522	$86,122	$86,122	$86,122	$86,122	$86,122
Medical Assistant	$35,000	$8,400	$3,227	$46,627	$173,600	$173,600	$217,000	$260,400
Receptionist	$35,000	$8,400	$3,227	$46,627	$43,400	$43,400	$52,080.0	$60,760.0
Billing Specialist	$55,000	$13,200	$4,757	$72,957	$72,957	$72,957	$72,957	$72,957
Ultrasound tech	$25,000	$6,000	$2,364	$33,364	$33,364	$33,364	$33,364	$33,364
Overtime/Misc.					$25,000	$25,000	$25,000	$25,000
				Total salary costs	$1,435,263	$1,435,263	$1,612,960	$1,790,657
Coder (contract)					$30,000	$35,000	$40,000	$45,000
Tax accountant (contract)					$5,000	$8,000	$11,000	$15,000

Lourdes Family Clinic Business plan completed by Patty-Jo Mantel, FNP-BC, on April 28, 2017

There are two common pitfalls that occur when writing the executive summary (Johnson, 1988). First, it is critical to avoid highly technical, complicated terminology and acronyms. Writing with simple, easy-to-understand terms makes it easier for potential investors to understand the thinking behind the business plan. Second, it is important to avoid writing an excessively long executive summary. Investors and top executives are extremely busy, and they value a crisp executive summary that clearly shows the promise and potential of the proposed business venture.

Package the Business Plan Professionally

While the content of a successful business plan is paramount, the reality is that packaging really matters. The "look and feel" of a business plan must be formal and professional and not conversational. The good news for new nurse executives is that there are many templates, samples, and software available on-line for writing business plans. However, every executive who is writing a business plan must make important aesthetic decisions about the plan's layout. There must be logic, consistency, and coherence throughout the document in the headers, footers, font choices, titles and subtitles, charts, tables, graphics, spacing, borders, and capitalization. The writing must be clear, concise, and free of any contractions, colloquial terms, and acronyms. The business plan should not include any of the "bells and whistles" available today with computer programs. This includes overly complex and distracting graphics, the use of any fluorescent or neon colors that appear unnaturally bright, and color spreading, which blurs the edges of a graphic. To ensure a typo-free, easily read document, it is essential that the final editing of a draft of a business plan (copied in black and white) be completed by a professional editor with extensive experience editing business documents.

Chapter Takeaways

1. This chapter provides the classic framework for building a C-Suite business case and includes the essential information that comprises a successful business plan.

2. DNP nurse executives who are inexperienced with business planning should consider developing partnerships with financial experts who can assist with the preparation of data reports and with professional editors who can prepare the final copy of the business plan.

3. The formatting of a business plan can enhance or distract from the content of a business plan.

Chapter Summary

In 2015, Health and Human Services Secretary Sylvia Burwell announced the agency's goal to shift 50% of payments to value-based models by 2018 (Rappleye, 2015). "Whether you are a patient, a provider, a business, a health plan, or a taxpayer, it is in our common interest to build a healthcare system that delivers better care, spends healthcare dollars more wisely and results in healthier people," said Burwell. These expectations characterize the business environment of health care today, in which new nurse executives have opportunities to leverage their business skills for improving the quality of patient care, the hospital's bottom line, and the health of the nation. The classic framework for business planning described in this chapter details the step-by-step process through which DNP prepared nurse executives can obtain support and funding for reform initiatives. For these C-suite executives, business planning provides the path for success—a path that uses innovation and large-scale organizational change to achieve business success. Appendixes A–J contain the abbreviated business plan for an ambulatory practice family clinic.

Chapter Reflection Questions

1. In what ways has health care today become big business?
2. Why do today's nurse executives need business skills?
3. What kind of skills are required for writing a successful business plan?
4. How can DNP prepared nurse executives continue to improve their business skills?

References

Abrams, R. (2015). *Successful business plans: Secrets & strategies*. (6th ed.). Palo Alto, CA: Planning Shop.

Amadeo, K. (2017, October 26). *The rising cost of health care by year and its causes*. The balance Retrieved from https://www.thebalance.com/causes-of-rising-health-care-costs-4064878.

American Association of Colleges of Nursing (2006, October). *The essentials of doctoral education for advanced nursing practice*. Washington, DC: Retrieved from http://www.aacn.nche.edu/dnp/Essentials.pdf.

American Organization of Nurse Executives (AONE) (2015). *Nurse executive competencies*. Retrieved from http://www.aone.org/resources/nec.pdf

Baker, J. J. & Baker, R. W. (2014). *Health Care Finance: Basic tools for non- financial managers*. (4th ed.). Burlington, MA: Jones & Bartlett Learning.

Barberio, J. A. (2010, July 13). Establishing an independent nurse practitioner practice. Retrieved from http://nurse-practitioners-and-physician-assistants.advanceweb.

com/Features/Articles/Establishing-an-Independent-Nurse-Practitioner-Practice.aspx.

Berry, T. (2016). What Is a SWOT Analysis? *BPlans*. Retrieved from http://articles.bplans.com/how-to-perform-swot-analysis/.

Benner, P., Sutphen, M., Leonard, V., & Day, L. (2009). *Educating nurses: A call for radical transformation*. San Francisco, CA: Jossey-Bass.

Carlson, K. (2015, February 13). Business education for nurses? Retrieved from http://exclusive.multibriefs.com/content/business-education-for-nurses/medical-allied-healthcare.

Carrier, E., Yee, T., & Stark, L. (2011, December). Matching supply to demand: Addressing the U.S. primary care workforce shortage. *Policy Analysis No. 7*. National Institute for Health Care Reform: Washington DC. Retrieved from http://www.kcnpnm.org/news/news.asp?id=118578.

Discover Business.us. (2016). How to write a business plan. Retrieved from http://www.discoverbusiness.us/business-plans/#7

Douglas, K. (2010). Taking action to close the nursing-finance gap: Learning from success. *Nursing Economics, 28*(4), 270-272. Retrieved from https://www.nursingeconomics.net/necfiles/staffingUnleashed/su_JA10.pdf

Entrepreneur. (2016a). How to write a business plan. Retrieved from https://www.entrepreneur.com/article/247575

Fontinelle, A. (2016b). Business plan: Your organizational and operating plan. *Investopedia*. Retrieved from http://www.investopedia.com/university/business-plan/business-plan6.asp

Fontinelle, A. (2016). Business plan: Your financial plan. *Investopedia*. Retrieved from http://www.investopedia.com/university/business-plan/business-plan7.asp

Jain, S.H. (2015, April 7). The skills doctors and nurses need to be effective executives. *Harvard Business Review*. Retrieved from https://hbr.org/2015/04/the-skills-doctors-need-to-be-effective-executives

Jain, S. H & Tsang, T. (2014, May 30). Health care becomes entrepreneurial (finally). *Harvard Business Review*. Retrieved from https://hbr.org/2014/05/health-care-becomes-entrepreneurial-finally

Johnson, J. (Ed.) (1988). *The Nurse Executive's Business Plan Manual*. Rockville, MD: Aspen Publishers, Inc.

Johnson, J. E. & Garvin, W. S. (2017). Advanced practice nurses: Developing a business plan for an independent ambulatory clinical practice. *Nursing Economics, 35*(3), 126–133,141.

Jones-Berry, S. (2017, May 30). Teach nurses business skills, urges leading US entrepreneur. Retrieved from https://rcni.com/nursing-standard/newsroom/news/teach-nurses-business-skills-urges-leading-us-entrepreneur-87851

Institute of Medicine. (2010). *The Future of Nursing: Leading Change, Advancing Health*; The National Academies Press, Washington, DC, 2011. Retrieved from www.iom.edu/Reports/2010/The-Future-of-Nursing-Leading-Change-Advancing-Health.aspx

Institute of Medicine. (2001). *Crossing the quality chasm: A new health system for the 21st century*. Committee on Quality of Health Care in America, Institute of Medicine. Washington DC: National Academies Press.

Larson, J. (2015, March 16). Chief nursing officers need new skill sets. *Healthcare Finance*. Retrieved from http://www.healthcarefinancenews.com/blog/chief-nursing-officers-need-new-skill-sets

Liu, N., & D'Aunno, T. (2011). The productivity and cost-efficiency of models for involving nurse practitioners in primary care: A perspective from queing analysis. *Health Services Research, 7*(2), 594-613. doi: 10.1111/j.1475-6773.2011.01343.x

Mantel, P.J. (2017) Lourdes Family Clinic (Summary) Business Plan. Unpublished manuscript. The Catholic University of America School of Nursing, Washington, D.C.

O'Sullivan, H. (2016, October 11). Required skills for today's nurses: Nursing leaders need to be able to tackle tomorrow's value-based care challenges. *Hospitals & Health Networks*. Retrieved from https://www.hhnmag.com/articles/7687-required-skills-for-todays-nurses

Paterson, M.A. (2014). *Healthcare finance and financial management: Essentials for advanced practice nurses and interdisciplinary care teams*. Lancaster, PA: DES Tech Publications, Inc.

Patient Protection and Affordable Care Act (ACA), 42 U.S.C. § 330A–1 (2010). Retrieved from http://www.oshpd.ca.gov/reform/PPACA_TitleV.pdf

Patrishkoff, D. (2015, March 29). A SWOT analysis of SWOT analysis. Retrieved from http://insurancethoughtleadership.com/swot-analysis-swot-analysis/

PR Newswire. (2012, June 22). Pharma execs continue looking for growth opportunities in spite of increasing regulatory challenges: KPMG Survey. [Press release]. Retrieved from http://www.prnewswire.com/news-releases/pharma-execs-continue-looking-for-growth-opportunities-in-spite-of-increasing-regulatory-challenges-kpmg-survey-159993345.html

Rappleye, E. (2015, December 3). On the record: 50 best healthcare quotes of 2015. *Becker's Hospital Review*. Retrieved from http://www.beckershospitalreview.com/hospital-management-administration/on-the-record-50-best-healthcare-quotes-of-2015.html

Rothausen, T. J. & Bazarko, D.M. (2014). Working paper: Business education for nurse leaders: A case study of leadership development in a vital, highly gendered industry. Retrieved from https://ir.stthomas.edu/cgi/viewcontent.cgi?referer=https://www.google.com/&httpsredir=1&article=1003&context=ocbmgmtwp

Rogers, E.M. (2003). *Diffusion of innovations*. New York: Free Press.

Sherman, A. J. (2016). Business planning: Building an effective business model. Entrepreneurship.org Resource Center. Retrieved from http://entrepreneurship.org/resource-center/business-planning-building-an-effective-business-model.aspx

Stevens, K. R. (2013, May 31). The impact of evidence-based practice in nursing and the next big ideas. *OJIN: The Online Journal of Issues in Nursing, 18*, (2). Manuscript 4. Retrieved from http://www.nursingworld.org/MainMenuCategories/ANA-Marketplace/ANAPeriodicals/OJIN/TableofContents/Vol-18-2013/No2-May-2013/Impact-of-Evidence-Based-Practice.html

Stoy, D. B. (1999). The link between entrepreneurial success and advanced skills in organization development. In J. Hommes, et al. (Eds.). *Educational innovation and economics and business IV: Learning in a changing environment*. Dordrecht, The Netherlands: Kluwer Academic Publications.

Taylor, N.F. (2016, April 1). SWOT Analysis: What it is and when to use it. *Business News Daily*. Retrieved from http://www.businessnewsdaily.com/4245-swot-analysis.html

U.S. Agency for Health and Human Services. (2016). Qualitative research methods in program evaluation: Considerations for federal staff. Retrieved from https://www.acf.hhs.gov/sites/default/files/acyf/qualitative_research_methods_in_program_evaluation.pdf

U.S. Agency for International Development. (2013). Technical note: Conducting mixed-method evaluations. Retrieved from https://www.usaid.gov/evaluation/technical-note/mixed-method

U.S. Small Business Administration. (2016). Developing a marketing plan. Retrieved from https://www.sba.gov/managing-business/growing-your-business/developing-marketing-plan

U.S. Small Business Administration. (2016). Executive summary. Retrieved from https://www.sba.gov/starting-business/write-your-business-plan/executive-summary

Van Dyke, M. (2008). CNOs and CFOs team up to teach nurses business skills. *Nurse Leader*. Retrieved from http://www.nurseleader.com/article/S1541-4612(08)00238-3/pdf

Wasserman, E. (2016). How to write the financial section of a business plan. *Inc*. Retrieved from http://www.inc.com/guides/business-plan-financial-section.html

Wilson, A., Whitaker, N., & Whitford, D. (2012, May 31). Rising to the challenge of health care reform with entrepreneurial and intrapreneurial nursing initiatives. *OJIN: The Online Journal of Issues in Nursing, 17*(2). DOI: 10.3912/OJIN.Vol-17No02Man05. Retrieved from http://www.nursingworld.org/MainMenuCategories/ANAMarketplace/ANAPeriodicals/OJIN/TableofContents/Vol-17-2012/No2-May-2012/Rising-to-the-Challenge-of-Reform.html

Wolters Kluwer. (2012, May 24). Product development must be an ongoing, intentional process. *BizFiling*. Retrieved from http://www.bizfilings.com/toolkit/sbg/marketing/product-development/product-development-an-ongoing-process.aspx

ROSEMARY VENTURA

10
Informatics for the DNP Nurse Executive

Chapter Objectives

- Discuss the importance of informatics for Doctorate in Nursing Practice (DNP) nurse executives.
- Describe the essential IT skills needed by DNP nurse executives.
- Describe the role of the DNP nurse executive in the selection, adoption, and utilization of health care information technology (HIT).
- Identify the impact of key federal legislation on DNP nurse executives and long-term utilization of HIT.
- Discuss two future trends in nursing informatics and their potential impact on nursing practice.

> KEY WORDS: chief nursing informatics officer, DNP nurse executive, health care technology, informatics skills, information technology, nursing informatics, and nursing leadership.

Introduction

The growth of information technology (IT), the complexity of today's health care environment, and the integration of health care information technology (HIT) in nursing practice have driven the need for informatics expertise at the executive level. The nurse executives who work in the C-Suite of today's hospitals must understand the value of informatics and its contribution to today's health care delivery ecosystem, and they must also address contemporary IT challenges that face health care organizations today.

During the past decade, the HIT market has grown to over $24 billion dollars, driven in part by government incentives and improved clinical technology (Office of the National Coordinator [ONC], 2016). Government incentives have targeted improving quality outcomes and increasing patient engagement in the management of their personal health. These incentives have included payments to eligible professionals, eligible hospitals, and critical access hospitals as they adopted, implemented, upgraded, or demonstrated "meaningful use" of certified electronic health records (EHR) technology (U. S. Department of Health & Human Services [HHS], 2016). As a result, the demand for advanced informatics skills in both clinical nursing practice and nursing leadership has increased. This is true for all nurse leaders, including C-Suite executives (Simpson, 2013). It is more critical than ever for C-Suite nurse executives to understand the increasing role of informatics at all organizational levels and in clinical care venues. Nurse executives must acquire advanced knowledge in HIT and develop a technically savvy skill set that is specific to their respective clinical arena. Advanced knowledge and a well-developed IT skill set will enable the DNP C-Suite nurse executive to leverage the technology that ultimately drives organizational goals.

Technological advances by nurses began in 1992 with the introduction of "nursing informatics" (NI) (Saba & McCormick, 2015). The American Nurses Association (ANA) ensured the term's place in the nursing lexicon by developing the specialty's "Scope of Standards" in 2015 (ANA, 2015). Since then, nursing informatics has become a foundation for clinical, academic, research, and administrative nursing practice. Today, NI is the field of study that integrates nursing science with multiple information and analytical sciences to identify, define, manage, and communicate data, information, knowledge, and wisdom in nursing practice. (ANA, 2015). Nursing informatics supports nurses, consumers, patients, the interprofessional health care team, and other stakeholders who focus on achieving improvements in clinical outcomes (ANA, 2015).

Competencies in NI have evolved in the changing health care environment through examination and the support of professional organizations, such as the American Academy of Nursing, the National Institute of Nursing Research, and the American Medical Association. Early informatics competencies for C-Suite executives focused on high-level use of technology. Skills included general knowledge of software applications, such as basic administrative software, use of electronic mail, and the ability to access information (Westera & Delaney, 2008). However, NI nursing competencies have evolved into a multi-disciplinary scientific endeavor of analyzing, formalizing, and modeling how nurses collect and manage data, process data into information and knowledge, and make knowledge-based decisions and inferences for patient care (The TIGER Institute, 2014).

Understanding and recognizing these distinctions enables the DNP-prepared C-Suite nurse executive to advance nursing's unique perspective and align with informatics competencies more familiar to non-nursing executives (Remus & Kennedy, 2012). Organizations such as the Technology Informatics Guiding Education (TIGER) Institute believe in leveraging technology and practice through transformational leadership (The TIGER

Institute, 2014). Although concepts in transformation leadership theory may be familiar to non-nursing executives, the transformational infomatics leader incorporates the concept of polarity thinking into their perspective and approach to change. Polarity thinking has been described as paradoxes, dilemmas, or tensions. Polarities are interdependent pairs that need each other over time to gain and maintain performance, and reach a higher purpose (Johnson, 1992). In essence, polarity thinking supplements traditional problem-solving "either-or" approaches, with "both-and" thinking which is necessary to overcome hurdles in complex environments inherent in technology implementation (The TIGER Institute, 2014). Through utilization of this skill, nursing informaticists are differentiated from other informatics specialties.

Many unique TIGER concepts have been acknowledged by the American Association of Colleges of Nursing (AACN) in the *2006 Essentials of a Doctoral Education for Advancing Nursing Practice* and in 2015 by the American Organization for Nursing Leadership (AONL) (formerly the American Organization of Nurse Executives) *Nurse Executive Competencies*. This chapter focuses on AACN *Essential IV*: Information Systems/Technology and Patient Care Technology for the Improvement and Transformation of Health Care, and the seven Information Management and Technology business skills necessary for today's DNP nurse executive (AACN, 2006). Relating these skills to key informatics topics will provide foundational information and recommendations in areas where many nurse executives face challenges related to the implementation, use, and optimization of technology. Such challenges, which are critical to the success and future of today's health care organizations, underscore the need for improved preparation and education of DNP-prepared C-Suite nurse executives in the rapidly changing field of information technology.

Essential HIT Skill Set for the DNP-Prepared Nurse Executive

Essential HIT Skill Set Evolution

Today's DNP nurse executive, who works in the C-Suite and who represents the technological needs of nursing, must have a global understanding of HIT and how it has changed the health care ecosystem. Although the definition of a health care specific ecosystem remains fluid and standardization has been difficult, the concept aligns with the traditional use of the term ecosystem, or as defined by Merriam-Webster "the complex of a community of organisms and its environment functioning as an ecological unit" (Merriam-Webster, 2018). The health care ecosystem has been described as a network of inter-connected stakeholders, or actors, who are charged with improving quality of care while lowering costs through use of advanced technology (*Becker's Hospital Review*, 2014). Key stakeholders might include clinicians, patients, health care organizations, and government agencies. Understanding a global concept, such as a health care ecosystem, goes beyond the current AACN's essentials skills for a modern DNP nurse executive. There is a need to update the informatics skills, originally introduced in 2006 and which have remained unchanged, to reflect modern day technology and its impact on the globalization of health care. Technology has driven health care services beyond traditional care settings, such as health care systems or academic settings, and into local communities and homes. This is relevant in today's global health care market where there is increasing movement towards remote patient monitoring (RPM) and home health care, particularly in rural settings. Nursing supports a technically savvy global health care consumer who brings knowledge and needs that extend well beyond the walls of traditional hospital settings. Developing a level of technological proficiency and understanding its impact on access to global health care is important for nursing at all levels, but especially for nurse executives whose aim is to improve patient outcomes by advancing clinical practice.

The Contemporary HIT Essential Skill Set

To support executive decision-making, essential HIT skills have morphed beyond basic computer skills and use of common software programs to expanded knowledge of sophisticated mobile environments, clinical technology beyond the EHR and traditional health care settings, and the use of social media platforms (Weaver, Lindsay, & Gitelman, 2012). Requiring these skills at the executive level of an organization demonstrates the organization's appreciation of the role of HIT in institutional processes and outcomes, its commitment to continual renewal of HIT platforms and products, and the utilization of technology as a key clinical and leadership tool in organizational operations (Poe, 2011).

The AACN's Essential IV distinguishes DNP graduates by their ability to use information systems and technology to support and improve patient care and health care systems, and their leadership within health care systems and academic settings (AACN, 2006). In a study by Choi and Zucker (2013), DNP students self-evaluated their informatics competencies in computer skills, informatics knowledge, and informatics skills. Computer skills included decision support, communication, basic desktop software, systems documentation, data access, monitoring, education, and administration. Informatics knowledge included impact, privacy/security, systems, and data. Informatics skills included data systems, clinical, administration, and privacy/security. These areas were consistent with the informatics competencies outlined by AACN DNP Essentials IV. The study results suggested that DNP students perceived themselves as not competent in any of the three categories. It is critical to acknowledge this gap and its impact on patient care and health care leadership. DNP executives must advocate for changes, such as increasing training in informatics in formal nursing education programs, and in practice settings through onboarding for new nurses and managers.

Although the AACN guidelines focus on five practical, concrete, informatics skills necessary for everyday executive decision-making, AONL (2015) advocates that DNP-prepared nurse executives demonstrate a global, high-level perspective of HIT and collaborate at the executive level on prioritizing HIT goals. One example is participating in an information technology strategic planning session to develop the future state HIT roadmap of an organization. This might include multiple and distinct components, such as infrastructure needs, needs for future clinical and financial applications, and all required device integrations. For the DNP-prepared nurse executive, participation in these conversations involves evaluating the technology by determining the impact on patient care; assessing the availability of appropriate clinical and technical resources necessary for the development, implementation and ongoing management of the system(s) for optimal clinical, operational and financial outcomes; and projecting how the data obtained through use of the technology provide new knowledge for the organization.

After recognizing that these skills may require an on-site specialist in nursing informatics, nurse executives might also consider forming a nursing informatics team to guide decision-making, develop and execute clinical workflow analysis, and provide implementation and operational support for all affected personnel. Reflecting on the 2011 Institute of Medicine (IOM) report, *The Future of Nursing: Leading Change, Advancing Health*, the Health Information Management and System Society (HIMSS), in collaboration with the ANA and Alliance for Nursing Informatics (ANI), established recommendations for informatics in the areas of leadership, education, and practice (HIMSS, 2011). This resource may be useful for DNP nurse executive as they develop their own informatics skills and teams.

The AONL (2015) recommends that all system-level organizational structures include the development of a nursing informatics plan and the creation of a CNIO position. Free-standing hospitals can also benefit from retaining a CNIO with expertise in advanced leadership and informatics. The CNIO works in tandem with other senior leaders, such as the chief medical informatics oficer and chief information officer, to drive transformational strategies that meet the needs of clinicians, and the organization's vision and goals. The CNIO is positioned to lead critical initiatives that influence improved clinical efficiencies, as well as operational, financial, and quality outcomes. With distinctive skills that combine clinical and technical knowledge and expertise in informatics, the CNIO has the operational and leadership skills to develop solutions that optimize organizational outcomes. Along with the chief nursing officer, the CNIO develops a comprehensive informatics strategy, which addresses the role of informatics in practice, policy development, leadership, and education, and which aligns and supports the organizational and nursing strategic plans (Tupper & Alexander, 2012). Tupper and Alexander outline the following core responsibilities that can serve as guidelines for DNP-prepared nurse executives (see Table 10.1).

These core responsibilities represent essential skills for executive practice. Table 10.2 outlines these skills and aligns each with a closely related HIT core function. Discussion of each core function provides an enriched understanding and appreciation of the CNIO and C-Suite DNP-prepared nurse executive who work together to leverage health care information technology, advance patient care, and improve clinical outcomes.

The Role of the DNP Nurse Executive in Technology Selection and Life Cycle

Information technology projects are often complex and expensive, and they require multiple financial, clinical, and operational resources (Schoville & Titler, 2015). Matching the right technology and vendor to the organization's culture and goals is a crucial component of long-term organizational success. *The Future of Nursing: Leading Change, Advancing Health* (IOM, 2011) emphasizes the need for health care organizations to engage nurses and other point-of-service personnel to work with developers and manufacturers in the design, development, purchase, implementation, and evaluation of medical devices and health information technology products. For DNP C-Suite nurse executives, this effectively means ensuring that nurses, at all levels and from different clinical settings, are directly and/or indirectly involved in the evaluation and selection of new information

Table 10.1 Chief Nursing Informatics Officer Core Responsibilities

Chief Nursing Informatics Officer	• Core Responsibilities • Build an infrastructure for evidence-based practice • Define competencies and provide mentorship • Partner for workforce readiness and development • Support and optimize evolving care delivery models • Blend business and clinical intelligence and analytics • Incorporates human factors concepts and usability for transforming care delivery • Educate organizations about informatics • Communicate and sustain the vision • Provide leadership in system design, selection, including future releases and upgrades, implementation, monitoring, and evaluation

Table 10.2 Crosswalk of HIT Core Functions to Organization-Based Essential Skill.

HIT Core Funtdon	AACN-Essential IV	AONL- Nune Executive- Information Management & Technology	AONL- System CNE-Information Management & Technology
General HIT Skills	• Design, select, use and evaluate programs that evaluate and monitor outcomes of care, care systems and quality improvement including consumer use of health care information systems. • Provide leadership in the ev-aluation and resolution of ethical and legal issues within healthcare systems relating to the use of information, information technology, communication networks, and patient care technology.	• Use technology to support improvement of clinical and f'mancial performance • Collaborate to prioritize for the establishment of information technology resources.	• Design and develop the use of new technology for clinical integration of the electronic health record. • Incorporate "human factors" concepts related to technology. • Implement, evaluate and lead the activities of a system \Vide nursing informatics plan the system the CNIO role.
Technology Selection	• Analyze and communicate critical elements necessaJy to the selection, use and evaluation of health care information systems and patient care technology.	• Participate in evaluation of enabling technology in practice settings.	
Technology Adoption & Utilization		• Provide leadership for the adoption and implementation of information systems.	
Big Data & Analytics	• Demonstrate the conceptual ability and technical skills to develop and execute an evaluation plan involving data extraction from practice information systems and databases.	• Use data management systems for decision making. • Demonstrate skills in assessing data integrity and quality.	
Legislation & EHR			
eHealth	• Evaluate consumer health information sources for accuracy, timeliness, and appropriateness.		
Future Trends			• Identify technological trends, issues and new developments as they apply to patient care.

systems technology. This is especially true for the organization's nursing informaticist and CNIO. Research suggests that the current HIT knowledge of nurses, nursing leadership, and nurse executives may be insufficient for effective technology selection and executive decision-making in today's complex health care environment (Simpson, 2013). Thus, the DNP nurse executive must proactively enrich his or her knowledge of contemporary HIT, provide appropriate education for other nurse leaders and project champions, and advance recommendations that will ensure solid system selection and implementation outcomes.

The DNP nurse executive must also be aware that technology selection extends beyond software applications such as the electronic health record. Although EHRs represent a fundamental component of HIT, nursing practice is influenced significantly by other technology and applications. For example, in today's health care ecosystem, advanced HIT improves the delivery of safe patient care by providing tools for early diagnosis, ongoing monitoring, and the treatment of patients (Schoville & Titler, 2015). Examples include wireless intravenous pumps and vital sign machines for greater workflow efficiencies, mobile smart phone devices for point-of-care decision support, and radio frequency identification devices (RFID) that monitor patients who may be at high risk for falls.

Table 10.3 Role of the DNP Nurse Executive During the System Life Cycle.

Project Phase	Role of DNP Nurse Executive
General HIT Skills	• Provide vision and goals as they align with the strategic plan of the organization • Communicate the business and clinical requirements
Planning-Design; Testing; Training; Support	• Lead and/or engage in a key stakeholder analysis to ensure appropriate nursing team of experts and resources are assembled throughout project • Participate in key governance meetings with senior project leadership • Ensure financial resources are mapped and allocated for each project phase • Assemble nursing structure alongside oroiect team for oroiect oarticioation
Implementation	• Participate in project update meetings and facilitate escalations as necessary
Evaluation	• Participate in the development of evaluation criteria including metrics for success that align to quality, financial and ooerational aoals
Monitoring	• Participate in review of ongoing reports on system performance, adoption and success metrics • Create necessary workgroups responsible for ongoing maintenance and monitoring, including project plans to address issues or system optimization

For DNP nurse executives to be effective in technology selection, the HIT essentials recommend "a working knowledge of standards and principles for health care system selection and evaluation, a cognitive awareness of technology integration and its impact throughout the health care delivery system" (AACN, 2006). This includes analyzing and communicating business and clinical requirements specific to the technology under consideration, such as the selection of new patient beds. The DNP-prepared nurse executive may require wireless data transmission capabilities and integration of data with the EHR, which creates efficiency for nursing process and documentation requirements. Another example is unit-based electronic tracking boards that reflect patient movement during the selection of a new patient tracking system.

For the DNP nurse executive, the goal of technology is to drive and support clinical practice, provide decision support for nurses and nurse leaders, and ensure compliance with regulatory requirements, hospital policies and procedures. To achieve these goals, the DNP nurse executive must engage fully in technology selection and the systems life cycle, which includes system/technology selection, implementation, monitoring, and evaluation. Table 10.3 outlines the role of the DNP nurse executive during the system life cycle from technology selection through project evaluation that will ensure that the technology meets the organization's intended goals.

Noteworthy Trends in Technology Selection and Tools for the DNP Nurse Executive

During the past 35 years, technology selection has evolved beyond the simple selection of an EHR. Although system selection continues to be the primary technology consideration that many DNP nurse executives will encounter, the selection process has become far more complicated, as it shifted from "best-of-breed" applications to highly integrated, all-encompassing, single vendor, enterprise systems (Fareed, Ozcan, & DeShazo, 2012). For the DNP nurse executive, this transition may require difficult decisions and consultation from nursing informatics specialists. Sometimes enterprise solutions may not sufficiently match existing functionality found in best-of-breed solutions. In this situation, the DNP nurse executive should collaboratively engage the CNIO, or other nursing informatics leadership, and complete a functional analysis or clinical evaluation for informed decision-making. These tools are important for every DNP executive. Table 10.4 is an example of a clinical evaluation for a single solution intended to satisfy current state barcoding technology as well as satisfy new clinical communication needs.

As the utilization of technology in clinical practice increases, the selection of these tools must be comprehensive and thoughtful. Organizations will rely heavily on the participation of the DNP nurse executive, as well

Table 10.4 Clinical Evaluation Parameters.

Clinical Functionality	Vendor 1	Vendor 2
Provides Bar Code Scanning/PPID		
Care Team identification		
Provides patient context w/features (e.g., text messages, alerts, alarms, etc.)		
Single sign-in (all apps) vs. multiple sign on's		
Simple navigation experience		
EMR integration • Can document data In EMR via handheld		
Provides critical test result alerts (display customizable)		
Displays clincal alarm waveforms (ECG)		
Supports single platform solution for various alarm systems/equipment devices (ventilators, fetal heart monitor, cardiac monitor, pagers, IV pumps, etc.)		
Permits hierarchy of features (alarms vs. phone calls) • Can critical alarms breakthrough other functions		
Provides clinical decision-support at point of care (with alarms and alerts)		
Links to clinical aides and materials (e.g., vessel anatomy chart, links to policies)		
Presence		
Shows presence (clincian working or not working)		
Displays clinician availability/unavailability (I.e., RN in a med pass—Zone of Silence)		
Communication		
Able to send broadcast text messages		
Able to assign dynamic roles/functions		
Can customize pre-programmed text messages		
Has desktop version		
Call bell response		
Escalates alerts/messages/calls		
Integrates with nurse call system		
Nolse level		
Can change ringtones/place on vibration		
Future state		
Supports one device/multifunction model		

as nursing informatics and other nursing leaders, to provide knowledge of clinical workflows and contributions to future state processes, including the integration of the technology throughout the entire health care enterprise. Tools such as these undoubtedly influence the delivery of nursing care, and they underscore the importance of nurse leader contributions in the process of technology selection and all phases of the system life cycle.

Overcoming Challenges in Health Care Technology Adoption and Utilization

The world of HIT is viewed as 5% technology and the remainder as *people and process*. To a large extent, the 2010 Patient Protection and Affordable Care Act (ACA) and the 2009 American Recovery and Reinvestment Act with the Health Information Technology for Economic and Clinical Health Acts (HITECH) advanced the implementation of EHRs, exceeded the target of 450,000 eligible providers and made payments to 464, 634 eligible providers as part of the meaningful use program, in fiscal year 2015 (Department of Health & Human Services, 2016). The meaningful use program required that basic EHRs include "patient demographics, patient problem lists, medications, clinical notes, prescriptions, ability to view laboratory results, and the ability to view imaging results" (Department of Health & Human Services, 2016). These requirements established a foundation for improved EHR interoperability and health data exchange.

During the positive surge in EHR implementations, some high-profile projects provided some valuable lessons. In 2017, it was reported that Banner Health's Cerner EHR replacement led to an increase in medical errors (Monica, 2018). Reports also surfaced that MD Anderson's 2015–2016 Epic EHR contributed to a 77% drop in adjusted income over a 10-month period (Becker's Hospital Review, 2016). These events offered important lessons about failed implementation efforts including the importance of executive leadership commitment and support, which when absent, can lead to a lack of clinician adoption, utilization, or technology rejection. These examples also demonstrate the importance of the client-vendor partnership, vendor flexibility, and vendor engagement.

According to the IOM (2011), the DNP-prepared nurse leader has the capacity to translate research, shape systems of care, potentiate individual care into population-health initiatives, ask the clinical questions that influence organizational-level research, and improve performance with informatics and quality improvement models. With these talents, the DNP nurse executive can effectively execute the HIT essential skill of providing leadership in technology adoption through the selection, implementation, monitoring, and evaluation of information systems in all care delivery settings and venues.

Technology Adoption Models and the Role of the Nurse Executive

To facilitate technology transitions and culture change, new methodologies and adoption models have evolved to consider factors beyond individual end users. These technology adoption models (TAMs) identify how users learn to accept and use innovations in technology (Schoville & Titler, 2015). Models such as the integrated technology implementation model (ITIM) emphasize the role of leadership in successful technology adoption. Specifically, the model describes the significance of the nurse executive, director, and frontline manger, who set forth the vision, goals, and strategies, and who participate in diverse activities related to project communication, effects on policy, and the establishment of performance expectations for the technology. Other HIT industry leadership groups, such as the TIGER Institute, reference the DNP prepared executive as a role that is critical in sponsoring and driving the implementation, adoption, and utilization of HIT that is capable of generating new knowledge as a natural byproduct of care delivery (The TIGER Institute, 2014).

Skills and Strategies for Building HIT Adoption

One of the most valuable skills a DNP nurse executive can bring to HIT adoption is the recognition of human factors in technology. As noted by the Office of the National Coordinator (2016) in their organizational responsibility guidelines, leadership responsibilities require attention to social and technical matters, especially in complex "sociotechnical" health care organizations. Recent studies have found that rapid implementation of new medical technology, EHRs, patient monitoring devices, surgical robots, and other tools can lead to adverse patient events when the implementation is not thoughtfully integrated into workflow (McGonigle & Mastrian, 2018).

The DNP nurse executive is well positioned to recognize the importance of human factors in two key areas. First, DNP nurse executives are aware of shifts in responsibilities that result from workflow redesign. These changes often require DNP nurse executives to negotiate relationships with other senior leaders. Second, since adoption begins at the inception of the project, it is important for nurse executives to champion the involvement of personnel who represent different parts of the organization throughout the entire process, including post-implementation, ongoing maintenance, and governance. This process of involvement develops subject matter experts (SMEs) who ultimately become unit level champions who drive culture change with peers and leadership. The DNP nurse executives must ensure that key stakeholders attend to these adoption activities which require sufficient budgeting and both short-term and long-term financial support.

Key Process Milestones for Successful HIT Adoption

System adoption and utilization are also dependent on key process milestones which DNP nurse executives must include in HIT project plans. The activities conducted as part of these processes are signature skills of the NI portfolio that executives can leverage. These include current and future state workflow assessments, mappings, and organizational readiness assessments. Workflow assessments and mappings are often used to support staff training and serve as a reference for staff, IT teams, support teams, and vendors. The key to IT adoption is appropriate vetting of the future state workflow and the final approval from the project leadership. This builds agreement and commitment from the organization. Figures 10.1 and 10.2 are examples of current state and future workflow maps for the implementation of new technology that supports specimen collection in an emergency department.

Organizational readiness assessment is an exercise that determines the state of readiness within an organization for the adoption and implementation of a new process. Unfortunately, this process is often overlooked and not considered as a key component of technology implementation. Excluding a readiness assessment as a key project component can lead to missed opportunities for addressing chronic organizational issues that must be addressed prior to the introduction of new workflows or new technology.

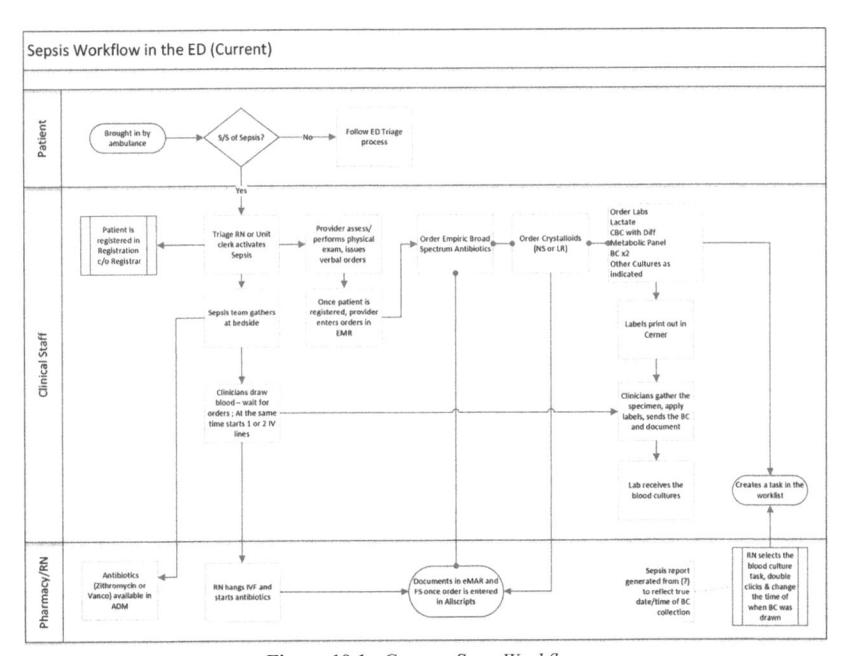

Figure 10.1. *Current-State Workflow.*

DNP nurse executives should anticipate and plan for resolving these issues which can be a chronic operational issue, such as a lack of computers, or a processes issue which lacks a clear owner. Left unresolved or ignored, these issues eventually resurface during the implementation phase.

The DNP nurse executive needs advanced leadership skills to navigate these chronic cultural or process issues to avoid lack of adoption, utilization, or even rejection of the new technology. An example is the implementation of Bar Code Medication Administration (BCMA) technology, which was considered a best practice for the safe administration of medications through the use of positive patient identification technology (PPID). In this example, the underlying issue was the lack of pharmacy resources for real-time loading of new bar codes into the system. Without this step, nurses were unable to scan during the BCMA process. In such a case, executive level leaders must intervene in order to negotiate delicate decisions that may have greater organizational effects beyond the specific technology project.

Important strategies for technology utilization and optimization include establishing governance and committee structures with membership that represents diverse clinical specialties, that along with clinical point-of-service staff, will receive sufficient practice, training and other educational resources. For the DNP nurse executive, it is important to create structure through a shared governance model or a well-established, highly

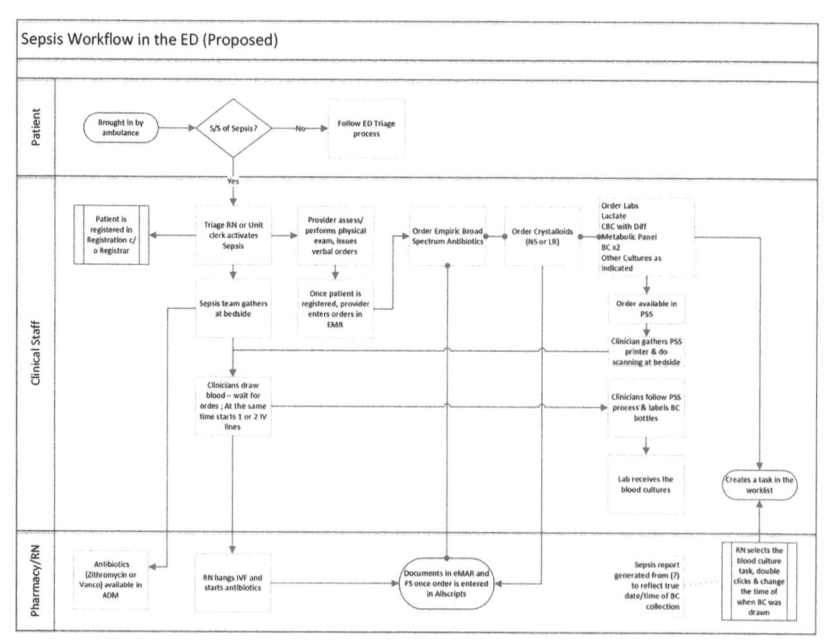

Figure 10.2. *Future-State Workflow.*

**Enterprise Nursing Informatics Council (NIC)
Governance Structure**

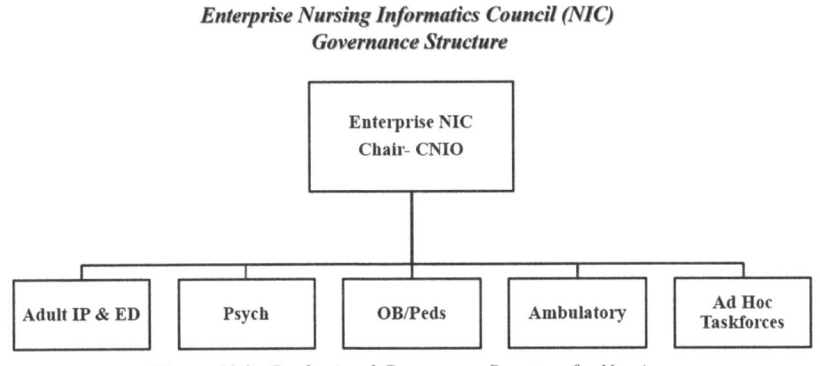

```
                    ┌──────────────────┐
                    │   Enterprise NIC │
                    │   Chair- CNIO    │
                    └────────┬─────────┘
      ┌──────────┬───────────┼───────────┬──────────┐
┌─────┴────┐ ┌───┴──┐ ┌──────┴──┐ ┌──────┴────┐ ┌───┴──────┐
│Adult IP  │ │Psych │ │ OB/Peds │ │Ambulatory │ │ Ad Hoc   │
│ & ED     │ │      │ │         │ │           │ │Taskforces│
└──────────┘ └──────┘ └─────────┘ └───────────┘ └──────────┘
```

Figure 10.3. *Professional Governance Structure for Nursing.*

visible governance process that has decision-making authority and support throughout the organization. This facilitates committee autonomy and builds a sense of point-of-service ownership in the technology and related processes. The DNP nurse executive supports these groups by effectively leading and engaging the various teams, leveraging motivational skills, and demonstrating the ability to energize and focus on knowledge transfer among a variety of professions. Success depends on effective collaboration among professionals who must work effectively toward common value-based goals and objectives designed to create a seamless continuum of health care delivery (TIGER, 2014). Table 10.3 is an example of a governance structure responsible for nursing technology.

With these strategies, the DNP-prepared nurse executive demonstrates leadership and support for HIT at a senior level. By influencing individuals, creating solid processes, and proactively implementing strategies to increase technology adoption, DNP-prepared nurse executives position the organization for success, not only in achieving technology and project goals, but achieving strategic goals supported by the technology such as best practices, new information, and workflow efficiencies.

Big Data and Analytics

Knowledge is power. In all industries, timely, accurate, and reliable data are key to effective decision-making and executive leadership. According to Simpson (2013), ". . . to productively contribute and ultimately, drive technology decisions, nurse executives need to be constantly updating and advancing their HIT knowledge (Saba & McCormick, 2015) beyond the basic understanding of one system (p. 277)." Building on the foundation of the nursing informatics' metastructures of data, information, knowledge, and wisdom (ANA, 2015), the HIT essentials call for the DNP nurse executive to use data management systems for decision-making and assessing data integrity and quality. The nurse executive must also be knowledgeable about new opportunities in big data, and be able to innovate and advocate for proactive analytics at all levels of the organization that allow real-time decision making and quality outcomes.

What are Big Data?

Gaffney and Huckabee (2014) describe "big data" in terms of data volume, variety, velocity, and veracity. Each component contributes a facet of big data, which are effectively datasets that are very large and cannot be analyzed with typical data management tools. There is the need for data warehouses that serve as repositories for clinical, administrative, and financial data. The abundance of data generated from multiple applications in a large health care environment has required organizations to create analytic strategies to turn the big data into information, knowledge, and wisdom (Saba & McCormick, 2015).

For the DNP nurse executive, understanding and managing big data may prove challenging. As a result of growing concern for better management and control of big data by HIT and health care leaders, the HIMSS CNO-CNIO Vendor Roundtable established the Big Data Principles Workgroup in 2015 (Delaney & Westera, 2016). This workgroup developed guidelines that could be used by nurse executives to incorporate HIT into their quality improvement or data analytics strategies. Relevant to the skills necessary for the DNP nurse executive is an understanding of the four key principles of big data: privacy and security of health information, data standards, interoperability, and immutability. Table 10.5 highlights the key attribute of each principle that is most relevant to the DNP-prepared nurse executive.

Table 10.5 Four Key Principles of Big Data.

Big Data Principle	Key Attribute for the DNP Nurse Executive
Privacy and Security of Health Information	• HIT standards and protocols must be implemented to ensure appropriate data privacy and protection
Data Standards	• Data standards, or a common language, must be implemented for data sharing and extraction
Interoperability	• The ability for multiple HIT systems to communicate, exchange and use data
Immutability	• Maintaining the integrity of all data by tracking changes and events in a fashion that can be discovered and maintains its history

Obtaining and Displaying Data

Today's HIT provides an opportunity to track individual patient data in real time to implement effective strategies for clinical issues before they advance to critical and costly levels (TIGER, 2014). These same tools allow nurse leaders to leverage reports that provide evidence of individual and aggregate patient trends over time. Emerging technologies have simplified real-time data collection in health care organizations through the Internet of Things (IoT) and Internet Connection Devices (ICD), devices such as radio frequency identification (RFID) sensors, cameras, and smart phones (Agbali, Trillo, Arayici, & Fernando, 2017). Specific to nursing data, documentation in the EHR is the most common data source for obtaining information.

The dilemma or opportunity for the DNP nurse executive is creating a strategy that merges data in a way that builds information, knowledge, and wisdom. Innovations in analytics, such as virtualization and cloud computing now make it easier to bring real-time, clinical and leadership decision support to the point of immediate need for maximum impact (Raghupathi & Raghupathi, 2014). In addition, milestones in nursing informatics have also built foundations focused on nursing sensitive data. Groups such as the Nursing Knowledge and Big Data Science Initiative have improved the focus on nursing data by sharing a framework for data gathering and sharing of nurse sensitive data, nursing education standards that reflect the nurse's role in technology and EHRs, and big data science that includes nursing's leadership and contribution to transforming health and health care (Delaney & Westera, 2016). Building on this work, DNP nurse executives need to engage with experts in informatics, business analytics and quality, and to collaborate, develop, and drive the analytical strategy for automated data and quality outcomes reporting via smart tools and dashboards.

Smart Tools

Smart tools account for two key areas important to a nurse executive: data capture, and data rendition and availability. DNP nurse executives must understand that most health care data originate from multiple sources. Data repositories and warehouses may not contain the appropriate data necessary for effective decision-making. To promote executive decision-making from reliable metrics, the DNP nurse executive must advocate, educate, and lead groups that understand clinical, operational, and technical landscapes, as well as groups that can work cohesively to develop necessary process and workflow mappings.

Smart tools for data capture must be automated and reside as close to the source point as possible. With the surge of mobile technology in health care, organizations are depending on mobile apps that make data capture easier, faster, and more reliable. This applies to nursing data traditionally found in EMRs. This approach eliminates paper data collection tools and manual entry into electronic formats for analyzing metrics and creating reports. For clinical data pertinent to the patient record, it is imperative that data captured through these tools interface with their appropriate location in the medical record. Too often, nurses are asked to capture data more than once and outside normal workflows. This places an extra burden on clinical staff, and increases the likelihood that the required data are not captured accurately or consistently.

Data rendition, availably, and visibility are also key areas where smart tools, such as knowledge dashboards, support the DNP-prepared nurse executive and the leadership team. One of the most effective approaches is driving dashboards that render information on multiple levels. A good example is monitoring catheter-associated urinary tract infections (CAUTIs). Using data from multiple source applications, including the EMR, the dashboard displays all patients with urinary catheters, along with other

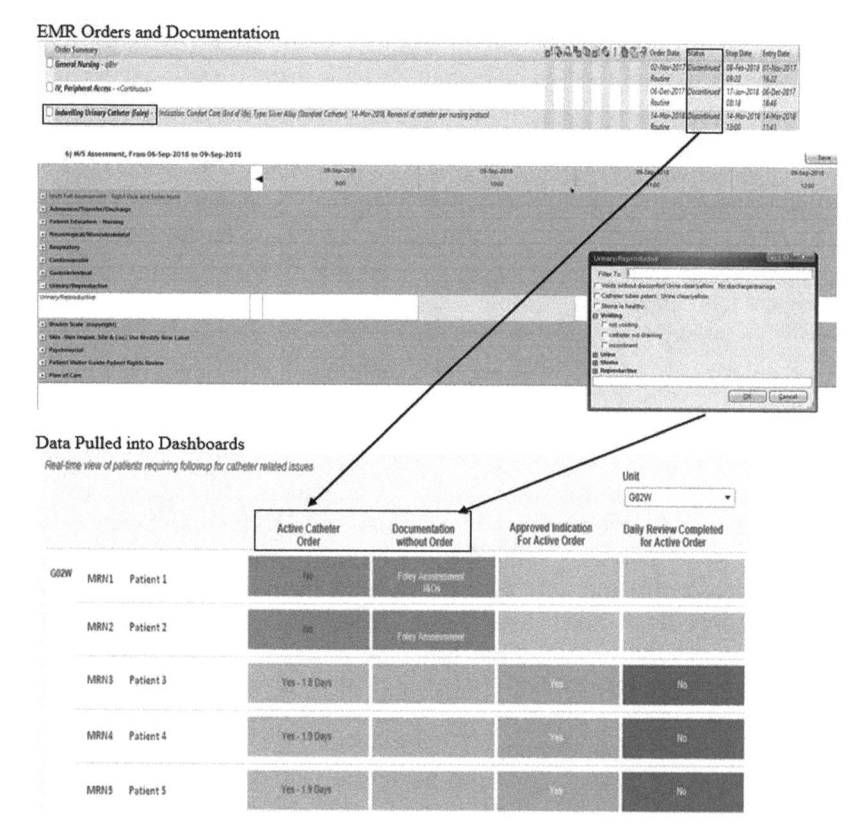

Figure 10.4. *Catheter- associated Urinary Tract Infection (CAUTI) Dashboard Process and View*

relevant points, which can then be filtered to the unit, service line, and facility level. The dashboard, which is readily available on the internal Intranet and can also be accessed through smart phones, also contains other key measures prioritized by the organization, in a central location, which in turn enables availability and visibility.

An example of the integration of dashboards into practice is their use during leadership or interdisciplinary rounds. Frontline managers or staff can quickly identify potential problem areas, such as those patients whose urinary catheter has been in for longer than the recommended time, discuss the concern with the care team, and engage in real-time decision making which leads to an improved clinical outcome. This approach has successfully driven down CAUTI rates and improved the overall organization's quality metrics. Figure 10.4 is an example of the CAUTI dashboard process and view from EHR documentation to a data visualization dashboard.

As a DNP nurse executive, understanding how to select the most appropriate tools for capturing and evaluating data is key. Partnering with informatics experts to utilize tools that bring knowledge to the right people at the right time is critical for achieving strategic goals. Using today's HIT capabilities effectively makes that possible.

Health Care Legislation and the Electronic Health Record

Executive leaders must monitor the activities of government agencies that fund and create legislation which affects health care. With HIT, the past decade has been revolutionary. As DNP nurse executives, knowledge of these regulatory changes and their effect on the health care industry are key to understanding the current HIT landscape. Although the HIT essentials do not specifically mention legislative effects on technology, this area offers future opportunities for expansion of the essential skills.

In 2004, the federal government created the Office of the National Coordinator (ONC), under the U.S. Department of the Health and Human Services (HHS). This branch of government provides oversight and establishes regulations related to HIT. The most significant pieces of legislation that have affected HIT and health care organizations were the American Recovery and Reinvestment Act (ARRA) and HITECH Act of 2009. The HITECH act allowed HHS to establish programs to improve health care quality, safety, and efficiency through the adoption of health information technology, including EHRs and private, secure electronic health information exchange. The ARRA included provisions that created incentives for the adoption and meaningful use of HIT, and also strengthened standards for maintaining the privacy and security of health information. The ARRA also provided grants to help state and local governments as well as health care providers in their efforts to adopt and use HIT (IOM, 2011).

The law included $19.5 billion for health information technology and authorized the Centers for Medicare & Medicaid Services (CMS) to provide reimbursement incentives for eligible professionals and hospitals which become "meaningful users" of certified EHR technology in three stages (2011, 2013, 2015). Medicare reimbursement focused on physicians, while Medicaid reimbursement also included dentists, certified nurse-midwives, nurse practitioners, and physician assistants (Martin, Monsen, & Bowles, 2011). The magnitude of this legislation was felt by every health care leader, organization, and department because its scope affected all areas of the health care delivery ecosystem.

Impact of Technology Legislation on the DNP Nurse Executive

What does this mean for today's DNP nurse executive? On many levels, the recent legislation changed the landscape of health care and affected health care organizations, clinicians, and patients by changing the delivery of care through the use of technology. The legislation also affected federal reimbursement and imposed penalties for non-adherence. Mandates from these laws are still active and are driving initiatives such as population health management, patient experience related to access and participation in health care decisions, and requirements for increased information sharing between organizations.

The DNP nurse leader must remain knowledgeable and participate in the development of a strategic approach for meeting the remaining regulatory requirements of meaningful use (MU). Although a majority of the technical requirements were implemented in past years, effects on organizations, the patient experience, and nursing practice continue. For example, hospital nurses must understand the law when discussing items such as the patient portal. Nurses should also be aware of how portions of a patient's records are shared among various level of care providers in the information exchange. This meant that hospitals should have received information on the patient from the patient's primary care provider, which they should be able to access and review upon the patient's admission. The DNP nurse executive must establish processes and programs for nursing education on these regulations. Policy education should be incorporated into the functional, technical training.

There are many lessons for nursing informaticists, as well as clinical and operational professionals in response to the new IT regulations. At the time the regulations were launched, many organizations did not have informatics experts or effective approaches to HIT project implementation. Fortunately, lessons learned have created new opportunities for improvement in these processes, which DNP nurse executives can now leverage for better results when using technology to meet regulatory requirements.

eHealth

As the health care ecosystem has evolved and new health care delivery models have generated costs reductions and increased access to care, new programs driven by advances in technologies have become increasingly popular with health care executives. Innovations in the areas of eHealth such as mobile health (mHealth) and telehealth are now incorporated into almost all areas of clinical practice (World Health Organization [WHO], 2016). eHealth, as defined by the World Health Organization (WHO), is the cost effective and secure use of information communication technologies (ICT) in support of health and health-related fields, including health care services, health surveillance, health literature, and health education, knowledge, and research (WHO, 2016). DNP nurse executives must understand the expanding role of nurses in eHealth and incorporate the HIT essential of evaluating consumer health information sources for accuracy, timeliness and appropriateness—a hallmark of this rapidly growing section of eHealth.

Mobile Health

Mobile health, or mHealth, is a technology that has opened opportunities for facilitating timely data access, communication, and clinical interventions (ONC, 2012). The WHO (2016) defines mHealth as "an area of electronic health; as the provision of health services and information via mobile technologies such as mobile phones and Personal Digital Assistants (PDAs)(p. 9)." The use of mobile devices, including smart phones and apps, is increasing in health care settings, including outpatient clinics, acute care hospitals, and the consumer space of HIT via mobile applications or apps. These devices and apps are used by frontline clinicians, operational and support staff, as well as leaders, for decision making, communication, and administrative functions. For the DNP nurse executive, it is imperative to understand the needs and requirements of mobility for nursing. As organizations build mobile workforces through the expansion of mobile solutions that leverage point-of-care opportunities, the DNP prepared nurse executive should be prepared to include this technology in their nursing strategic plan. Smart phones also represent the opportunity to consolidate and retire multiple devices and functions commonly used by nurses.

Mobile Nursing Information Systems

Inclusion of mobile nursing information systems (m-NISs) are quickly becoming one of the most vital applications of mobile health care. Hsiao and Chen (2012) found that m-NISs have the potential to increase the speed, quality, and efficiency of bedside nursing. However, introduction of an m-NIS presents a tremendous change for any health care institution because it affects both individual daily tasks and organizational management strategies. The Hsiao and Chen (2012) study found that using a m-NIS had a significantly positive effect on nursing performance by improving exchanges between health care professionals, facilitating communication with patients, increasing efficiency of patient care duties, improving quality of care, increasing the professional image of nursing, and improving the overall performance in nursing practices. These results are promising, although there are limited studies on the use of this technology and its effect on nursing practice. Therefore, the DNP nurse executive, along with the CNIO or nursing informatics team, must carefully evaluate the effects on nursing workflow and practice before implementing these solutions.

Telehealth

Another extension of eHealth which has demonstrated growth is telehealth, which is defined as the use of electronic information and telecommunication technologies to support and promote long-distance clinical health care, patient and professional health-related education, and public health (Health Resources and Services Administration [HRSA], 2015). Improvements in digital communications and decreased costs of devices such as laptops, tablets and smart phones have increased the opportunity for organizations to use telehealth as a way to expand their services (WHO, 2016). For DNP nurse executives, this represents an opportunity to promote the expansion of nursing that also requires deep knowledge, organizational support, and commitment. According to the TIGER Institute (2014), the innovative nurse leader will be functioning in an environment where patients are treated well beyond the traditional care setting. Care will be delivered remotely with mobile monitoring that uses innovative communication solutions. These require expanding nurse leaders' accountability and expanding HIT into practice.

Remote Patient Monitoring

Traditional telehealth models that involve nurses include remote patient monitoring (RPM). The use of RPM is growing rapidly and being facilitated by the growth of biometric devices (indwelling heart or blood sugar monitors) that collect, monitor, and report information from the patient in real time, in either an institution or the home (IOM, 2011). Some of these devices can also provide direct digitally mediated care such as the automated insulin pump and implantable defibrillators. Common use cases are eICUs, where critical care trained nurses provide cardiac and hemodynamic monitoring of patients in intensive care units or home telehealth with daily tele-monitoring of vital signs by patients and subsequent transmissions of those data to offsite nurses who monitor and address significant changes. These models, along with opportunities for telenursing, where nursing services are delivered using telecommunications and information technology, are examples for DNP nurse executives to consider as part of the organization's HIT strategy (McGonigle & Mastrian, 2018).

Barriers to Implementing Telehealth

Although these new programs are often used as organizational initiatives and strategies to decrease readmissions, avoid ED admissions, increase patient throughput, and decrease length of stay, DNP nurse executives should be aware of the common barriers to implementing telehealth programs. Solutions can have large implications on many facets of an organization because they require funding, a great deal of technology infrastructure, and they often compete with other health care priorities and are governed by tight regulation and legislation (WHO, 2016). These programs also rely on patient engagement. A robust telehealth program must include a strategy to target and enroll patients who are often considered high risk. This requires careful consideration and planning. Overall, executives must carefully consider these challenges before embarking on these programs.

Future Projections

Growth in HIT and its growing impact on improving the delivery of health care is recognized by industry leaders. As noted by the IOM (2011), there is perhaps no greater opportunity to transform practice than through the use of technology. As part of the HIT essentials, the DNP nurse executive must have the ability to identify technological trends, issues, and new developments as they apply to patient care (AONE, 2015). As nurse executives participate in long-term strategic planning, the demand for more sophisticated HIT—such as personalized medicine, artificial intelligence and machine learning—will continue to grow. This is especially true as health care delivery models pivot to focus on patients as health care consumers, including technology consumers. Expectations of patients and clinicians are increasing for health care organizations to utilize better technology that facilitate care. In prior decades, organizations have struggled to remain current with consumer technology because of financial constraints and technology that did not support clinical workflow. It is important for the DNP nurse executives to understand the value of informatics to identify technological trends, issues, and new developments as they apply to patient care, and to advocate for HIT that decreases costs while improving the work environment and patient safety (Tupper & Alexander, 2012).

Emerging Technologies

Along with artificial intelligence (AI) and machine learning, the literature suggests that emerging technologies such as genetics and genomics, 3-D printing, cloud computing, robotics, biometrics, predictive analytics, and sensors for integration of patient provided health information will change nursing practice (Huston, 2013). The impact of these technologies and the degree of their utilization in clinical practice remain unknown. Acknowledging the rapid nature and evolution of HIT is necessary for DNP nurse executives who must remain vigilant and attentive to emerging technologies. This can be achieved through the relationship with the CNIO and nursing informaticians. Leveraging these partnerships ensures that the DNP nurse executive will possess the required knowledge of current technology features, future roadmaps for technology vendors, and the latest industry trends.

Chapter Takeaways

1. HIT skills necessary for C-Suite DNP nurse executives encompasses a series of technological components.
2. The C-Suite DNP nurse executive plays a key role in technology selection, implementation, monitoring and evaluation.
3. Key standard processes for HIT adoption form the framework for implementation success.
4. C-Suite nurse executives must develop proficiencies in managing big data and fluency in constructing strategies for the use of smart tools for data analysis and display.
5. The impact of ARRA, HITECH, and MU on the current state of HIT dramatically changes leadership functions and dynamics.
6. The nurse executive must develop a keen understanding of eHealth, mobile health and telehealth and their impacts on a health care organization.
7. C-Suite members assume responsibility to understand and strategically-plan to access best-fit options as future HIT trends become a reality.

Chapter Summary

To lead in today's health care ecosystem, DNP nurse executives must have strong skills in informatics and knowledge of HIT. The need to maintain and further develop these skills will continue to grow as use of technology drives new health care delivery models, best practices, and improved outcomes. The DNP C-Suite nurse executive must understand the process of technology selection and their role in providing the vision and structure to ensure alignment with the organization's strategic goals. It is also essential that DNP-prepared nurse executives recognize the importance of people and process because these technologies are implemented to maximize user adoption, utilization, and optimization.

Leveraging information through the proliferation of HIT is also critical for the DNP nurse executive. Developing strategies for using analytics at all levels of the organization will position nurse executives for success by driving real-time decision support that begins with frontline clinicians through to the senior leadership level. A DNP C-Suite nurse executive must also understand effects on the health care environment from changes in legislation. Mandates from key HIT legislation continue to affect clinical practice and health care organizations today. There will be pressure to improve population health management and the exchange of health information that requires new knowledge for clinicians and better technology solutions. However, the benefits of improved access to health information will be important for clinicians and patients.

Finally, there is great opportunity to affect health care delivery through solutions such as eHealth. Improvements in telecommunications and other technology tools have opened doors for the delivery of health services at a distance. This provides a means for improved access to health care, clinicians, and closer monitoring for patients at high risk who require additional health management. Informatics will continue to grow and support nurse executives. Through improvements in HIT, today's DNP C-Suite nurse executives have a unique opportunity to drive new, innovative ways to deliver care, create and manage data, and improve clinical patient outcomes.

Chapter Reflection Questions

1. What HIT or informatics skills does today's DNP nurse executive need?
2. How can DNP nurse executives drive the use and adoption of HIT?
3. How is HIT used to support nursing practice?
4. What internal structure should a DNP nurse executive have to support nursing informatics and the leadership team?

References

Agbali, M., Trillo, C., Arayici, Y., & Fernando, T. (2017). Creating smart and healthy cities by exploring the potentials of emerging technologies and social innovation for urban efficiency: lessons from the innovative city of Boston. *International Journal of Urban and Civil Engineering, 11*(5), 618–627.

American Association of Colleges of Nursing (2006, October 1). *American Associa-*

ton of Collages of Nursing DNP essentials. Retrieved from American Associaton of Colleges of Nursing : http://www.aacnnursing.org/DNP/DNP-Essentials.

American Nursing Association (2015). *Nursing informatics 2nd edition scope and standards of practice*. Silver Springs, MD: nursesbooks.org.

American Organization of Nurse Executives (2015). *AONE Nurse leader competencies*. Retrieved from American Organization of Nurse Executives: http://www.aone.org/resources/nurse-leader-competencies.shtml.

Becker's Hospital Review. (2014, October). *Becker's Hospital Review—Leadership*. Retrieved from The new healthcare ecosystem: 5 emerging relationships: https://www.beckershospitalreview.com/hospital-management-administration/the-new-healthcare-ecosystem-5-emerging-relationships.html

Becker's Hospital Review. (2016, August 26). *Becker's Hospital Review; Legal and Regulatory*. Retrieved from MD anderson points to epic implementation for 77% drop in adjusted income: https://www.beckershospitalreview.com/finance/md-anderson-points-to-epic-implementation-for-77-drop-in-adjusted-income.html

Choi, J., & Zucker, D. (2013). Self-assessment of nursing informatics competencies for doctor of nursing practice students. *Journal of Professional Nursing, 29*(6), 381–387.

Delaney, C., & Westera, B. (2016). 2016 nursing knowledge big data science initiative. *CIN: Computers, Informatics, Nursing, 34*(9), 384–386.

Department of Health & Human Services. (2016, February). *FY 2017 Annual Performace Plan and Report—Goal 1 Objective F*. Retrieved from HHS.gov: https://www.hhs.gov/about/budget/fy2017/performance/performance-plan-goal-1-objective-f/index.html#analysis

Fareed, N., Ozcan, Y., & DeShazo, J. P. (2012). Hospital electronic medical record enterprise application strategies: do they matter? *Health Care Manage Rev*, 4–13.

Gaffney, B., & Huckabee, M. (2014, July 4). *What is big data?* Retrieved from Health Information Managment and Systems Society : www.himss.org/ResourceLibrary/genResourceFAQ

Health Information Managment and Systems Society: (2011, June 17). *Position statement on transforming nursing practice through technology & informatics*. Retrieved from Health Information Managment and Systems Society: www.himss.rog

Health Resources and Services Administration (2015, November 1). *Health Resources & Services Administration Telehealth Programs*. Retrieved from Health Resources & Services Administration: https://www.hrsa.gov/rural-health/telehealth/index.html.

Hsiao, J., & Chen, R. (2012). An investigation on task-technology fit of mobile nursing information systems for nursing performance. *CIN: Computers, Informatics, Nursing, 30*(5), 265–273.

Huston, C. (2013). The impact of emerging technology on nursing care: warp speed ahead. *OJIN: Online Journal of Nursing Informatics, 18*(2).

Institute of Medicine (2011). *The future of nursing: leading change, advancing health*. Washington: National Academy of Science.

Johnson, B. (1992). *Polarity managment: identifying and managing unsoluable problems*. Amhurst : HRD Press.

Martin, K., Monsen, K., & Bowles, K. (2011). The omaha system and meaningful use applications for practice, education, and research. *CIN: Computers, Informatics, Nursing, 29*, 52–58.

McGonigle, D., & Mastrian, K. (2018). *Nursing informatics and the foundation of knowledge*. Burlington, MA: Jones & Bartlett Learning.

Merriam-Webster. (2018, September). *Merriam-Webster*. Retrieved from Merriam-Webster: https://www.merriam-webster.com/dictionary/ecosystem

Monica, K. (2018, July 23). *Banner health $45M cerner EHR replacement led to medical errors*. Retrieved from EHR Intelligence : https://ehrintelligence.com/news/banner-health-45m-cerner-ehr-replacement-led-to-medical-errors.

Office of the National Coordinator (2016, Novermber 1). *Health IT.gov*. Retrieved from Health IT.gov Safer Guides : https://www.healthit.gov/

Poe, S. S. (2011). The Chief Nursing Information Officer's Impact on Electronic Health. *iHealth Connections*, pp. 61–63.

Raghupathi, W., & Raghupathi, V. (2014). Big data analytics in healthcare: promise and potential. *Health Information Science and Systems, 2*(3), 1–10.

Remus, S., & Kennedy, M. (2012). Innovation in transformative nursing leadership: nursing informatics competencies and roles. *Nursing Leadership, 25*(4), 14–26.

Saba, V., & McCormick, K. (2015). *Essenials of nursing informatics, 6th Edition*. New York: McGraw-Hill Education.

Schoville, R., & Titler, R. (2015). Guiding healthcare technology implementation a new integrated technology implementation mode. *CIN: Computers, Informatics, Nursing, 33*, 99–107.

Simpson, R. L. (2013, November). Chief nurse executives need contemporary informatics competencies. *Nursing Economics, 31*(6), 277–287.

The TIGER Institute. (2014). *The leadership imperative: TIGER's recommendations for integrating technology to transform practice and education*. The TIGER Institutue. Chicago: Health Information and Managment Systems Society. Retrieved from Health Information Managment Systems Society: http://www.himss.org/professionaldevelopment/tiger-initiative

Tupper, S., & Alexander, D. (2012). Leading from the future; the nursing informatics exectutive. *CIN: Computers, Informatics Nursing*, 123–125.

Weaver, B., Lindsay, B., & Gitelman, B. (2012). Communication technology and social media: opportunities and implications for healthcare systems. *The Online Journal of Issues in Nursing*.

Westera, B., & Delaney, C. (2008). Informatics competencies for nursing and healthcare leaders. *AMIA 2008 Symposium Proceedings* (pp. 804–808). Washington: American Medical Informatics Association.

World Health Organization. (2016). *Global diffusion of eHealth: making universal health coverage achievable*. World Health Organization. Geneva: WHO Document Production Services. Retrieved from World Health Organizaiton .

KEVIN RULO

11

Disseminating Knowledge Through Mastering Writing Competency

Chapter Objectives

- Identify the diverse functions of writing in the nursing field, in the health professions, and in the C-Suite environment.
- Demonstrate improved writing skills in academic and professional genres.
- Engage in high order thinking through technical writing.
- Employ principles of rhetorical analysis to communicate effectively in any situation.

> KEY WORDS: technical writing, doctoral writing skills, writing proficiency, business writing, and rhetoric and composition

Introduction

"Their papers demonstrate a lack of knowledge about basic aspects of writing—sentence and paragraph structure, logical progression of facts and ideas.... References are often missing or from inappropriate sources; formatting isn't systematic; length requirements are ignored" (Kennedy, 2014, p. 7). This litany of lament from Maureen Shawn Kennedy (2014), Editor-in-Chief of the *American Journal of Nursing*, which refers to DNPs but which attests just as much to the poor quality of writing so widely prevalent in the broader field, might surprise you. Why all the fuss? Sure it would be wonderful to be a great writer, you might be thinking, but isn't nursing as a profession rather far removed from literary endeavors? Recent guidelines from the World Health Organization (2016), American Nurses Association (2013), and others (Regan and Pietrobon, 2010) suggest that nurses, irrespective of their specialty or practice setting, need to know the principles of effective communication and need to be able to make wide and various use of those principles in the concrete situations of the work

315

environment. The American Association of Colleges of Nursing (AACN) (2006) has recognized writing among its essentials of doctoral education for advanced nursing practice, while the American Organization for Nursing Leadership (AONL) (formerly the American Organization of Nurse Executives) (2015) has noted the absolute necessity of strong communication skills in the executive context. The AACN specifically emphasizes "consultative and leadership skills to create change in health care and in complex healthcare delivery systems" (AACN, 2006). Employing effective communication strategies in the development and implementation of such systems inevitably requires clear, concise, and effective written communication. DNP nurse executives who lack technical writing skills reduce the impact of their work and may fail to engage interprofessional colleagues essential to the analysis of "complex practice and organizational issues" (AACN, 2006). Likewise, although AONL stresses strong business skills and acumen, its nurse executive competencies equally stress effective communication specific to the executive's responsibility to "produce written materials for diverse audiences" (AONL, 2015). Effective writing can influence behaviors, build credibility with physicians as a champion for patient care and quality, and foster a trusting environment by advancing relationships and maintaining credibility. The consensus couldn't be stronger.

Why might these leading bodies place such an emphasis on writing and communication? The reasons are many. For one, the work of nurses, particularly nurse executives in the C-Suite, depends upon efficient and seamless sharing of information. Writing is necessary to accomplish many of the activities integral to the profession, such as those related to documentation, teaching, planning, and decision making (McQuerrey, 2017). Nurses must also be able to write persuasively and informatively about what they do and to advocate for innovations in practice and procedures (Hill, 2012). As a field, nursing has a duty to communicate new research via the methods and venues of academic and professional scholarship. To this end, nursing professionals with advanced degrees in leadership roles, and particularly those in the C-Suite context, find themselves in a unique position and have even greater responsibilities (Morrison, 1960; Davis, 1991). Imagine for a moment that you are a Chief Operating Officer (COO) in a major metropolitan hospital. As part of your responsibilities, you send routine email communications to your nurses and to the wider medical staff. What would be the impression given if these messages were littered with misspellings, typos, and grammatical errors? True or not, such messages would implicitly convey to your readers a lack of care, or worse, incompetence. No less important, errors can cause confusion and result in misunderstanding. Even the small details can have a big impact. They can shape in significant and unconscious ways how people view you and your organization. To the staff under your charge, these errors can communicate that you don't value doing a job well in the particulars. With such errors, you establish a culture of mediocrity and sloppiness.

As a COO, however, you will face much bigger writing challenges than the avoidance of typos or the proper placement of a comma. You will need to formulate policy reports, respond to patients (often in difficult and delicate circumstances), and generate strategic plans. Crafting successful written compositions will require the ability to analyze, synthesize, and persuade. You must be able to convey complex information clearly and concisely. You will need to consider your audience carefully and how your writing can best influence them. You will be required to become practiced in communicating to both specialists and non-specialists. You will have to provide a compelling vision that will inspire and spur to action. Without the ability to write, you can do none of these things (Johnson, 2017).

Becoming a good writer, however, takes time. Apprentice writers often struggle to appropriate unfamiliar modes of discourse. Nursing educators have acknowledged that both undergraduate and graduate curricula have neglected to address writing skills adequately (Johnson, 2017). But even for experienced, highly skilled writers, learning how to write in new genres can be a difficult, sometimes lengthy process. In this chapter, we will discuss, with specific reference to DNP prepared nurse executives working in the C-Suite environment, the strategies and best practices that good writers adopt for their communications, and to ensure continuous growth and development.

What Writing Is

Human beings speak. They always have. They have not always written. The technology of writing is a relatively recent invention, first appearing in its earliest forms roughly 6,000 years ago (Ong, 1982, p. 2). The earliest formal reflection about what makes for effective writing is more recent still, dating from less than 2,500 years ago, and was closely tied to a system of theory and praxis about oral communications known as rhetoric, a term which in its original Greek form, denoted the art of speechmaking. Ancient rhetoricians, first Greek then Latin, studied how to invent, compose, and deliver persuasive speeches to be given in the assembly, at the tribunal, and on the occasion of funerals or other events of pageantry. As the written word became more pervasive, studies were devoted to oral speeches that had been transcribed into text. Eventually, lexigraphical documents came to be analyzed as rhetorical acts and rhetoric itself came to mean the activity and study of purposeful communication of whatever kind (Bazerman, 2013, p. 17–20; Kennedy, 1999, p. 127–136; Ong, 1982, p. 9–10). This transition took time but was already in process in antiquity, where its formal instruction began to emerge in the Trivium of language arts that included logic, grammar, and rhetoric (McLuhan, 2006). Already firmly entrenched in curricula, rhetoric rose in importance in the Early Modern period, partly as a result of the rediscovery of classical authors like Cicero (Lynn, 2010, p. 15). It has continued to be an influential discipline even into the contemporary period, with a new flourishing in the twentieth century as rhetoricians like Kenneth Burke and Wayne Booth came to prominence (Herrick, 2012).

An interest in composition has been a part of grammar and reading instruction from classical times, but as a distinct discipline, it grew out of the study of rhetoric only in the nineteenth century. Composition studies examine the concrete reality of writing as both a process and product widely prevalent in daily life (Lynn, 2010, p. 29). Composition distinguishes itself from rhetoric in this focus on the intricacies and significance of the act of writing, as well as on the practical pedagogical challenges of improvement and development. Even with this distinction, however, the two areas of study are closely linked in the joint field of rhetoric and composition, which became increasingly prevalent in the 20th century, as efforts to teach writing at the college level intensified. The result has been a wealth of new research on all aspects of writing, including everything from how writers learn to write to the way writing can differ by purpose or discipline to the uses of writing in the classroom (Fulkerson, 1987; Fulkerson, 2005). Although this reflection on writing has produced a rich variety of thought on the major questions of the field, a strong consensus has emerged related to the significant dimensions of purposeful communication and best practices for writing process and improvement.

What is writing, conceived as a uniquely human act, and what are some of the acknowledged challenges encountered in understanding and practicing it? The answers are more complex than you might imagine. For example, we might be tempted to say that writing is the communication of thought through a specific medium. Certainly, that would be true in part, but this formulation omits much importance. It implies an understanding of the writing process that is basically stage to stage: We think and then we write to convey our thoughts on the page. But is that really how writing works? Although it is undeniably correct to say that the act of composition is almost always preceded by preparation of one kind or another, often writing stimulates our thinking in such a way as to provide a means for cognitive development about the subject on which we are writing (Bazerman, 2005; Lawrence, 1996). The early medieval theorist of rhetoric Augustine of Hippo (2015) puts it thus: "I endeavour to be one of those who write because they have made some progress, and who, by means of writing, make further progress" (p. 293). Awareness of this principle should affect writing practice. We should be cognizant of the ways in which writing can be used to think through an issue or problem and of how macro-level revisions can aid in the refinement not only of clarity of expression, but also of the ideas themselves.

Such awareness is needed because writing embraces the multifarious and ubiquitous activities of our daily lives. We write and respond to emails and text messages often on an hourly basis. We craft reports and plans. We jot notes to ourselves about tasks to be accomplished, chores to do, and groceries to be bought. In doing so, we compose in different genres, to a variety of different people (including ourselves), for various reasons and to achieve countless ends. Our writing helps us to think and to organize our thoughts. It sets goals and brings people together to achieve them. It conveys information. It mobilizes for action. In short, writing is a chief means by which the work of this world is done.

This ubiquity and variety inevitably means that principles of successful written communication can be difficult to define in the abstract. Will this argument persuade? The only sensible answer is to say that it depends on whom you are trying to persuade. Is it appropriate to use the first person in this piece? To answer this question, we would have to know something about *what kind of writing* it is that you are engaged in, the genre, and its conventions. Rather than focusing on abstract rules that may or may not hold in your particular writing circumstance, it is often more helpful to think about frameworks that you can use in any situation to determine the most appropriate and effective means of communication.

Technical Writing Basics

Imagine again that you are a new DNP prepared Chief Nursing Officer (CNO) of a major hospital. Among your initial duties, you are tasked with writing a strategic plan. In thinking about how you will achieve success in this assignment, your initial concern might be about the document itself. You might find yourself wondering what a strategic plan is exactly. What purposes does it serve? What does it do for you, for your unit, for the hospital? You may also need to think about the more practical aspects of strategic plans. How long are they generally? Is there a conventional format that they tend to follow? Are there required components for your hospital? With these concerns, it becomes clear to you that you will also need to put some thought into your readership. Who will be examining this document? In what contexts? What is the mindset and the values of your likely readers? What do they think is important? These are not random questions. Each is crucial to the success of your strategic plan. They each have to do with specific functions or aspects of written communication. Comprehending these dimensions of communications better can help you to more easily identify and address the unique challenges of any and all writing tasks that you face.

We could call this type of questioning the analysis of rhetorical situation. As a writer, one of your most critical tasks, in whatever circumstances you find yourself, will be to analyze the audience of your potential readers in view of your purpose and context. Your readership in any given rhetorical situation will be comprised of persons who have their own unique assumptions, understanding, and facility with your topic. They may have specific expectations or desires about how information should be presented or about what arguments are best. In order to be successful in your communication, you must anticipate the needs of your readers and reflect upon which strategies of persuasion best fit this group. This way of thinking about your discourse and its effects makes it possible to know with confidence what strategies are best to employ in your particular circumstances.

The systematized means by which you formulate strategies for successful communication counts for a good definition of rhetoric as a mode of inquiry. As Mailloux (2017) has suggested, rhetoric is not strictly speaking a discipline as we typically understand the term. It is more properly an "interdiscipline" that operates through disciplinarities to facilitate "critical work in various intellectual spaces" (p. 2). The critical work of this interdiscipline grounds itself in the way of thinking that we previewed in the previous paragraph and that was best summed up by Aristotle (1926) to be "the faculty of discovering the possible means of persuasion in reference to any subject whatever" (p. 15). Rhetoric transcends the disciplines or applies itself to each of them in that it provides a means for thinking through what happens when we communicate, how our communications work (and sometime don't work), and what we can do about it. Mastering the transdiscipline of rhetoric will help you to recognize what matters as a writer in the specific compositional task before you, what writer choices you have, and how to assess which of those choices would be best in this given case.

The Rhetorical Triangle, Figure 11.1, is derived from Aristotle's (1926) thought about the main appeals of persuasive communications. It illustrates the basic components of all acts of communication and aims to represent

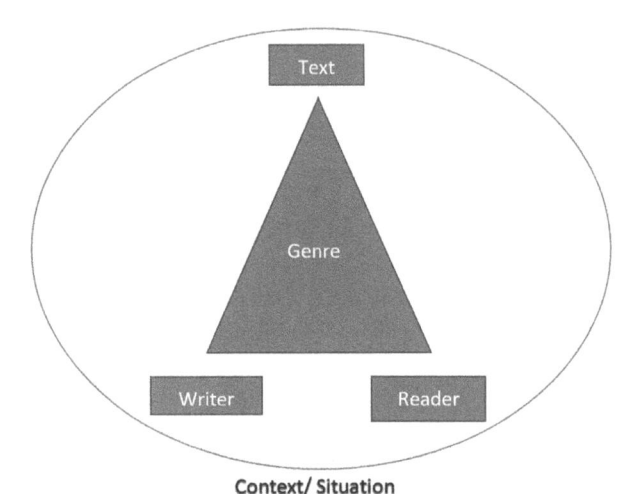

Figure 11.1. *The Rhetorical Triangle.*

the many diverse and complex kinds of interaction among them. The language of the triangle above assumes specifically written communications.

A writer or writers generate(s) text. They compose this text intentionally for a reader or a group of readers. Their composition occurs within a specific situation. Successful communications take all of these factors, and how they interact variously, into consideration. In so doing, the successful writer reflects on the *text* in order to *understand what needs to be said*; on the *reader and context* in order to *know how to say it*; and on the *writing self* in order to *think about how he or she will be perceived*.

The writer-text-reader triad, above all, points to the integral nature of communication as a rhetorical act. Isolating one element of the triangle is only useful to the extent that it illumines the other two dimensions. Reflecting on the sides of the triangle helps to bring into relief various aspects of a rhetorical act as they relate to each other. For example, focusing on the *audience or reader* will only underline the extent to which the basic message needs to be shaped for the addressee. Thinking about your readership will clarify for you the level of specificity appropriate for your text, as well as the most persuasive strategies to employ. Communicating patient care protocols to the nursing staff, for example, may require and can assume the use of more technical jargon of the nursing discourse community, while conveying those same protocols to executives within the corporate hospital structure would require the use of less specialized vocabulary and greater care on the writer's part to ensure that the information is fully explained, as the ability of the more general audience to make inferences about patient care practices would be much more limited.

Thinking about *your own rhetorical stance* can also move you to alter your communication. Someone writing from the authority of the executive will have a particular set of advantages and challenges that he or she must negotiate. Generally speaking, having less authority may translate to your feeling the need to explain your position more and with greater deference and tact. Having more authority may necessitate protecting against heavy handedness. Whatever the case, you should be in the habit of thinking about where you stand in relation to what you are communicating and how others will interpret what you say.

Likewise, understanding the *context* of your communication is vital to success. Context involves all the situational elements that separate your specific communicative act from all others. More generally, context includes two related concepts: purpose and genre. Purpose can be defined as your reasons and motives for writing. You have to know with clarity what you want your writing to accomplish in this specific circumstance. Only then can you hope to structure your communication to meet the identified goals (for the simple reason that the goals have to be clearly identified before they can be met). Closely related to your purpose is the genre in which you are writing. If we reflect on genre, the question of appropriateness can be clarified in many areas. Genres are "ways of doing things" (Bazerman, 2013, p. 24) that often include set patterns for organizing and presenting our information, as well as conventional stylistic modes of discourse that will condition levels of formality, phrasing, and citation practices. As "ways of doing things," genres cannot be disentangled from the purposes that give rise to them and that they themselves re-establish. The 20th century philosopher Ludwig Wittgenstein (1953) introduced in another context the concept of the "language game," which helps us to think of speech and writing acts as rule-governed operations. The idea can be a useful way of thinking about genres. Recognizing the expectations and rules of the game ensures efficacious communication.

To illustrate how these principles of the triangle can come together in situations faced regularly by the DNP nurse executives in the C-Suite, consider the case of fictional Mary Jones:

Case Study—Mary Jones

Mary Jones recently completed her DNP degree and had just been appointed CNO of Midwest Memorial, a major metropolitan hospital in the middle of the country. She had previously worked as director of a division within a similar-sized hospital in the general region. Midwest Memorial faces challenges related to the changing health care industry that are not uncommon to most contemporary hospitals, but amid these difficulties, it remains financially stable. The previous CNO, however, did not manage the nursing division effectively. As a result, working conditions were not good and morale was low. In her first few months on the job, Mary was tasked with writing a five-year strategic plan for the entire nursing division. It was to be, she understood from her conversations with superiors, her vision for reform. It was clear to Mary even from her initial interview that because of the general state of disarray that she inherited, her superiors were looking for someone to present a fresh approach and revamp the unit. They were willing to take her lead on how best to do that. Mary reviewed applicable AONL Nurse Leadership Competences in preparing herself to undertake what she considered to be a monumental task. She centered on the competency of effective communication and reviewed foundational thinking skills necessary to promote nursing leadership as both a science and an art (AONL 2015). Quickly, she found herself reminded of the importance of solid writing skills and writing mastery as a critical component of her work and professional success.

Mary's rhetorical situation was such that she could, and even would be expected to, propose a bold new vision that broke with her predecessor's outlook and practice. She knew that her audience would be willing to listen to new initiatives and new directions. She was also aware of the genre of the strategic plan and had read many before. But importantly, she had never written one herself. She knew they were documents that presented a broad vision for units and that determined long and mid-term actions. She also knew that it would be used formally and informally within Midwest Memorial as a charter for resource allocation, hiring, and assessment. But it was her first effort at writing one and she puzzled over many of the details. So, she decided to look at past models of plans from her division and from adjacent operational divisions within the hospital to get a sense of expected format, length, and general tenor. She also consulted with trusted colleagues at neighboring hospitals who could provide more helpful examples of successful strategic plans. From these, she was able to get a good sense for the conventions and rules of the "language game".

It was clear that Mary's audience would be disposed to give her ideas a full hearing and would lend her the benefit of the doubt when it came to her credibility for conceiving and enacting a new plan for the unit. Even so, she spent some time thinking about what might best persuade the most likely and most important readers of her plan, namely her superiors. They were looking for a new vision but given the recent past experience with the failure of leadership in the division, Mary thought that they would also be looking for a coherent, realistic plan that seemed achievable. Mary was new to the institution and felt that she needed to demonstrate expertise to establish for her audience that her plan was properly informed as to what would work best for Midwest Memorial at this particular moment. So, Mary decided that she would add a section detailing the institution and the nursing division's history, with special emphasis on the last ten years. She would then spend some time in her plan identifying issues of concern that would be addressed by her plan. Although this was to some extent a usual way of structuring a strategic plan, Mary highlighted and placed greater emphasis on this institution-specific approach and also spent more time on it than she might otherwise have because she deemed it uniquely important for her rhetorical context.

Writing the strategic plan flummoxed Mary. Even with using the AONL Nurse Executive Competencies (AONE, 2015) to guide her thought process, she ruffled at the thought of addressing a variety of audiences all at once: her nursing staff, her superiors, the nursing and health care field as a whole. Along these lines, one particularly daunting challenge for her was finding ways to talk about best practices in the field and difficulties particular to nursing in a way that was easily digestible for a less-specialized audience. Mary was also sensitive to the fact that she needed to find ways to express herself in short declarative statements through genre conventions like objectives. Condensing complex problems and practices into short pithy sound bites proved difficult. But Mary knew that many of the most powerful people in the hospital would not have time to pore over the more detailed portions of the plan, so she spent extra time on this headline discourse and made sure the document's overall message could be understood just from reading these portions. Mary also went back to her trusted colleagues asking them to read drafts of her work. She found their experience and feedback invaluable. Sparing no effort, she also tapped her husband, Joe, who was an online newspaper reporter, for editing and proofing.

Her plan was well-received by all levels of the hospital and the main tenets were accepted unanimously by the board. Mary's success had much to do with her field experience and abilities, but without her rhetorical and compositional sophistication, she would have had a difficult time convincing her audience to accept her views and to believe that she was competent enough to entrust the future of the nursing division to her and her plan. What did Mary do? First, she reoriented herself to cogent nurse executive competencies to better frame her understanding of the strategic plan she envisioned developing. Then, she analyzed and understood well all aspects of the rhetorical triangle: namely, the audience that she was trying to persuade, the rhetorical situation and context in which she found herself, the type of document that she was writing, and her own position as the writer/proposer.

Techniques for Writing Improvement: A Ten-Point Plan

How do you gain the expertise that Mary has? The key to your success will be your use of the rhetorical triangle as a means of crafting persuasive texts. However, beyond these context-dependent factors, you will need to nurture attitudes and mentalities conducive to the consistent production of quality writing. You will also need to grasp and learn how to apply the near-to-universal principles of good writing—correct grammar and mechanics. Mastery of these aspects of writing is essential to effective communication. Writing excellence is a matter of habits of practice as much as know-how. Following this norm, we suggest a long-term plan for writing improvement along the following ten points:

1. Pledge to Do What it Takes to Grow as a Writer

Jack Kerouac (1995), the twentieth-century American novelist, who authored classics like *On the Road*, once wrote that "Writers are made, for anybody who isn't illiterate can write; but geniuses of the writing art like Melville, Whitman or Thoreau are born" (p. 488). Kerouac's statement should be consoling. So often we hear students and apprentice writers express their certainty that writing is an innate ability, one they don't have. This idea is reinforced by the talk we encounter throughout our education in our English classes and no less in our broader culture that centers on "great literature," the net effect of which is to make us think that writers are certain types of people, people on whom have been bestowed particular gifts of language and expression. If we are not the types of people who have supposedly been those types of people ever since they first picked up a pen, then we think we must not be writers. Kerouac's proposal, however, won't let us off the hook so easy. Maybe we're not geniuses of the writing art, but we shouldn't take that to mean that we can't be good writers. Good writers are the product not of birth or of some obscure genius gene. Good writers are the product of work: smart work, hard work, and long work.

Developing your abilities as a writer will create opportunities for you in the nursing profession that you would not have otherwise. Your ability to move into leadership roles and to advance in the field will be directly impacted by the extent to which you can make use of the technology of writing to collect and present information, think through problems, and persuade others that they should think the way you do about the issues that matter. In a word: writing matters for you, for your short and long-term success. The good news is that you can improve. The first step in that process of development—however, in some ways the most crucial step—requires you to understand the importance of writing and to recognize your ability to grow as a writer. The second step is to make a pledge to put in the time and the tears to make it happen.

2. See Writing as a Process

A strong commitment to writing development represents a necessary beginning toward putting yourself on the path to becoming the writer that you should be. But without a proper understanding of the act of writing as a process, your efforts at improvement will sputter. Our schooling and our experiences with writing growing up sometimes lead us to conceive of it as a product-oriented activity. Much of the writing done by students across the ability spectrum, in primary and secondary schools and even in college, could be called "binge writing", i.e., papers composed in one swoop a few hours before the due date (Brookshire and Brundage, 2016). With these habits of practice, we can easily fail to consider the discrete moments or stages involved in composing. The tradition of classical rhetoric, developed in ancient Greece and Rome, schematized the process of composition in the terms of invention, arrangement, and style, in which invention stood for the initial generation of material; arrangement, for the organization of that material into an ordered whole; and style, for the refinements made at the level of sentence and texture (Kennedy, 1999, p. 102). This model helps us to see the folly of compositional binging in that it points to the many pivotal moments of writing from the first spark of an idea to the final polishing of prose. More modern approaches have supplemented these canons by emphasizing the recursive nature of their relation, how, in other words, the moments of inventing, arranging, and styling are replayed and refigured as we draft and revise. Rather than a stage-to-stage model, contemporary composition studies underlines the messiness of the writing process, whereby we find ourselves arranging and styling even as we invent and inventing as we arrange and style (Perl, 1994; Bean, 2011). Appreciating the process of composing can help especially apprentice writers to value the power of revision for enhancing writing quality. Certainly, revision can be an opportunity to correct smaller errors or to perfect sentence structure or clarity. But it can be for more experienced authors and often is a more dynamic process of reconceiving matters of argument, evidence, organization, and overall approach (Sommers, 1980). It is not uncommon for seasoned writers to have eureka moments about their overall research or its value for readers, even at the very late stages of composition. A good sense of the writing process can also help you to experiment in useful ways to discover what approach works best for you both more generally and for the different genres and tasks that you undertake.

My pencils outlast their erasers.—*Vladimir Nabokov*

Invention	Arrangement	Style
• Initial conception • Content creation	• Dividing • Ordering	• Polishing • Editing

3. Read as a Writer

We tend to read passively. We mine the text for its information and content, for what it can tell us about our subject. In other cases, we may read for pleasure, for the delight of the style, or for the way the story is told. These kinds of reading serve their purpose well, but writers in particular benefit from another kind of reading, which should be done in addition to, rather than in place of, the more usual consumptive reading. When we read passively, we read as readers. Our attention is focused on the process of understanding and interpretation that comes with the effort of comprehension. Another form of reading locates us in the position of the writer. We read this way when we seek to revise or edit our own texts or the texts of our peers and colleagues. But reading as a writer can be beneficial also for published works or finished documents, especially when they are of a high quality. As a writer of scholarly articles, you should take note of well-written papers when you encounter them. Set aside some time regularly to re-read such articles, carefully observing the rhetorical strategies and genre conventions that the writer uses to express his or her thought well. Keep a notebook of effective strategies and sentences. The same can and should be done for other types of writing that you engage in, whether it be strategic plans, annual reports, or simple emails. Each of these genres has its own internal logic and observing how others have successfully navigated that form of communication, given their specific situations and aims, will help you to broaden and enrich your own repertoire of what is possible for your writing.

4. Get the Fundamentals Right.

Good writing is more than correctness, but without a solid grasp of usage and grammar, it is difficult to be effective as a communicator. The results of poor command in the fundamentals can be miscommunication of ideas, the ultimate failure in writing; even when meaning is not affected, your credibility as a writer surely will be. So, make every effort to know and master the basics of English prose, a few of the more important aspects of which are considered below.

Active and Passive Voice. We live in a world of action, and we appreciate and respond best as readers to active voice writing, which tends to be crisper and more engaging. When writing is in the active voice, the subject of the sentence is the doer of the action.

ACTIVE: The nurses helped the patients.

(The subject of the sentence is "nurses," who are also the doers of the verb "helped.")

PASSIVE: The patients were helped by the nurses.

(The subject of the sentence is "patients," who are the object of the verb "were helped." The doer of the verb, those who helped, is part of a prepositional phrase "by the nurses.")

Sometimes the doer of the action in passive voice sentences is omitted.

PASSIVE: The patients were helped.

To avoid passive voice, make sure that the doer of the verb is in the subject position. To use passive voice, put the object of the action in the subject position of the sentence.

Despite its defects, the passive voice can sometimes be useful. You may not know who the doer of the action is, or you may want to de-emphasize the doer and/or emphasize what was done. (For example a sentence like "The project was considered a success" would emphasize the project and its success, not the evaluator.)

Parallelism. Parallelism strives to achieve a symmetry between form and content at the sentence level; multiple ideas, expressed in words or in word groups, are balanced with a corresponding grammatical structure.

Parallel structures can be of many kinds depending on the number of ideas and their relationship. One common form is *items in a series*. Below is an example of faulty parallelism followed by another corrected sentence, for items in a series.

Dr. Edwards spoke to the patient's husband, reviewed her chart and vital signs. (*Faulty parallelism*)

Dr. Edwards spoke to the patient's husband, reviewed her chart, and checked her vital signs. (*Proper parallelism*)

Notice in the second, correct sentence all three actions of Dr. Edwards are presented with verbs: *spoke, reviewed, checked*.

Coordination and Subordination. The grammatical structure of your sentences should reflect the relation between the various ideas being communicated. If ideas are equal to each other in importance, you should use coordinating conjunctions to connect them (coordinating conjunctions are for, and, but, or, yet, so). If certain ideas should be emphasized over others, you can use subordinating conjunctions to connect them (e.g., that, because, when, after, if, although, while, etc.).

Coordination

Francis is an internist, and Karen is a neurologist.

Subordination

While Francis is an internist, Karen is a neurologist.

The first sentence above relates the two ideas equally. We have two facts connected but on the same level of emphasis. The second sentence, however, subordinates Francis's being an internist and emphasizes Karen and her job.

Subordination can be particularly well-suited to academic writing, because it allows you to situate yourself within a larger conversation or data set. Here is an example:

While we have made a lot of advances in the study of brain tumor development, there is still much that we do not know.

A sentence like this one allows the writer to indicate where current research is and what it has accomplished while also emphasizing that there still remains a lot of work to do. The emphasis in the sentence is on that work to done. If the two clauses were reversed—i.e., if the sentence read "While there is still much that we do not know, we have made a lot of advances in the study of brain tumor development."—the entire thrust of the meaning would be changed. The sentence would be conveying a strong sense of the advances and strides accomplished in this area of research. The effect is partly a matter of placement; the final clause generally carries more emphasis in English, but it also, and chiefly, has to do with grammatical structure.

Subject-Verb Agreement. Subjects and verbs should agree in number and person. Plural subjects take plural forms of the verb, and vice-versa. While this seems like a straightforward principle, there are several difficult instances that trip writers up and therefore need to be addressed here.

One problem is that sometimes the subject that should determine the form of the verb is difficult to locate. Consider the following sentence:
The test tubes on the tray in the backroom are high quality.

The word "tubes" is the simple subject that in this case determines the form of the verb. Both "on the tray" and "in the backroom" are prepositional phrases between the simple subject and the main verb. Do not be confused by words placed between subjects and verbs.

The test *tubes* on the tray in the backroom *are* high quality.

In the case of a plural subject (e.g., conjoined with "and") use a plural form of the verb.

Drs. Edwards and Smith agree on the prognosis.

There are cases where two nouns joined with a conjunction may be a single subject and would need to take a singular verb (e.g., peanut butter and jelly, Johnson & Johnson).

Indefinite pronouns and collective nouns are generally singular.

This class likes the professor.

Each nurse is individually responsible for the care given.

Avoiding Weak Verbs. Weak verbs tend to be those that indicate states of being or that do not carry much action. They zap your writing of its flare and verve. Forms of "be," "have," and "do" are some of the most common weak verbs.

Often weak verbs result from a desire to sound sophisticated or overly formal. When we try to do that, we have a tendency as writers to put actions in the noun position and leave the grammatical action to a place-holding weak verb. For example, take a look at the following sentence:

The institution of the new policy by the medical team was a success.

The writer here has overloaded the whole subject and left the verb with not much to do. The real action being described ("institution") is placed in the subject position as a noun. By shifting the real action to the verb position, the sentence springs to life and loses a good deal of its clunk.

The medical team instituted a successful policy.

If you find yourself using weak verbs disproportionately, try looking for where the real action of the sentence can be found and shift that to the verb position.

5. Answer the "So What" Question.

Much of the writing that we do on a daily basis does not need to come with an explanation of its value and *raison d'être*. An email to your supervisor or a memo to the nursing team may be self-evident in its aims, scope, and relevance. Academic writing, however, when it comes in the form of scholarly articles, dissertations, and seminar papers, usually does require an explicit effort on the author's part to provide the larger contexts of the argument and how it contributes to current research on the topic. Your reader needs to know how your work relates to the work of others and how it changes our understanding of the issue being studied. A good article or dissertation chapter will demonstrate that our current knowledge is in some way incomplete or unsatisfactory and therefore that there is cause for exploring the issue further. Ultimately, you have to answer the "so what" question. Why should we care? It may seem obvious to you, but the rationale and the results of your research need to be justified fully for your readers. Below is a template that can be helpful in getting you started thinking about these issues:

The current conversation around my topic is _____.

This conversation is (incomplete/incorrect) in the following way _____.

My work changes/supplements the current conversation in the following way(s)_____.

My project will have the following impact(s) _____.

6. Begin Well.

The art of the introduction can be a challenge for even the most seasoned of authors. At the same time, the beginning is among the most important parts of a piece, precisely for the ways in which it provides a unique opportunity to convey the contributions and value of your project as outlined in the previous point. A good opening should interest your reader, provide him or her with a basic context for your argument, and forecast what can be expected in the pages that follow. For engaging your reader, it can be helpful to begin with an anecdote, an illustrative narrative, or an artfully phrased question that touches on the problem your paper will try to solve. When it comes to the composition process, the introduction should be written (or at least substantially re-written) last. It can sometimes be useful to begin with writing the introduction as a way of getting going, but it is likely that you will not know how best to introduce your argument and research until you have completed the body of the paper. Because writing is a thought process as much as a process of communication, your thinking will often advance and sharpen as you draft. Any introduction written at the outset of your composing may very well need some reconsideration. At the very least, you should review your introduction carefully as a final step before submission.

> The last thing one knows in constructing a work is what to put first.
> —*Blaise Pascal*

7. Take Care With Your Words

It might seem commonplace to say that you should be careful with your choice of words. All the same, it's worth saying again. *You should be careful with your choice of words.* The poet John Milton (2014) once wrote, "Apt words have power to swage/the tumors of a troubled mind" (p.49). The power of words can indeed be a soothing force for good, and amazingly so, but it can also be a just as potently destructive power if used poorly or to a bad end. Words used well can have all manner of positive effects and, most importantly, ensure that they will have your intended effect. Words used poorly or unjustly will obfuscate and damage your credibility. Take care with your words. In writing, they're all you have.

Write with a dictionary on hand. Do not use words with which you are unfamiliar. Avoid jargon whenever possible. If you can say it in fewer words, do it. If you can use a simpler word, there is no reason to use a big wordy word.

At the same time, cultivate a wide and rich vocabulary. Wittgenstein (1922) has said that *"the limits of my language* mean the limits of my world." Don't limit yourself. See to it that your world is capacious.

8. Fight Writer's Block

Writer's block is a problem for writers of all levels. Sometimes we find that the power of the blank page paralyzes us. At other times, we just don't know where to start. At still other times, our problem turns out to be less about being blocked from writing as about being distracted by the gazillion other things that compete for our attention (email, kids, spouses, email, the siren song of the internet, chores, and did I mention email?). The old Greek maxim "know thyself" can be a good starting point for conquering blocks. Each of us has our own personality, work style, and life circumstances; these will translate into a unique set of solutions for enhancing productivity. A few of the basic principles for achieving regular, high-quality writing productivity include the following:

Give yourself the right kind of time:

You need to make time for writing. It should be a regular time. It needs to be a well-defined portion of more than 45 minutes, and it needs to be a time for what productivity theorist Cal Newport (2016) calls "deep work." In other words, turn off the email, the internet, and the phone and immerse yourself in the research and the writing. Soundproof your room if you have to.

Set goals and plan ahead:

Goal setting is an important part of getting work done. If we can't get started, sometimes it's because we don't know where to start. Setting goals is not just about having a benchmark of hours logged or words written. It's really about turning your writing sessions into tasks that produce writing (e.g., "Today I will get started on the first part of my literature review section and try to solve the problem of how to divide it up. I will make progress in this goal by producing a semi-formal outline of that section."). At the end of your session, you should set goals for the next session (e.g., leave yourself some time to write notes before you end your session, notes about where you are and what issues you are struggling with). This is important because you probably will not remember what was preoccupying you by the time you return to your writing desk and you don't want to spend twenty minutes just getting back to where you were). Set goals for the week, the month, the semester, and the year, with a strategy for achieving them. Periodically check in on your long- and mid-term goals.

Categorize the kinds of work that need to be done:

Sometimes, we're just not ready to write that section that is sequentially the next to be written, because we need to either think about it more or do more research. That's okay. Write your sections in whatever order lends itself to continuous composition. Understand that different kinds of writing tasks may be easier to do at different times. For example, for many writers, mornings are a great time for first drafting and deep conceptual thinking, whereas the more sluggish afternoons may be better for the less cognitively intense bibliographic work, or for polishing and editing.

9. Have a Writing Improvement Plan

Planning is important for writing productivity. It is no less essential for writing improvement. Anyone can improve as a writer, but your growth rate will be substantially increased by a systematic approach. The first step is to assess your own strengths and weaknesses as a writer. Where do you feel strongest and most comfortable? In what areas do you feel you could improve? Consider all aspects of writing, from the sentence level style and grammar issues to organization, argument, style, and use of research. Once you have a sense for which areas need work, prioritize and focus on one or two key areas at a time. Every three or four months, do a check-in on yourself and reassess.

10. Get a Second Opinion.

Getting a second opinion: it can be a good practice of health care and of writing. We think of the writer as a solitary figure, hauled up in his chamber, scribbling away in solitude. In practice, however, writing looks much different. Professional authors vary in their disciplines, topics, and processes; one thing they almost all have in common is that they share their work with other experts on a regular basis. If the published authors are doing that, you should too. Make a point to share your work with your colleagues and mentors, even when it isn't required. When you do, be sure that you get a clear sense from them how they understood your writing and review very carefully the feedback they give. Show your work to different types of readers—editors, experts in your field, and educated non-experts—for various kinds of feedback. Doing this will help you to identify weaknesses in your writing and will provide much food for thought on how to improve.

Chapter Takeaways

1. Understanding the basic components of all communications can help you to determine the best strategies for persuasion in any given writing situation that you may face. The rhetorical triangle—with its emphasis on writer, reader, text, and context—provides a vocabulary and framework for analyzing your composition tasks and making decisions as a writer.
2. Your professional success as a DNP prepared nurse executive depends to a great extent on your writing success. Writing is a key competency for all nurses. Developing your communication skills should therefore be among your highest priorities. Fortunately, with time and effort anyone can develop as a writer. Make a commitment now to a consistent program of writing development. Create an action plan, review it regularly, and track your progress.
3. Make the most of the writing process. Use writing as a tool for thinking as well as a means of communicating your thought. Leave time for large-scale revision as well as more local edits. Collaborate with trusted colleagues by sharing and receiving feedback on your work.
4. Ensure that you have a thorough knowledge of the tools and rules of English, including grammar and usage. Include in your revision attention to correctness, as faulty mechanics conveys inattention to detail and even incompetency.

Chapter Summary

Writing is a key competency for the nursing profession. Nursing leaders, especially DNP prepared nurse executives, are charged in a particular way with the dissemination of knowledge in the field and are held to the highest expectations, which makes writing of even greater importance for them. At the same time, there is widespread recognition that nurses often do not have strong writing skills. Fortunately, research in writing studies has a long tradition of reflection on the methods of effective textual communication and the burgeoning field of rhetoric and composition offers sound advice for growth in writing for authors of all levels at any stage of their career. Making use of the best practices of this field can aid in writing mastery for DNP nurse executives in the C-Suite.

Effective communication cannot be completely standardized because circumstances vary so greatly. Every rhetorical situation is unique. Having a mode of analysis that allows a writer or speaker to determine what would be the best tactics for his or her specific task provides the highest learning impact for future success. The rhetorical triangle gives us such a methodology in that it can help us to see how all communications share key components and how we must carefully consider each component in relation to each other in order to craft communications that are optimally effective for each unique and unrepeatable writing situation in which we find ourselves. It is only through reflection on the interaction of elements, such as our audience, our text, our rhetorical stance, the genre, and our context, that we can come to trustworthy conclusions about persuasive and compelling writerly choices.

Beyond these context-dependent aspects of writing, however, there are also those habits that lead to high productivity and those principles of writing that are near to universally applicable, namely, those related to grammar and mechanics. Mastery of these aspects of writing is essential to effective communication. But, in all these areas, improvement takes time. Long-term commitment to a clear program of writing development based in full understanding of how the writing process works is needed from all nursing leaders.

Chapter Reflection Questions

1. What is your writing process like? In what ways has your process changed over time? How does it change from project to project?

2. What do you think are your current strengths and weakness as a writer? What kinds of writing are you most comfortable and most uncomfortable with? Where can you improve, and how might you do so?

3. Think about the writing situations that you will encounter in the C-Suite contexts as a nursing professional. What are some of the reasons for communicating in writing in this context? What does writing do in these contexts? To what different audiences might you be asked to communicate? How might your communications change based on the different audiences?

4. Review the ten-point plan for writing improvement presented in this chapter. What are some concrete changes in behavior that you can enact now to ensure that you implement the plan? (e.g., "I need to start writing earlier to have more time for pre-writing and revision.").

References

American Association of Colleges of Nursing (2006, October). *DNP essentials: The essentials of doctoral education for advanced nursing practice*. Retrieved from http://www.aacnnursing.org/Portals/42/Publications/DNPEssentials.pdf.

American Nurses Association. (2013, August). *Competency model*. Retrieved from https://learn.ana-nursingknowledge.org/template/ana/publications_pdf/leadershipInstitute_competency_modelbrochure.pdf.

American Organization of Nurse Executives. (2013). Nurse executive competencies. Chicago, IL: American Organization of Nurse Executives. Retrieved from http://www.aone.org/resources/nec.pdf

Aristotle (1926). *The "art" of rhetoric*. (J.H. Freese, Trans.) Cambridge, MA: Harvard University Press (Original work published 4th Century B.C.E.)

Bazerman, C. (2005). Genre and cognitive development: Beyond writing to learn. In C. Bazerman, A. Bonini, & D. Figueiredo (Eds.), *Genre in a changing world*. (pp. 279–94). Fort Collins, CO: Parlor Press.

Bazerman, C. (2013). *A rhetoric of literature action: Literate action, Volume 1*. Anderson, SC: Parlor Press.

Bean, J. C. (2011). *Engaging ideas: The professor's guide to integrating writing, critical thinking, and active learning in the classroom*. (2nd ed.). San Francisco, CA: Jossey-Bass.

Brookshire, R. H., & Brundage, S. B. (2016). *Writing scientific research in communication sciences and disorders*. San Diego, CA: Plural Publishing.

Davis, J. K. (1991). Professions, trades and the obligation to inform, *Journal of Applied Psychology, 8*(2), 167–176. Retrieved from http://hssfaculty.fullerton.edu/philosophy/johndavis/documents/Davis-Professions,%20Trades,%20and%20the%20Obligation%20to%20Inform.pdf.

Fulkerson, R. (2005). Composition at the turn of the twenty-first century. *College Composition and Communication, 56*(4), 654–687. Retrieved from http://www.jstor.org/stable/30037890

Fulkerson, R. (1990). Composition theory in the eighties: axiological consensus and paradigmatic diversity. *College Composition and Communication, 41*(4), 409. doi:10.2307/357931

Herrick, J. A. (2012). *The history and theory of rhetoric: An introduction*. (5th ed.). New York, NY: Routledge.

Hill, K. S. (2012). The art of communicating outcomes. *JONA, 42*(10).

Johnson, J. E. (2017). Advanced practice nurses: Developing a business plan for an independent ambulatory clinical practice. *Nursing Economics 35*(3), 126–141.

Kennedy, G.A. (1999). Classical rhetoric and its Christian and secular tradition from ancient to modern times. (2nd ed.). Chapel Hill, North Carolina: The University of North Carolina Press.

Kennedy, M. S. (2014). Getting writing right. *Am J Nursing, 114*(3), 7. Retrieved from http://journals.lww.com/ajnonline/Fulltext/2014/03000/Getting_Writing_Right.1.aspx

Kerouac, J (1995). *The portable Jack Kerouac*. New York: Viking Press. (Original work published in 1962.)

McLuhan, M. (2006). *Classical trivium: The place of Thomas Nashe in the learning of his time*. (Reprint ed.). T. Gordon (Ed.). Berkeley, CA: Gingko Press. (Original work written in 1943).

Lawrence, M. S. (1996). *Writing as a thinking process*. (2nd ed.). Ann Arbor: University of Michigan Press.

Lynn, S. (2010). *Rhetoric and composition: An introduction*. Cambridge, UK: Cambridge University Press.

Mailloux, S. (2017). *Rhetoric's pragmatism: Essays in rhetorical hermeneutics*. University Park, PA: The Pennsylvania State University Press.

McQuerrey, L. (2017). The importance of writing as a nurse practitioner. *Chron*. Retrieved from http://work.chron.com/importance-writing-nurse-practitioner-18156.html

Milton, J. (2014). *Samson Agonistes and other poems*. Ontario: Broadview Press. (Original work appeared in 1671).

Morrison, L. J. (1960). *Steppingstones to professional nursing*. St. Louis. MO: The C.V Mosby Co.

Newport, C. (2016). *Deep work: Rules for focused success in a distracted world*. New York: Grand Central Publishing.

Ong, W. J. (1982). *Orality and literacy: The technologizing of the word*. New York: Methuen.

Perl, S. (ed.). (1994). *Landmark essays on writing process*. Davis, CA: Hermagoras Press.

Regan, M., & Pietrobon, R. (2010). A conceptual framework for scientific writing in nursing. *J Nsg Education, 49*(8), 437–443.

Sommers, N. (1980). Revision strategies of student writers and experienced adult writers. *College Composition and Communication 31*.4, 378–388.

St. Augustine of Hippo (2015). *The letters of St. Augustine*. Jazzybee Verlag. (Original work written around 412.)

World Health Organization. (2016). Nurse educator core competencies. Geneva, Switzerland: WHO. Retrieved from http://www.who.int/hrh/nursing_midwifery/nurse_educator050416.pdf?ua=1

Wittgenstein, L. (1922). Tractatus Logico-Philosophicus. Edinburgh: Edinburgh Press.

Wittgenstein, L. (1953). *Philosophical investigations*. Oxford: Basil Blackwell.

CAROLYN K. ROOT
JEFFREY A. JOHNSON
ROBIN WIKLE

12

C-Suite Soft Skills and the Diverse Workforce

Chapter Objectives

- Appreciate the importance of "soft skills" in managing a wide range of challenges in the executive environment.
- Build a "personal brand," develop a rich personal network, and identify trusted advisors.
- Acknowledge the power of effective storytelling and the value in developing positive charisma.
- Appreciate the strength of strategic planning, the importance of pivoting, and learning how to fail fast and recover quickly.
- Describe organizational structure alternatives associated with rapid and agile practice teams.
- Apply soft skills to lead a collaborative, effective multi-generational workforce.

KEY WORDS: strategic planning, C-Suite soft skills, networking, trusted advisor, personal brand, generational diversity, workforce pipeline

Introduction

This chapter addresses the diverse American workforce and the skills needed to be a successful executive managing today's workforce. Today's workforce includes five generations of workers: (1) the Silent or Greatest generation, also referred to as "Traditionalists," born in 1945 or before; (2) the Baby Boom generation, born between 1946 and 1964; (3) the Gen-X or Generation-X, born between 1965 and 1980; (4) the Millennial generation, born between 1981 and 1996; and (5) the Post-Millennial generation, also referred to as Gen-Z, born in 1997 and after (Fry, 2018). Each generation has different life experiences that affect their world views, values, opinions, attitudes, and biases. The C-Suite executives who are leading today's diverse workforce need skills that will enhance their abilities to lead diverse teams of employees.

This chapter provides DNP nurse executives with an opportunity to consider the relationship between soft skills: and their success as C-suite executives. A well-developed set of soft skills, along with a record of trustworthiness and other leadership competencies, helps to assure success in the C-Suite. Such success requires a well-equipped personal skills toolbox, which is explored in this chapter. The chapter concludes with a case study designed to further expand industry knowledge with content based on a successful contemporary firm. The case study concludes with discussion questions and key takeaways designed to enable learners to personalize experiences and test knowledge.

The Leadership "Soft Skills" Toolbox

The concept of soft skills as a critical leadership characteristic is not new. The concept was identified in 1985 by Geneen, the former president and chief executive officer (CEO) of the International Telephone and Telegraph Corporation, when he noted that leadership was practiced in words but also in attitude and actions. Geneen's decades of C-Suite experience and his thoughtful analysis linked leadership and soft skills together as the successful combination for effective leadership and mastery in the executive suite. The role of the executive includes creating a vision for the organization, addressing the issues that affect the organization, making strategic hiring and policy decisions, and setting the tone for the organization and its future.

In recent years, providing excellent medical care, which has become the assumed norm in health care, has not been sufficient to ensure the viability of a hospital. Patient satisfaction has grown in importance. Patient satisfaction comes from the customer experience, which is influenced by the soft skills of all hospital employees, from the top to the bottom of the organization chart.

The ability to influence patient satisfaction begins when the patient enters the doors of the hospital and continues throughout the duration of the patient's treatment. This "whole care experience" is challenging for hospital employees and the patient and their family who are stressed by a serious medical condition that may have an unknown outcome. The hospital staff, from the individuals who conduct patient intake to the team of medical professionals who treat and support the patient, all contribute to the patient's view of their hospital experience. The hospital leadership creates and promotes the organizational brand that must be expressed by all who work in the hospital. High ratings in patient experience are synonymous with a brand that reflects excellence, compassion, respect, and responsiveness, as demonstrated by the hospital leadership and all the hospital staff.

Vision flows from the executive suite to the entire hospital organization. Survey research from the Center for Talent Innovation found that 67% of surveyed senior executives stated that gravitas is what really matters in an executive position. Over 28% of these executives ranked communication as a top leadership soft skill, and only 5% considered appearance as a key to the C-Suite (Hewlett, 2014). Nationwide, recent studies report the lack of soft skills as the most significant skill gap across all industry sectors. The most surprising outcome of these studies is that soft skills have become more important than technical skills in workforce development. Most employers now identify communication, collaboration and teamwork, time management, ethics, customer relationships, and problem-solving skills as skills critical to their work environments, and also report difficulty finding health care workers with these skill sets.

A hospital staff's lack of soft skills, whether in ethical standards, communication, or basic etiquette, has a direct, negative effect on the patient experience and ultimately, on the hospital's bottom line. All new and experienced C-Suite executives face a myriad of challenges that play a crucial role in their own success and the overall performance of their hospital. These include internal challenges (e.g., financial and performance metrics, culture, employee engagement, talent management, strategic direction, and vision) and external challenges (e.g., competition, suppliers, and customers). To face these complex challenges, C-Suite DNP prepared nurse executives must be competent in the "soft skill" essentials.

As of September 2018, there are no national standards for soft skills. Researchers are actively working to define the critical capabilities. Tarasovich (2015) identified the following competencies as skills and abilities that contribute to exceptional leadership in the finance industry:

1. Communicate a vision and a path.
2. Assess the competitive environment with an external orientation.
3. Foster breakthrough thinking.
4. Develop outstanding financial talent.
5. Build team commitment.
6. Propel to action.

Professional organizations are also working to define the seminal list of soft skill competencies that can guide the professional development of their members. The National Association of Colleges and Employers (NACE) competencies are as follows: critical thinking/problem solving, oral/written communications, teamwork/collaboration, digital technology, leadership; professionalism/work ethic, career management, and global/intercultural fluency. The American Organization for Nursing Leadership (AONL) (formerly the American Organization of Nurse Executives) core competencies include communication and relationship management, professionalism, knowledge of the health care environment, business skills and principles, and leadership (AONL, 2015).

As an example of the importance of soft skills, consider the following situation. A new hospital CEO was facing a challenging issue that would involve costs that are well beyond the existing budget. The CEO directed the staff she inherited from her predecessor to identify solutions in a very short period of time. The staff, who wanted to impress the new CEO, worked late nights and through the weekend to identify possible solutions and present data-based possibilities. At the Monday meeting with the CEO, the staff presented these options. During the presentation, the CEO was texting on her phone, not paying attention to the presentation, and not appearing to be very engaged. At the end of the presentation, the CEO concluded the meeting by announcing that her previous hospital had faced a similar issue, and that the current staff needed to pursue the same solution.

Although this CEO may have experienced success at her prior job, this experience with her new staff was negative with numerous problems with soft skills.

- *Communication*: The CEO did not pay attention to the staff's presentation. It is likely that she had already decided on a course of action but had not relayed it to her staff. The CEO's working on other issues during the staff presentation devalued the staff's efforts.
- *Motivation*: The staff was motivated initially by a desire to impress their new CEO. This desire motivated them to work the extra hours needed for identifying new, data-based solutions. Given the CEO's reaction, the staff would be unlikely in the future to invest the same time, effort, and diligence into resolving the next problem.
- *Etiquette about technology use in the meeting*: There are some who equate texting at a meeting or even at a meal to reading a newspaper. The newspaper creates a wall between the reader and the others who are present. Although there is no visual barrier to texting on a cell phone, the CEO's posture (with eyes and head down) sent a clear message that involvement with the phone was more important than involvement with the staff.

There could have been a different outcome. This time, at the meeting, the CEO announced that cell phones would not be allowed at any staff meetings. Anyone who was expecting an important call could leave their phone with a staff member outside who would notify them if necessary. During the staff's presentation, the CEO was engaged and asked thoughtful questions the staff had not considered. The CEO viewed the work the staff had completed, recognized their effort, and expressed appreciation to the team. The CEO suggested an additional solution, entertained questions, received feedback from the staff on the alternative, and made a commitment to have it investigated and presented at another meeting the following day.

This concluded the meeting. This scenario illustrates a CEO's action that defines a leader who sets boundaries, listens with the intent to understand, respects her team and recognizes their contributions, and in the end, has her staff aligned to investigate her suggestion and report back to the group.

The C-Suite executive with competency in soft skills has the potential to align his or her staff and the entire hospital and to motivate them for success. This chapter provides guidelines for building unique soft skills into the DNP prepared C-Suite nurse executive's personal toolbox.

Toolbox Soft Skill #1: Personal Brand

Most individuals understand the concept of a brand as a slogan, name, or symbol associated with a product or services provided by companies such as Apple, Nike, Amazon, Coach, or 3-M. Businesses strive to develop and maintain these brands to increase the perceived value of their products or services. As a result, customers determine the value of these products or services, which in turn informs buying decisions.

With a personal brand, we have the same actual and perceived value association as we apply to any company, institution, or business product. Jeff Bezos, the founder of Amazon, suggested that "Your (personal) brand is what people say about you when you're not in the room." (Lim, 2017). A personal brand is authentic and is the sum total of "what you do, how you do it and why you do it" (Lim, 2017). For a C-Suite leader, a "personal brand" conveys an individual leader's identity and reflects the types of attributes upon which a leader bases their executive leadership work and aspirations (Ulrich & Smallwood, 2007). This is defined by AONL as a reflection of personal and professional accountability or "professionalism at the executive level" (AONE, 2015).

Congruence between an individual DNP nurse executive's day-to-day work and their perceived personal brand can enhance their leadership success, whereas dissonance between the two can lead to failure. For example, developing a handbook on ways to improve clinical outcomes measures increases a nurse executive's perceived value as an executive leader who is committed to quality improvement that benefits the organization. Advancing this publication throughout one's hospital and the health care system further enhances a DNP nurse executive's perceived value to the organization and leadership team.

Ulrich and Smallwood (2007) identified five key steps in personal brand development. The first step requires the executive to focus on results or become value-focused, which means identifying the executive's ultimate goal. Identifying the goal is critical to showcasing any personal brand to customers, investors, employees, and stakeholders within and outside an organization (Ulrich & Smallwood, 2007).

There is a struggle that many new DNP-prepared nurse executives face upon promotion to the C-Suite. Difficulties in transitioning from a clinical practice position to an executive leadership role demands that the new nurse executive adjust to delivering direct patient care through the work of many others who are located in different organizational layers with varying numbers and types of clinicians, ancillary personnel, and outsourced personnel. Transition success requires expert skills in delegation, strategy development, and effective communication. The DNP nurse leader in a new executive position must rapidly adjust to new position responsibilities, readily demonstrate effectiveness, and prepare for the next level of leadership opportunity.

The second step suggested by Ulrich and Smallwood (2007) in building a personal brand involves identifying those attributes for which you want to be known. Table 12.1 provides a list of soft skill attributes from which a new DNP C-Suite executive can select based on past experience and personal leadership counseling (Ulrich & Smallwood, 2007).

Some soft skills align directly with the DNP's work experience, whereas others may seem completely foreign. Selecting new, less comfortable but "fit best" attributes, referred to as "stretch-attributes," enables continued growth and development if such attributes align with overall personal goals. For example, becoming *a passionate quality-oriented pragmatist*

Table 12.1 List of Soft Skill Attributes.

Accepting	Curious	Innovative	Pragmatic
Accountable	Decisive	Insightful	Prepared
Action-oriented	Dedicated	Inspired	Proactive
Adaptable	Deliberate	Integrative	Productive
Agile	Dependable	Intelligent	Quality-oriented
Agreeable	Determined	Intimate	Reality-based
Analytical	Diplomatic	Inventive	Religious
Approachable	Disciplined	Kind	Respectful
Assertive	Driven	Knowledgeable	Responsible
Attentive	Easygoing	Lively	Responsive
Benevolent	Efficient	Logical	Results-oriented
Bold	Emotional	Loving	Satisfied
Bright	Energetic	Loyal	Savvy
Calm	Enthusiastic	Nurturing	Self-confident
Caring	Even-tempered	Optimistic	Selfless
Charismatic	Fast	Organized	Self-oriented
Clever	Flexible	Outgoing	Sensitive
Collaborative	Focused	Passionate	Sincere
Committed	Forgiving	Patient	Sociable
Compassionate	Friendly	Peaceful	Straightforward
Competent	Fun-loving	Pensive	Thorough
Concerned	Good listener	Persistent	Thoughtful
Confident	Happy	Personal	Tireless
Confrontative	Helpful	Playful	Tolerant
Conscientious	Honest	Pleasant	Trusting
Considerate	Hopeful	Polite	Trustworthy
Consistent	Humble	Positive	Unyielding
Creative	Independent		

focused on *independent innovation* may enable the achievement of the stretch-goal of establishing an independent nurse-run ambulatory practice within a health care system.

The third step of brand development combines several attributes to form more complex descriptions that support a DNP nurse executive's personal brand and also identify specific actions necessary to reach an overall goal (Ulrich & Smallwood, 2007). For instance, *action-oriented, analytical*, and *inventive attributes* may enable *innovations* in IT integration that benefit the organization, the health care providers, and the community they serve.

The fourth step suggests that a DNP nurse executive combine complex descriptors to form a single statement that links these descriptors directly to a goal, which then effectively codifies the personal brand. An example might be "I want to be known for being *adaptable* and *accountable* so that I can deliver *value-driven* and *disciplined* clinical outcomes" (Ulrich & Smallwood, 2007). Once documented, the executive reviews this statement and verifies their ability to execute the daily activities required for goal achievement. The executive also ensures that the statement reflects the identified personal goals and, most importantly, that it aligns with expected organizational goals.

The fifth and final step in brand development requires identification of actionable steps that can help the executive further develop the personal brand. This requires periodic re-evaluation to be sure that the personal brand is aligned with the DNP executive's career aspirations. For instance, a DNP nurse executive may have entered nursing as a second-degree student with a computer science degree. With a *personal branding strategy* and the daily attention to practicing these soft skills, this nurse executive could achieve a career aspiration goal of entering the C-Suite as an IT executive.

Toolbox Soft Skill #2: Charisma and Story-Telling

Developing Charisma

The more an individual can develop, nurture, and promote his or her personal brand, the greater opportunity there is to become a desired colleague, staff member, supervisor, leader, or neighbor. This involves forming and nurturing the key collaborative relationships necessary to create and produce a shared vision (AONE, 2015).

In the first few minutes of meeting someone, each of us inevitably determines if we could "spend an hour eating lunch with this person" (Ferrazzi and Raz, 2014). Becoming charismatic involves developing the ability to be engaging with those we work with and work for, all in the quest of creating solid collaborative relationships. Preparing to engage others includes simple preparatory steps. For instance, read the newspapers and periodicals, and listen to interesting podcasts or the latest news prior to heading off to work. Reflect on any important or amusing event, even a funny failure, and share it when engaging others. These can be is first steps to becoming charismatic.

Equally important to having interesting points to discuss is the ability to convey a specific viewpoint or establish oneself as a subject matter expert. Expertise differentiates the DNP nurse executive from others. As a subject matter expert, the C-Suite nurse executive effectively becomes the go-to person for specific information and situations that require intervention. In the process of brand-building, the executive becomes more valuable to others (Ferrazzi and Raz, 2014). One practical example is the nurse executive's ability to understand the underlying algorithm(s) that drive Hospital Consumer Assessment of Healthcare Providers and Systems (HCAHPs) scores. Recognition of the importance of nurse courtesy, nurse friendliness, and staff collaboration as key to improving ratings (Press Ganey, 2017) and developing training programs that enhance staff performance may easily establish the DNP nurse executive as an action-oriented subject matter expert in the C-Suite.

Storytelling

Another key method of engaging others is storytelling. For example, a serious patient issue may have surfaced that must be addressed immediately. Rather than solely focusing on the issue's technical aspects, it might be more helpful to share how a corrective initiative will not only address the technical components, but will improve work flow, the patient environment, and clinical outcomes. By engaging colleagues in a discussion of *impact* rather than the *technical, procedural* aspects of problem-solving, the nurse executive draws colleagues into achieving broader goals, and support for the original initiative.

One example of this strategy is the chronic problem of emergency department (ED) over-crowding caused by the lack of inpatient beds needed to accommodate newly-admitted ED patients. Rather than focusing on the size and structure of the emergency department or the requirements of The Emergency Medical Treatment and Labor Act (EMTALA) and/or local ambulance hospital travel patterns, a nurse executive can use storytelling to describe patient flow improvements that provide a safe patient environment outside of an over-crowded ED. One nurse executive advanced the notion that instead of ED-admitted patients lining the hallways of the ED awaiting transfer, it might be better to place the patient in the hallway of the assigned in-patient unit where specialized nurses and physicians can readily address their diagnostic and clinical needs. After carefully engaging all stakeholders by retelling stories of other institutions that enacted similar strategies, the initiative was piloted, eventually endorsed and accepted, and

Table 12.2 Summary of Different Story Types.

Story Type	Focus
Who I Am	Stories that provide evidence and the right to influence a person or group of people
Why I'm Here	Stories that inform the audience of the benefit of having a conversation
Vision	Stories that describe a large big picture for an audience to rally behind
Values in Action	Stories that bring core values down to real tangible examples
Teaching	Stories that describe a previous experience to teach a specific outcome
I Know What You're Thinking	Stories to help bring along a reluctant audience

ultimately garnered multiple advantages for the institution. These included patient care delivered in a safer, clinically-expert in-patient environment that drove earlier in-patient discharge decision-making, improved working relationships and professional engagement between emergency room personnel and in-patient unit personnel, and the ability for the ED to triage and treat additional patients (Johnson, personal communication, January 3, 2018).

Storytelling also enables colleagues and peers to remember and associate stories with the person sharing the tale, the more interesting and differentiating the better. Simmons (2017) summarized different story types, as illustrated in Table 12.2.

Focusing on these five story types can enable the nurse executive to effectively describe real situations or challenges, promote engagement, and eventually create solutions that lead to a positive outcome. Stakeholders more readily relate to real life examples and case studies, particularly if the story applies to their own experience. To increase storytelling success, the DNP executive must do the homework necessary to know the audience, as described in the next section.

Toolbox Soft Skill #3: Know Your Audience

Conducting research on the challenges that colleagues, staff, and supervisors face and how they have dealt with past challenges helps the executive to relate to pressing issues and saves all the involved parties time spent on understanding each other. The DNP nurse executive's knowledge of care at point-of-service can best facilitate both high-level strategic thinking and health care economic policymaking because of the clinical practice knowledge required for both strategy and policy development (AONE, 2015). First, however, one needs to know their audience. Today, securing that knowledge is far easier with online resources such as LinkedIn,

Google, and Twitter. These resources assist in understanding the career paths of individuals with whom the nurse executive plans to meet, including their common interests and organizations, company history, and recent events. For example, when applying for a new job with a health care facility actively undergoing a merger with a large conglomerate system, the wise applicant must understand the impact of this event on the existing organization. Accessing financial reports and publicly available company information enables the sharing of personal insights with the interviewer and builds interviewer confidence in the nurse executive's ability to understand the job context. Without doing this background work, a nurse executive essentially walks into an important or a high-level discussion unprepared. This can be avoided by learning about the audience members in advance. Researching personal and professional information about each key member enables the executive to enjoy a rich, valued discussion.

Toolbox Soft Skill #4: Grow Your Network

Developing a large, diverse professional network is key to career advancement. This network should be sufficiently diverse to include work-related colleagues, friends with common interests, former classmates, fellow board members, and others with shared interests or experiences. A wide range of individuals provides network breadth and offers unique perspectives that equip the nurse executive with the ability to affect other people's professional and non-professional lives and underscore the importance of giving rather than taking.

However, developing a network requires a steady focus, and nurturing that network demands an investment of time and energy to remain an active network member. This means contacting individuals, meeting for coffee, or joining LinkedIn groups in order to comment on other people's ideas. These activities remind network members of unique relevant skills that one has honed over the long-term (Long, 2015).

One of the best ways to begin developing a professional network is to find a mentor, a trusted advisor. This begins with selecting an individual who aligns with and complements values that resonate with the DNP nurse executive, as well as being someone who already has a richly cultivated network. Mentors can help mentees with connecting with professionals and future colleagues. Networking is a long-term plan (Kumok, n.d.), and in the process of continuous network development, network traps exist. These include the wrong structure, the wrong relationships, and the wrong behavior. In 2011, Cross and Thomas summarized these traps and the associated managerial behavior types, as illustrated below in Table 12.3.

Effective networks provide support but more importantly, they challenge thinking (Cross & Thomas, 2011), and present new opportunities, broadened skill sets, forced reflection on current belief systems, and deepened expertise. However, network size often fails to correlate with overall personal success or performance (Cross & Thomas, 2011). Top performers exhibit higher-quality, deeper network relationships within smaller networks and they avoid establishing shallow alliances. Deeper relationships extend industry geography and can increase a DNP nurse executive's market perception and perspective. Cross and Thomas (2011) set forth a four-step process that can assist in bolstering an existing network, as shown below in Table 12.4.

Thinking through these steps reconnects with *building a personal brand*. *Analyzing* network participants can result in identifying opportunities for goals to align with network members who can support and assist in goal and brand achievement. A decision to jettison unproductive relationships—*de-layering*—frees the C-Suite DNP nurse executive to pursue more reciprocal associations. *Diversifying* or selecting the most helpful and influential network members and selectively choosing a close circle of individuals to act as trusted advisors and mentors becomes critical to long-term professional success. *Capitalizing* on those contacts with supportive engagement further advances the promise of personal brand achievement.

Table 12.3 Summary of Traps and the Associated Managerial Behavior Types.

Network Traps	Managerial Types	Description
1: The Wrong Structure	The Formalist	Focuses too heavily on his company's official hierarchy, missing out on the efficiencies and opportunities that come from informal connections
	The Overloaded Manager	Has so much contact with colleagues and external ties that she becomes a bottleneck to progress and burns herself out
2: The Wrong Relationships	The Disconnected Expert	Sticks with people who keep him focused on safe, existing competencies, rather than those who push him to build new skills
	The Biased Leader	Relies on advisors much like herself (same functional background, location, or values), who reinforce her biases, when she should instead seek outsiders to prompt more fully informed decisions
3: The Wrong Behavior	The Superficial Networker	Engages in surface-level interaction with as many people as possible, mistakenly believing that a bigger network is a better one
	The Chameleon	Changes his interests, values, and personality to match those of whatever subgroup is his audience and winds up being disconnected from every group

Table 12.4 Network-Bolstering Four-Step Process.

Step 1:	*Analyze*: Identify the people in the network and the rewards netted from the interactions.
Step 2:	*De-layer*: Make hard decisions to back away from redundant and energy-sapping relationships
Step 3:	*Diversify*: Select the right kind of people—energizers who assist in goal achievement.
Step 4:	*Capitalize*: effectively use contacts.

Toolbox Soft Skill #5: Identify Your Trusted Advisors

Trusted advisors are indispensable resources to one's growth as a C-Suite DNP nurse executive. These advisors should challenge and offer a fresh perspective that enriches original assumptions (Riper, 2016). Achieving the level of a trusted advisor is no easy task, and although many boast of achieving the status, few successfully navigate the scaffolding (Noonan, 2016). In Figure 12.1, Maister, Green, and Galford (2001) suggest that the evolution begins at the transactional level wherein a product or service of interest leads to the completion of a specific task as a subject matter expert. Extending an earlier example related to the inevitable C-Suite discussion of the Hospital Consumer Assessment of Healthcare Providers and Systems (HCAHPS) score performance and who should assume responsibility to address falling ratings, the nurse executive often assumes the role of subject matter expert.

To effectively address falling ratings, the nurse executive must include other members of the health care team and may engage industry experts as well. Such steps mirror the next level where affiliated personnel and

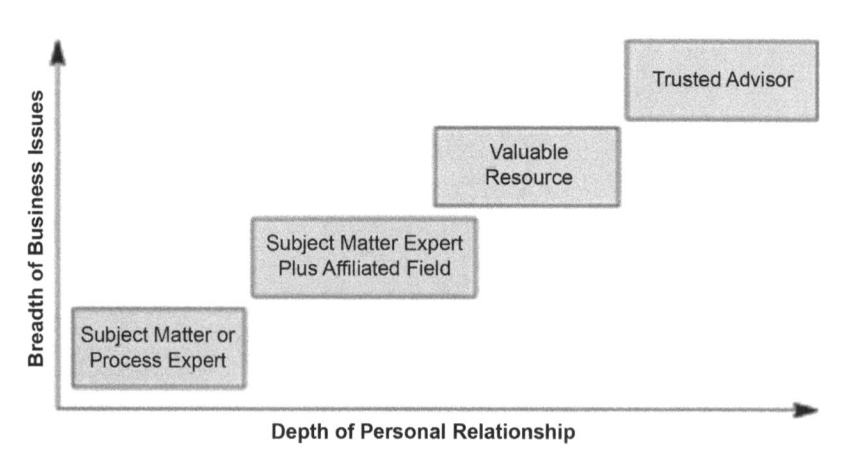

Figure 12.1. *Evolution Begins at the Transactional Level.*

experts participate in problem-solving (Maister, Green, & Galford, 2001). This step may link patients, services, and products in order to solve a complex set of tasks designed to improve patient ratings. Engagement expands detailed knowledge of the issues and promotes the development of relationships necessary to address them. The DNP nurse executive assumes a lead role in orchestrating this transition and solidifies the role of subject matter expert as the process unfolds. Here, the organization realizes that the nurse executive's skills extend far beyond the prototypical clinical nursing skill set noted at the outset.

The third type of advisor (the valuable resource) enables the C-Suite nurse to frame these complex issues and provides a wide perspective on a range of strategic problems that may affect the organization's ability to achieve HCAHPS score improvement. Lack of employee training and support, a rigid organizational culture, and the absence of leadership engagement are examples of strategic problems that require executive C-Suite attention. Here, the DNP nurse executive provides advice proactively while focusing not only on the definitive problem, but also on the broader organizational context (Maister, Green, & Galford, 2001). Once established as the subject matter expert who successfully engages and advances a strategy for addressing the broader HCAHPS score problem, and having reached the fourth level in the process, the nurse executive becomes the trusted advisor. At this level, proactive advice to address problems at a personal and a professional level are the hallmarks of its attributes. As a result, key organizational members now begin viewing the trusted advisor as a close confidant. Table 12.5 summarizes these four evolutionary types (Maister, Green, & Gulford, 2001).

Trusted advisors need not work to sell professional value. Instead, the ability to listen, reason, imagine and proactively solve issues sets these individuals apart (Noonan, 2016). Becoming a trusted advisor enlarges a

Table 12.5 Summary of Four Evolutionary Types.

	Focus Is On:	Energy Spent On:	Client Receives:	Indicators of Success:
Service-based	Answers, expertise, input	Explaining	Information	Timely, high quality
Needs-based	Business problem	Problem-solving	Solutions	Problems resolved
Relationship-based	Client organization	Providing insights	Ideas	Repeat business
Trust-based	Client as individual	Understanding the client	Safe haven for hard issues	Varied; e.g. creative pricing

$$\text{Trustworthiness} = \frac{\text{Credibility + Reliability + Intimacy}}{\text{Self-Orientation}}$$

Rational Components (numerator) / *Emotional Components* (denominator)

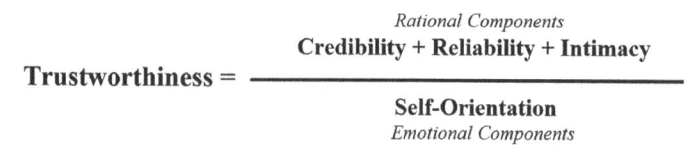

Figure 12.2. *Interrelationships between Credibility, Reliability, Intimacy, and Self-orientation.*

nurse executive's network tenfold as close connections form bonds that attract individuals from each of the prior transitional tiers. Finding close confidants who comprise a nurse executive's inner circle—where proactive challenging occurs, where advice is exchanged—increases the value of the DNP C-Suite nurse executive. However, to understand how professionals become trusted advisors, one must appreciate the components of trust that include credibility, reliability, intimacy, and self-orientation. Figure 12.2 illustrates their interrelationship (Maister, Green, & Galford, 2001).

The subtleties within this simple equation suggest that as the rational components of credibility, reliability and intimacy increase, trustworthiness increases. However, any increase in selforientation decreases trustworthiness. The more the DNP nurse executive becomes a subject matter expert (credibility), the easier it becomes to build trust within an organization. When the nurse executive delivers on promises (reliability), trustworthiness also increases. These two components form the basic rational components of the trust equation; both represent elements conducive to daily practice and overall outcome evaluation (Maister, Green, & Galford, 2001).

These two components also form an emotional context that matures over an extended period of time. Evaluating the worth of a solution requires vetting time to ensure that all issues related to problem resolution are properly addressed in the client's or customer's best interest (Maister, Green, & Galford, 2001).

The third numerator, intimacy, refers to the context of being safe, secure, and willing to openly discuss the topics at hand. If a relationship fails to fully developed, one may be less likely to openly discuss all aspects related to a given challenge, which in turn diminishes the probability of a successful outcome. The denominator, self-orientation, demonstrates personal intent to work with the client or customer. For example, if a nurse executive focuses solely on their own best interest, such as the nursing profession, trust diminishes. One example is advancing full practice authority for advanced practice nurses (APRNs) based on competency, nurse practice acts, and the 2011 Institute of Medicine report recommendations. Such an interest suggests an inward self-aggrandizing orientation rather than advancing the APRN role to better meet the health care needs of the served community. Such a position inevitably diminishes the nurse executive's trustworthiness.

To emphasize its importance, the denominator outweighs all other three components individually. This means that one can have the best accolades (credibility), does what one says one will do (reliability) and be very open with others (intimacy). However, if the initiative intent is for the wrong reason (oneself), trustworthiness plummets.

In developing a strategy to build trust, consider the following guiding principles:

1. *Check Your Ego at the Door.* Listen to the audience. Do not pretend to know everything (credibility) and be honest when you fall short. Follow-up with the audience on areas that require research (reliability).
2. *Care About the Audience and their Business Interests.* Always make sure that previous experiences and areas of expertise are used solely for the betterment of the audience and not oneself (self-orientation).
3. *Be Transparent.* When the timing is right, open up to your client. Bring in some non-professional aspects to your conversations (personal interests, children) to connect with the audience on a personal level to build a level of intimacy with the audience.

One final component in building trust includes ensuring that trusted advisors have the correct mindsets to foster close relationship development. Ferrazzi (2009) proposes four core mindsets evident in a true trusted advisor. These include the following:

1. *Generosity*: The commitment to mutual support that begins with the willingness to show up and creatively share our deepest insights and ideas with the world. It's the promise to help others succeed by whatever means one can muster. Generosity signals the end of isolation by cracking open a door to a trusting emotional environment—a "safe space." This type of environment is necessary for creating relationships in which the other mind-sets can flourish.
2. *Vulnerability*: Letting one's guard down so mutual understanding can occur. Here one crosses the threshold into a safe space after intimacy and trust have pushed the door wide open. The relationship engendered by generosity then moves toward a place of fearless friendship where risks are taken and invitations are offered to others.
3. *Candor*: The freedom to be totally honest with those in whom one confides. Vulnerability clears the pathways of feedback so that one may share personal hopes and fears. Candor allows one to begin to constructively interpret, respond to, and grapple with that information.
4. *Accountability*: Refers to the action of following through on the promises one makes to others. It's about giving and receiving the feet-to-the-fire tough love through which real change is sustained.

Toolbox Soft Skill #6: Pivoting

Core to the American Association of Colleges of Nurses' essentials for advanced nursing degrees is the concept of organizational and systems leadership for quality improvement and systems thinking (Nursing, 2006). Short and long-term strategic planning is essential to achievement. Systems thinking underpins successful strategic planning efforts. Several components of systems thinking include the development of sound business cases and developing a prioritized set of initiatives to enable plan achievement. Equally important is the ability to mitigate risk by planning against unpredictable history-defying events, the "black swan," and integrating "sustainability" to drive transparency, longevity, and stakeholder value. Soft skills relate to inevitable missteps and/or failures. AONL's core business skills and competencies align with this soft skill in focusing on human resource management, building optimal organizational structures, and creating a strategic management plan that mitigates risk, while infusing information technology and promoting innovation (AONE, 2015).

However, executing even the most thoughtful plan requires risk-taking behaviors and a willingness to fail. So, what is the key to achieving success after failure? Be nimble: fail fast and recover quickly. In industry terms, be able to pivot. To illustrate how a DNP C-Suite nurse executive might embrace the concept of failing fast, consider other industry approaches to dealing with outside market forces, risks, and challenges.

The market landscape today is highly competitive and complex, and change is inevitable. To make the planning process even more challenging, today's markets overlap with each other. For instance, advancement in technology causes constant disruption with new market entrants, all in an effort to press clients to purchase and expand a new vendor's market share (Page, Rahnema, Murphy, & Mcdowell). To compound the issue, large organizations are unfortunately the same monolithic structures of yesterday and have not adapted to the more agile and nimble new entrant/entrepreneur upstarts. In the 1950s, the average lifespan of a Standard and Poor (S&P) 500 company was 60 years. Today a company's lifespan is closer to 15 years and steadily shrinking (Page, Rahnema, Murphy, & Mcdowell). As a result, smaller companies that can be created and operational in days without the complexities of larger organizations now reshape markets; this includes the health care market. One example is remote monitoring technology that has rapidly expanded as a method to more closely monitor patients in rural locations and that offer hospitals an alternative way of providing patient care off-site (Solway, 2016; Takahashi, 2009).

Thus, the strategic plan a C-Suite executive puts in place today, probably won't survive the year in its original form. As a result, any strategic business plan must also include strategies to quickly rebound from a misstep or outright plan failure. This is known as pivoting. The executive's ability to pivot in the face of change or initiative failure represents a soft skill that differentiates winners from losers. Trusted advisors become crucial to helping executives appreciate the impact of new ideas, innovations, opportunities, challenges, competitors, and customers. A trusted advisor should challenge your current way of thinking, the content of your strategic business plan, and press you to remain alert to potential risks, and prepare for a nimble response.

Becoming a Nimble Pivoter

To become and remain nimble, companies must embed an agile or lean component into their organizational structures. The agile or lean component structure should be as flat as possible in order to proactively address customer concerns, advance initiatives, and revise strategies. It is a structure designed to expect failure and rapidly respond at a minimal cost (Kedar, 2017). The DNP prepared C-Suite executive might consider separating innovative strategic plan initiatives into rapid and agile practice teams. For smaller newer companies, this could involve the entire organizational structure. For larger companies, a multi-speed organization that incorporates both traditional and agile practices at the same time may prove advantageous. Regardless of the structure, rapid and agile practice teams should execute the more innovative initiatives.

According to Deloitte (Page *et al.*, n.d.), building a more rapid, agile organization to respond to change can be completed in four specific steps. First, it's important to understand which organizational areas can benefit from a rapid operating environment to embrace innovation and agility. Completely separate work from initiative development. Identify target markets with intense competition as prime candidates for a rapid and agile organizational team structure. The advantage of this model is that while the new edge team structure rapidly innovates, the core business remains intact. An example is Google. This company reorganized under the overall umbrella, Alphabet Inc., and separated into the more traditional Search, Ads, Maps, and YouTube business and the more long-term pursuits that include driverless cars, and robotics (Page *et al.*, n.d.). A health care example includes health care systems that create urgent care feeder facilities that are separate ambulatory care-focused organizational components with a focus on new provider ventures.

Step 2 involves operating in an environment that utilizes networked teams that stretch across core functions and eliminate traditional organizational silos. Step 3 immediately requires these teams to develop and embrace a collaborative system mindset (Page *et al.*, n.d.) With appropriately assigned roles and resources, these self-managing and autonomous teams rapidly move forward to achieve a specific outcome. Another operating method to consider is stepping away from large organizational structures charged with a very specific operating task and passing a completed task segment to another team to complete the next step and the next steps. Instead, take individuals from all those teams and develop "network service teams" An example of this method is the "2-pizza team" principle, developed by Bezos, CEO of Amazon.com. Bezos' principle is founded on the belief and practice that smaller teams get more done in a faster timeframe, and that these teams should be sized to the number of participants that can be fed with two pizzas (Deutschman, 2004). These small teams can operate more nimbly than a larger organization if the team includes the correct talent. However, they must be sufficiently autonomous to own, plan, build, and operate all project timeline components.

Step 4 is the most crucial and final step that requires the executive to create the conditions for a flexible organization. The organization's vision, mission, and values provide the foundation for the organization to adapt change quickly. This vision must be unified across the organization and be embraced by energizing leaders who guide and encourage the networked teams. Redesigning the traditional workforce begins with leadership executives, and includes flexible insourced employees, outsourced specialists or vendors, and experienced consultants who can engage and be organically embedded to solve problems (Page *et al.*, n.d.).

The Workforce in 2020 and Beyond

With five generations in the workforce, an organization's ability to create functioning teams is challenging. Generational differences can create barriers through biases that one generation has toward the others. Although generalizations are born from behavioral observations of a group, applying them to an individual is inappropriate in any context. Not all Millennials are entitled, and not all Baby Boomers are "My way or the highway." However, the Millennial and Post-Millennial generations have had access to more information than earlier generations, and this has influenced their worldviews. They have instant contact and connectivity with individuals in their networks. They have no concept of waiting for their turn on a party line or dialing a rotary phone only to find a busy line with no ability to leave a message. These small differences may highlight why the younger generations get frustrated when they have to wait for something they expect to be instantly available, whereas older generations are generally more patient waiting for websites and even laptops to load. A recent interaction between a Greatest Generation individual (who will be called Bob), and a Millennial (Andy) highlight this. Bob had retired but continued as a consultant to National Oceanic and Atmospheric Administration (NOAA) on weather satellite systems. He was recently asked to give a presentation on the new weather satellite constellation under development by a joint NASA/NOAA venture for the local state college guest lecture series. Bob arrived with his laptop and was introduced to Andy, who was the school's IT specialist for the lecture. Bob turned his five-year old laptop on and patiently waited the minutes for his old system to come up. Andy, in the meantime, paced while watching the excruciatingly slow process and finally saids, "Dude, you need a new laptop."

From Bob's perspective, his current laptop is a wonder of technology. Bob started programming back when computers were built with vacuum tubes and a "bug" taking the system down was literally a moth. He spent his career welcoming each technology improvement that improved his productivity. From having to submit decks of punched cards to a computer center and retrieving the deck with a printout that summarized the results of a run and usually took overnight, to having a display on his desk where the deck of cards was replaced with a file of lines of software and the ability to replace batch processing with interleaved and then parallel processing with relatively immediate results, Bob was very happy with his current system. Andy, on the other hand, viewed Bob's ancient 5-year old system as a brick. With access to high speed systems, Andy did not have the patience to wait for a long boot. His system was usually available as soon as he punched a key and entered his password. Bob had the advantage of perspective and knew why Andy's impatience existed. Andy, if he had insight into Bob's history with computers, could have used that knowledge to be much more understanding of this older gentleman's situation. When asked to speak again at the lecture series, Bob brought his presentation on a thumb drive instead of using his laptop.

Millennials now make up the largest generation in the workforce as shown by the Pew Research Center's graph (Figure 12.3) (Fry, 2018).

The DNP prepared C-Suite nurse executive must understand how this

Millennials became the largest generation in the labor force in 2016

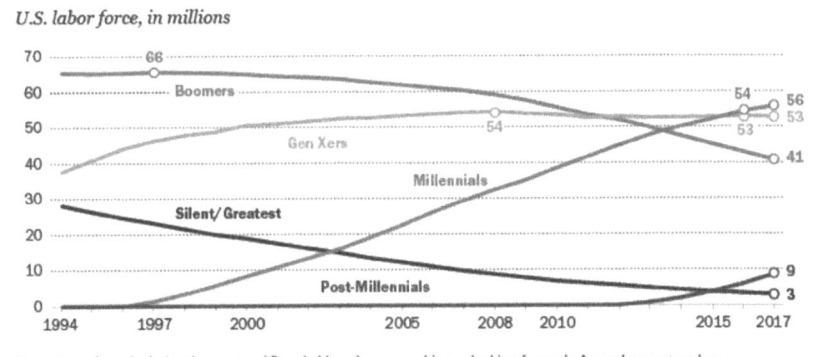

U.S. labor force, in millions

Note: Labor force includes those ages 16 and older who are working or looking for work. Annual averages shown.
Source: Pew Research Center analysis of monthly 1994-2017 Current Population Survey (IPUMS).

Figure 12.3. *Distribution of the Generational Workforce. Reproduced from Fry 2018.*

generational diversity affects the workforce. Nurses on the floor interact with patients and families of all ages and will be working with and managing employees of vastly different ages.

Diversity adds positively to an organization. Awareness of diversity differences provides the ability to build strong teams. Consider the range of ages, beliefs, and cultures of patients and family members that hospital staff personnel interface with on a daily basis. Expanding work teams that represent a wide range of the community provides an individual in the team with a resource when confronted with a new situation. However, managing this diverse mix can be challenging. How does the DNP nurse C-Suite executive learn this skill?

Bechervaise (2015) developed a list for managing an age-diverse workforce that the DNP nurse can utilize:

1. Facilitate strong networks of communication
2. Resolve conflicts quickly and effectively
3. Invest in time for nurturing employee relationships
4. Promote team work
5. Celebrate achievements

Communication, and the way staff are engaged and heard have a dramatic impact on the harmony of the workplace. Good communications is needed in all directions within an organization, horizontally and vertically. A process that is organization-wide can help with establishing expectations across that organization and minimize generational differences. One generation may be more comfortable with a face-to-face meeting to transfer data, while another would rather send a text. If these two generations need to share information between themselves, their preferred communication styles further create an impediment to communicating information. A directive that critical information be transferred via email or technology can be appropriate for your organization. This creates accountability by imposing a common methodology.

Tightly coupled with networked communication is the ability to recognize and address conflict quickly and effectively. Since you have learned to establish a trusted advisor network, why not become a trusted advisor to your work teams? That will provide you with access to the information you need to remain current on issues before they blow up into major crises, and allow you to lead by example because those you are advising and who are sharing these issues with you will be paying attention to how you resolve them. Exercise your nimble pivoting skills. If a problem arises that you don't have experience with, seek guidance and advice from your own network of advisors. Chances are someone has dealt with a similar problem in the past and can help you develop the appropriate resolution.

It can be difficult to create environments that allow interpersonal relationships to grow from the workplace. However, strategic grouping of individuals in committee work, establishing mentorships, maintaining work teams to allow relationships to develop, as well as providing opportunity for off-work engagement are all approaches that foster an environment of understanding and respect across diverse workforces. This is another area to reach out to your advisor network to explore. This is one area that highlights the benefits of having advisors from a variety of business sectors in your network.

There is nothing more demoralizing than working for an organization that pushes you to work better, harder, faster, but does not recognize the efforts of the individuals to achieve efficiency and innovation in the workforce. Don't let this happen to your workplace. Take the time to recognize individual and group contribution to goals. There are many means available for providing the recognition appropriate for the achievement. For incremental milestones, announcements at department meetings, emails identifying positive outcomes attributed to an individual or a team, a newsletter or posting to the internal message board to share recognition are effective when used appropriately. A successful leader recognizes that recognition shared is more beneficial than that claimed for themselves.

Chapter Takeaways

1. Mastering C-Suite "soft skills" underpins the successful nurse executive and enables the development of foundational leadership qualities.
2. Developing one's personal brand promotes an executive's image, values, and enables knowledge transfer.
3. Successful networking requires a long-term commitment and attention to developed relationships.
4. Failing fast, remaining nimble and learning to pivot underpins a DNP nurse executive's success and C-Suite survival.
5. The five-generational workforce mix challenges novice and seasoned C-Suite nurse executives; understanding each cohort and developing relational skill sets enables workforce harmony and productivity.

Chapter Summary

As nurse leaders progress through leadership ranks toward the C-Suite, mastering soft skills becomes critical to executive success. This chapter focused on a series of soft skills that are associated with successful executives. Without these foundational skills, success in the C-Suite becomes increasingly difficult. Presented as a leadership toolbox skill series, new and seasoned nurse executives learn that building a personal brand begins with the identification of goals and values, and transfers to expanded skills that focus on delegation, strategy development, and effective communications. Storytelling is one method of advanced communication that assists in the development of charisma, which is critical to personal brand development and the formation of collaborative relationships.

To learn the art of storytelling, one must understand the audience. Knowing the audience requires research—doing the homework—prior to engaging in any high-level discussion. Completing such research becomes easier if the executive develops a rich personal and professional network. However, network development requires a long-term commitment and continuous attention to network members. From one's network, a trusted advisor may emerge to offer support and guidance that challenges one's thinking, all in an effort to continually advance one's competencies. Along the way, the nurse executive can emerge as a subject matter expert and achieve trusted advisor status who assists less experienced leaders to achieve. Key to these roles and relationships is establishing trust and underpinning it with credibility, reliability, intimacy, and a limited orientation towards one's own self-interests.

If there is an art to contemporary success, it invariably includes the early realization of the inevitably of missteps or failures, and that remaining nimble in the face of failure drives ultimate success. Failing fast and recovering quickly must underpin the DNP-prepared nurse executive's skill set. Further, implementing new age team structures—the "2-pizza team"—can assist organizations in embracing non-traditional operating methods that can rapidly achieve specific outcomes.

The current workforce pipeline is a challenging mix of five generations that is weak in soft skills. The DNP nurse executive must use all the skills in his/her toolbox to address these generational challenges and foster a healthy work environment. This comes through team building, skilled conflict resolution practices, and strong lines of communication.

Resolving challenges in the workplace will draw heavily on a DNP nurse's ability to develop strong soft skills. The next decades will see significant changes in the traditional workforce. DNP prepared C-Suite nurse executives will need to pivot and create conditions for a flexible organization that can survive and thrive in such conditions.

Case Study: 5G Power Skills

Industry surveys have identified a critical lack of soft skills in the workforce pipeline. Coupling this lack of soft skills in the workforce with the unprecedented five generations in the workforce today creates a very challenging environment for business success, and one that challenges executive suites across all industry sectors.

Alpha UMi LLC, in direct response to this industry skill crisis, has developed its 5G Power Skills Certification to address the top soft skills necessary in the workforce today. '5G' refers to the five generations in the workforce. Power Skills indicates that mastery in the soft skills will empower one to sustain or advance in one's career. The 5G Power Skills Certification aligns with the National Association of Colleges and Employers (NACE, 2017) competencies.

This researched-based and empirically driven program focuses on six soft skills sectors. Five sectors are delivered with a facilitated workshop, engaged learning environment: Diversity and Collaboration, Interpersonal Communication, Adapting Thinking, Principles of Professionalism, and Leadership and Management. The sixth, Critical Thinking, is addressed with an interactive online course. Beginning with Diversity Awareness, which explores generational differences from the perspective of worldview, the workshops guide personal development through a very introspective experience using large and small group discussion and large and small group and individual exercises, and culminating in a final discussion in which all competencies come together to create the ultimate Customer Experience.

The conclusion that hospital executives may draw from the data are that soft skills must be part of human capital development initiatives within their organization. From screening for hiring, to onboarding, to grooming for promotion, opportunities to assess, develop and exercise these skills need to be planned to ensure a positive patient experience and result in a successful business outcome.

To build an effective toolbox of skills, consider the structure an innovative small company, Alpha UMi LLC, has used to develop soft skill talent across all levels of the workforce, from executive to entry-level. Omitting the industry specific hard skill requirement and focusing on soft skills, Alpha

Table 12.5 NACE (2017) and AONE (2015) Competencies.

5G Power Skills Pillars	NACE Competency	AONE Competency
Diversity and Collaboration	Global/ Intercultural Fluency; Teamwork/ Collaboration	Communication & Relationship Management
Interpersonal Skills	Oral/ Written Communications	Communication & Relationship Management
Adaptive Thinking	Career Management	Business skills and Principles
Principles of Professionalism	Professionalism/ Work Ethic; Digital Technology	Professionalism, Business Skills and principles
Leadership and Management	Leadership; Career Management	Professionalism, Leadership
Critical Thinking	Critical Thinking Problem Solving	Business skills and Principles

Reproduced from NACE, 2017.

Table 12.6 Summary of Research and Research-based Articles that Demonstrates Why these 5G Power Skill Pillars are Significant.

5G Power Skills	Research Shows:	Source:
Diversity and Collaboration	Individuals from a wide spectrum of dimensional diversity challenge each other more, driving innovation and productivity: • 57% better team collaboration, • 45% more likelihood of improving market share, • 70% more likelihood of success in new markets.	Harvard Business Review, November 2013
Interpersonal Skills	Communication is: • 55% non-verbal • 38% tone of voice • 7% words	Psychology Today, 2011
Adaptive Thinking	A winning mindset has a huge impact on the workplace: • Trust is 47% higher • Engagement is 34% likelier • Innovation is 65% stronger • Ethics are 41% stronger	Delaney, S., 2014
Principles of Professionalism	No matter the size, industry or level of profitability of an organization, leadership, employee and business ethics are some of the most important aspects of long-term organizational success.	Investopedia, 2017
Leadership and Management	Companies with leadership development programs achieve increased return on investment from 147% to 633%	Byham, W., 2017
Critical Thinking	If a decision is made relying on data rather than pure intuition, the chances of succeeding are 79% higher. Outcomes resulting from decisions that are influenced by cognitive biases range from the mundane to catastrophic.	Tiwari, N., 2013 Psychology Today, May 2013

Reproduced from AONE, 2015.

UMi's 5G Power Skills product has grouped its 25 soft skill competencies into five pillars. These pillars are aligned as follows with the NACE (2017) and AONE (2015) competencies as shown in the Table 12.5 and Table 12.6.

The Table12.6 provides a relevant summary of research and research-based articles that demonstrates why these 5G Power Skill Pillars are significant.

Chapter Reflection Questions

1. Does your organization have rules of business etiquette that address the use of personal, portable, and/or hand-held technology within your workplace? If so, what are they and what impact do they have on work practice? What rules would you write to improve your workplace environment?
2. What is your organization's culture? How does your organization identify whether a potential new hire will fit within the its culture?
3. What are ethical organizations? Identify several ethical and non-ethical companies and discuss the impact of those companies' ethics on their long-term viability.
4. How does a positive patient experience affect the overall health of the hospital organization and environment? How might the executive suite nursing professional contribute to a positive patient experience? How are negative trends in customer experience identified early and mitigated?
5. Identify traits of individuals or teams you have worked with that collaborated well. How has your work experience been changed by having the opportunity to work in a positive collaborative environment? Identify traits of a poor collaborator with whom you have worked. How would you seek to improve those traits so that a more positive collaborative experience is created for that individual and those who interface with him/her?

References

Accenture *(2017). Technology vision 2017: Technology for people.* Accenture.

American Organization of Nurse Executives (AONE) (2015). *Nurse executive competencies.* Chicago, IL: AONE. Retrieved from http://www.aone.org/resources/nec.pdf.

Bechervaise, C. (2015). *5 Best tips on managing age-diversity in the workplace.* Retrieved from: https://takeitpersonelly.com/2015/07/02/5-best-tips-on-managing-age-diversity-in-the-workplace/.

Bonini, S. & Gorner, S. (2011). The business of sustainability: Putting it into practice. McKinsey & Company. Retrieved from https://www.mckinsey.com/~/media/mckinsey/dotcom/client_service/sustainability/pdfs/putting_it_into_practice.ashx

Bower, J.L. & Christensen, C.M. (1995). Disruptive technologies: Catching the wave. *Harvard Business Review, 73*(1), 43–53.

Byham, W. (2017). *The business case for leadership development.* Retrieved from: http://www.clomedia.com/2017/08/17/business-case-leadership-development/.

Cross, R., & Thomas, R. (2011). A smarter way to network. *Harvard Business Review, 89*(7/8), 142–153.

Delaney, S. (2014). Why fostering a growth mindset in organizations matters. *Stanford University*. Retrieved from: http://knowedge.senndelaney.com/docks/thought_papers/pdf/standford_agilitystudy_hart.pdf

Deutschman, A. (2004, August 1). Inside the mind of Jeff Bezos. Retrieved from https://www.fast.company.com/50661/inside-mind-jeff-bezos

Erskine, R. (2016). 22 Statistics that prove the value of personal branding. *Entrepreneur*. Investopedia, LLC. 2017. *Business Ethics*. Retrieved from: http://www.investopedia.com/terms/b/business-ethics.asp.

Eccles, R., Ioannou, I., & Serafeim, G. (2012, January 6). Is sustainability now the key to corporate success? Retrieved from https://www.theguardian.com/sustainable-business/sustainability-key-corporate-success

Ellison, A. (2017). Hospitals and health systems move forward with value-based payment models amid uncertainty over healthcare reform. *Becker's Hospital CFO Report*. Retrieved from https://www.beckershospitalreview.com/finance/hospitals-and-systems-move-forward-with-value-based-payment-models-amid-uncertinty-over-healthcare-reform.html.

Ferrazzi, K. (2009, July 4). Who's got your back: The four mind-sets of a successful leader, Part 1 of 5. Retrieved from *Huffington Post*: https://www.huffingtonpost.com/keith-ferrazzi/whos-got-your-back-the-fo_b_210954.html

Ferrazzi, K., & Raz, T. (2014). *Never eat alone: And other secrets to success, one relationship at a time.* New York: Crown Publishing Group.

Forum, W. E. (2017). *The Global Risk Report 2017*. Geneva, Switzerland: World Economic Forum.

Fry, R. (2018, April 11), Millennials are the largest generation in the US labor force. Retrieved from www.pewresearch.org/fact-tank/2018/04/11/millennials-largest-generation-us-labor-force/

Geneen, H., (1985). *Managing*. Geneen and Moscow, Granada Publishing Ltd.

Hewlett, S. A. (2014). As you start your career, focus on people skills. *Harvard Business Review*. Retrieved from https://hbr.org/2014/04/as-you-start-your-career-focus-on-people-skills

Hewlitt, S.A., Marshal, M., & Sherbin, L. (2013). How diversity can drive innovation. *Harvard Business Review*. Retrieved from: https: hbr.org/2013/12/how-diversity-can-drive-innovation]

Kedar, P. (2017). Why 75% of startups fail? Retrieved from: https://canwilltech.com/startups/why-75-of-startups-fail/

Kumok, Z. (n.d.). Making connections: How to create and cultivate your professional network. Retrieved January 1, 2018, from: https://www.goodcall.com/career/professional-network/

Lim, C. (2017). 5 steps to building your personal brand from scratch. Retrieved from https://www.entrepreneur.com/article/298513

Long, J. (2015). 8 tips to help grow your professional network. Retrieved from: https://www.huffingtonpost.com/jonathan-long/8-tips-to-help-grow-your-_b_7562332.html

Maister, D. H., Green, C. H., & Galford, R. M. (2001). *The Trusted Advisor*. New York: Touchstone Publishers.

Mendix. (2016). An interview with Geoffrey Moore on disruptive technologies and innovation. Retrieved from: https://www.mendix.com/blog/interview-geoffrey-moore-disruptive-technologies-innovation/

Mordechai, G. (2015). The innovation S-Curve. Retrieved from http://www.galsinsights.com/the-innovation-s-curve/

Mosher, M. (2016). Sustainability incorporated: Embeddinig sustainability into a company's core business strategies. Retrieved from: http://www.csrwire.com/blog/posts/1701-sustainability-incorporated-embedding-sustainability-into-a-companys-core-business-strategies

National Association of Colleges and Employers (NACE) (2017). Career readiness and competencies. Retrieved from http://www.naceweb.org/career-readiness/competencies/career-readiness-defined/

Noonan, P. (2016). Becoming the trusted advisor. Retrieved from: https://blog.commonwealth.com/becoming-the-trusted-advisor

Nursing, A. A. (2006). *The essentials of doctoral education for advanced nursing prcatice*. Washington, DC: American Association of Colleges of Nursing.

Page, T., Rahnema, A., Murphy, T., & Mcdowell, T. (n.d.). *Unlocking the flexible organization: Organizational design of the an uncertain future*. Retrieved from https://www2.deloitte.com/content/dam/Deloitte/global/Documents/HumanCapital/gx-hc-unlocking-flexible-%20organization.pdf

Press Ganey. (2018). HCAHPS regulatory survey. Retrieved from http://www.pressganey.com/solutions/service-a-to-z/hcahps-regulatory-survey

Riper, P. V. (2016, Feburary 23). Finding a trusted advisor. Retrieved from http://cloud-4good.com/announcements/finding-a-trusted-advisor/

Simmons, A. (n.d.). *The six kinds of stories*. Retrieved December 31, 2017, from http://annettesimmons.com/the-six-kinds-of-stories/

Sobol, I. (2017). Integrating sustainability into your core business. Retrieved from https://www.conference-board.org/retrievefile.cfm?filename=sustainability-rwg-project-brief.pdf&type=subsite

Solway, Lucy. (2016). *Bosh Health Buddy® for Monitoring Cancer Patients on Chemotherapyand Biological Therapy*. Retrieved from https://wmhin.org/wp-content/uploads/2016/02/Solway_Health-Buddy_WIN2016.pdf

Takahashi, D. (April 28, 2009) Bosh enters remote healthcare electronic market with Health Buddy®. Retrieved from https://venturebeat.com/2009/04/28/bosch-enters-remote-healthcare-electronics-market-with-health-buddy/

Taleb, N. N. (2010). *The black swan: The impact of the highly improbable*. New York: Random House LLC.

Tarasovich, B. M. (2015, March 2). *What's in your leadership toolbox*? Retrieved from http://sfmagazine.com/post-entry/march-2015-whats-in-your-leadership-toolbox/

Taylor, J., (2013). Cognitive biases are bad for business. *Psychology Today*. Retrieved from: https://www.psychologytoday.com/us/blog/the-power-prime/201305/cognitive-biases-are-bad-business

Thompson, J. (2011). Is nonverbal communication a numbers game? *Psychology Today*. Retrieved from: https://www.psychologytoday.com/blog/beyond-words/201109/is-nonverbal-communication-numbers-game

Tiwari, N. (2013). Business intelligence, helping data driven decision making. Helical IT Solutions Private Limited. Retrieved from: https://yourstory.com/2013/04/business-intelligence-helping-data-driven-decision-making-2/

Ulrich, D., & Smallwood, N. (2007). Five steps to building your personal leadership brand. *Harvard Busines Review, 85*(7/8), 92–100.

Zimmerman, B. (2017). 3 quality measures that most influence overall HCAHPS scores- *Becker's Hospital Review*. Retrieved from https://www.beckershospitalreview.com/quality/3-quality-measures-that-most-influence-overall-hcahps-scores.html

JEFFREY A. JOHNSON

13

The Executive Leadership Role in Transforming Health Care: Journey into the Executive Suite

Chapter Objectives

- Understand the new business climate of health care today.
- Appreciate the central role that learning plays in a hospital executive's success.
- Define and describe different types of learning that are important for leaders.
- Utilize case studies that illustrate new ways of working and thinking as a health care executive.

KEY WORDS: black swans, block chain, branding, sustainability, transparency, whitewater

Introduction

The first 12 chapters of this textbook focused on the critical compendium of knowledge, skills, attributes, policies, and processes that DNP nurses will need to master as they begin and advance new executive careers in their hospital's C-Suite. The textbook chapters, with diverse topics such as data and financial analysis, business planning, technical writing, health policy development, and informatics, reflect the 2015 AONL Nurse Executive Competencies and leave no doubt about the breadth and depth of the leadership portfolio that DNP nurses need for success.

In this final chapter, we take a totally different journey, one in which we walk with a new nurse executive into a hospital C-Suite. Here we offer a sampling of current topics of concern for hospital executives—from considering blockchain technology, improving transparency and sustainability, to purchasing a robot who will work side-by-side with humans in a busy hospital department. Here is a snapshot of the daily reality in today's C-Suite: the scope, diversity, uncertainty, and sheer complexity of issues that face a hospital's executive team—the new language of business today, the short shelf life of ideas, the difficult business decisions that must be made in hospitals every day, and the steep, very challenging learning curve that is anticipated for all hospital leaders who work in the current whitewater climate of health care today. For DNP prepared nurse executives and virtually all leaders, this journey includes traveling through a tough, uncomfortable terrain that was simply not part of their prior professional education. Although it is impossible to predict the future, it is certain that the work that lies ahead in the C-Suite will include many challenges, plenty of discomfort, and new excitement about growth opportunities as well.

The chapter concludes with two real-life case studies that will challenge your thinking and provide an opportunity for you to explore new ways of learning and working.

The C-Suite Agenda

On any given day, members of a hospital's executive team take their usual seats in the hospital's C-Suite conference room, roll up their sleeves, and begin their work on a long agenda. No item on the agenda is simple, and all are complex and challenging.

Blockchain

New DNP nurse executives who anticipate working on the ongoing integration of electronic medical records at their hospitals may be surprised to learn that blockchain technology may soon send shock waves through the entire health care industry. According to Sharma (2017), blockchain technology is a "game-changer" that which will change the complete landscape of how business is done (p.1). Sharma warned that ". . . The healthcare industry is on the verge of disruption in its digital infrastructure" because the current system does not fully support the required security or interoperability of medical records (p. 1).

What is Blockchain Technology? Writing in the NEJM Catalyst

Gordon, Wright, and Landman (2017) reported that blockchain technology, the distributed database technology based on advances in cryptography and network science that enables the bitcoin digital currency, was first described in a 2008 paper by Satoshi Nakamoto (believed to be a pseudonym for multiple authors) as a decentralized, public, cryptographically empowered currency system, a way for financial transactions to go "from one party to another without going through a financial institution" (p.1). Peters, Till, Meara, and Afshar (2017) added that ". . . The proposed system eliminates trusted third parties, such as banks and credit card companies, from online financial transactions and replaces them with secure, peer-to-peer financial networks" (p. 1).

Blockchain technology is very complex, but is basically a shared database, a decentralized, encrypted way of distributing, sharing, and storing information. Reporting for *Healthcare ITNews*, Miliard (2017) offered a simpler description:

> Blockchain transactions are logged publicly and in chronological order. The database shows an ever-expanding list of ordered "blocks," each time-stamped and connected to the block that came before it — thereby constituting a blockchain. Crucially, each block cannot be changed, deleted, or otherwise modified: it's an indelible record that a given transaction occurred. That's exactly what has many in healthcare excited about blockchain's potential for data security. Its open and decentralized nature could lend itself well to managing health records and proving identity. Rather than a central database, the blockchain record can be distributed and shared across networks, with credentialed users able to add to—but not delete or alter—the transaction log. Transactions are encrypted and must be verified by the network. (p. 1)

Gordon *et al.* (2017) emphasized that blockchain technology is a great deal more than a traditional database. Instead of central ownership:

> . . . data are managed by the consensus of participants in a network, who work together (with the help of cryptography) to decide what is added, while each participant maintains an identical, full copy of all transactions. The network can be public (like bitcoin, open to anyone) or private (restricted to certain members). When new information needs to be added, every computer on the network is notified and updates its copy accordingly. The result is an expansive and distributed source of truth — built not from trust, but through cryptographically enforced consensus. The information stored can be anything: financial transactions (à la bitcoin), land-title deeds, personal identity, intellectual property, even 'smart contracts'—computer code that executes when certain conditions are met. (p.1)

In their primer on blockchain technology written for surgeons, Peters *et al.* (2017) identified three major advantages of blockchain technology over centralized banking systems: (1) *transparency*—In contrast to centralized financial ledgers that are subject to fraud and misuse, blockchains offer transparent, verifiable records for every transaction, which validate the underlying currency and protect holders from counterfeit coins, pyramid schemes, and other forms of fraudulently duplicated value; (2) *immutability*—Centralized ledgers can be rich targets for hackers, who regularly attack such IT systems, at a global cost of billions of dollars each year. With blockchain technology, an attack on a single node has little network-wide effect because each member of the network, or node, holds an identical copy of the shared ledger, and efforts to hack or change the ledger will be

Table 13.1 Potential Benefits of Blockchain in Healthcare.

- *Clinical data sharing.* Advance directives, genetic studies, allergies, problem lists, imaging studies, and pathology reports are some data elements that could be distributed. Alternately, instead of storing actual patient data, blockchain could store access controls—like who a patient has authorized to see their health data—even if the clinical data itself is stored by the EHR.
- *Public health.* A shared, immutable stream of de-identified patient information could more readily identify pandemics, independent of governmental bodies currently aggregating this data—for example, an influenza reporting system.
- *Research and clinical trials.* Distributing patient consent or trial results could foster data sharing, audit trials, and clinical safety analyses.
- *Administrative and financial information.* Insurance eligibility and claims processing workflows could benefit from blockchain, which would decrease transactional costs.
- *Patient and provider identity.* National (or international) patient or provider identities could be secured in the blockchain, which would provide the basis for health data portability and security.
- *Patient-generated data.* Personal health devices, "wearables," "Internet of Things" (IOT) devices, and patient-reported outcomes are some examples of patient-generated data that could leverage the blockchain for security and sharing. (Gordon *et al.*, 2017, p. 1)

rejected by the broader network. The historical record on a blockchain is immutable and cannot be changed since blockchains provide a common history or shared truth that cannot be altered; and (3) *anonymity*—The data in the blockchain are anonymous and encrypted, which makes the information of little value for coercion, extortion, or corporate espionage (p. 1).

Is blockchain technology relevant in hospitals today? Gordon *et al.* (2017) identified some compelling benefits of blockchain that are specific for the health care industry, as shown in Table 13.1.

In their summary of the potential benefits, Peters *et al.* (2017) said that ". . . Blockchain technology stands to revolutionize the interoperability, security, and accountability of electronic health records (EHR) and health information technology (HIT), medical supply chains, payment methodologies, research capabilities, and data ownership" (p. 1).

Gordon *et al.* (2017) acknowledged that blockchain technology empowers patients to own and gather their own data, although they believe that the greatest promise of blockchain "lies outside the current health information technology framework—by directly challenging the siloed, centralized data stores that dominate healthcare data today" (p. 1). They also acknowledge that there are challenges ahead that could hamper the spread of blockchain throughout the industry. These include the vulnerability of being discovered because, despite being cryptographically hidden, blockchain is anonymous and also public; the challenge of duplication because blockchain relies on a unique identifier to link events together (similar to patient IDs in EHRs), which requires that different patient IDs in the blockchain must be deduplicated somewhere; and the reality that the sheer volume of clinical data generated far exceeds the practical storage capabilities of the current blockchain.

In addition, the authors emphasized that the blockchain is immutable because it works by consensus; if a majority of the network decides to move in a different direction, the blockchain could split (2017, p. 1). However, these challenges can be overcome by storing data off the chain or using a private blockchain, a network of trusted nodes in which only certain, permissioned entities are allowed to participate. Gordon *et al.* (2017) remind us that with a private blockchain, participants must trust other entities on the network: "If you have trust, blockchain is less necessary, and more just like a standard distributed database," they added (p. 1).

What lies ahead for the future of blockchain technology in the transformation of health care? Experts are simply unsure. Sharma (2017) predicted that blockchain technology will promote greater data sharing among health care providers without risks to data security and integrity, improve the accuracy of diagnoses and the effcicacy of treatments, and enhance the ability of health care instiutions to deliver high quality, cost-effective patient care. Looking ahead, Sharma reported that in a survey of 200 American healthcare executives, 16 percent expected to have a commercial blockchain solution at scale in the near future (p. 1).

The federal government is expected to play a role in the advancement of blockchain technology. In 2016, the U.S. Department of Health and Human Services (HHS) held a contest to elicit innovative ideas about the use of blockchain technology (Office of the National Coordinator, 2016). The contest submissions (CCC Innovation Center, 2017) described a variety of potential uses in clinical trials, claims processing, patient-reported outcome measures, records, and alternative payment methods. Peters *et al.* (2017) added that HHS will have a critical role in "developing administrative policy objectives that clearly define how the HHS Health Insurance Portability and Accountability Act [HIPPA] policy rule might govern over the distributed networking essential to a blockchain health record system" (p. 1). Meanwhile, hospitals and others interested in building the health care blockchain will face considerable challenges, particularly with electronic health records, said Peters *et al.* (2017). These challenges include adopting common data standards, building appropriate software or "middleware" capable of interfacing with blockchain ledgers, aligning incentives to attract the processing power for the network, and deciding how much data will be fully incorporated into an individual's electronic health chain.

Despite the many challenges, most technology experts suggest that we are now witnessing just the beginning of the blockchain revolution. Others, such as Das (2017), warn that blockchain "may not be the universal solution for managing conflicting data standards with disparate terminologies in the healthcare industry" (p. 1). In this rapidly developing phenomenon, what is clear is that health care leaders, including new nurse executives, must be actively engaged in determining the critical risks vs. rewards of this promising, but very complex new technology development.

Transparency

At any C-Suite meeting, a new nurse executive will soon realize that transparency is very much on the minds of health care leaders. But what is transparency, why is it so important in health care today, and what are the challenges?

Reporting for the American Health Policy Institute, Wetzell (2014) defined the key elements that comprise transparency in health care, see Table 13.2.

It is no secret that American health care suffers from extremely high costs and significant variations in quality. In his 2014 landmark research study, Wetzell detailed the reasons that greater transparency is important in American health care today. Transparency informs health care consumers, group purchasers, and policymakers about price and quality information, information that permits better decision-making about health care choices and ultimately creates a more rational marketplace. Wetzell (2014) said that improved transparency helps employers better manage their resources, improve benefit design strategies, make choices about plans and providers based on the best value, influence health care reforms, and work to eliminate the price and quality discrimination that continues to haunt the American health care system.

Writing in *Health Catalyst*, Brown and Skelley (2017) emphasized that the definition and perceived importance of transparency vary with different stakeholder groups. For example, to make informed health care decisions, consumers need easy-to-decipher, essential information about both the price and quality of health care services. Throughout the country, consumers have complained loudly about the difficulty of finding such information and their inability to determine the best choices for their care, their insurance coverage, and their out-of-pocket costs.

Table 13.2 Key Elements of a Fully Transparent Healthcare Marketplace.

	Cost Measures	Quality Measures	Customer Experience Measures
Healthcare exchange vendors	✓	✓	✓
Insurers and health plan administrators	✓	✓	✓
Pharmacy benefit managers	✓	✓	✓
Hospitals	✓	✓	✓
Doctors	✓	✓	✓
Other providers and facilities (chiropractors, mental health providers, nursing homes, ambulatory surgery centers)	✓	✓	✓
Treatments	✓	✓	✓

Not surprisingly, physicians often have a different perspective. In the fee-for-service system of the past, Brown and Skelley (2017) point out that physicians had no financial responsibility for the quality of care delivered by referral partners. However, that has changed in the new era of accountable care organizations, in which physicians are accountable for the care they provide and the care delivered by their referral partners. According to the Centers for Medicare and Medicaid Services (CMS) (2017), these organizations are groups of physicians, hospitals, and other care providers who voluntarily join together to provide coordinated, high quality care for Medicare patients. The goal is ensuring that the chronically ill receive "the right care at the right time"—that unnecessary duplication of services is avoided—and that medical errors are prevented. There are mutual benefits from success: patients receive better care and providers who participate in value-based contracts share in the savings for Medicare.

The emergence of value-based care has also begun to affect the expectations about transparency between payers and providers, which have been very problematic in the past. According to Brown and Skelley (2017), these major decision makers in health care "have guarded their proprietary information jealously to maintain their competitive positions in price negotiations, . . ." (p. 1). However, they report recent progress in which payers and providers have begun to agree on the metrics for quality, efficiency, and patient satisfaction that they will be prioritizing and tracking. Brown and Skelley (2017) suggest that this type of collaboration can improve cost and quality scores, overall medical costs, and use of the emergency department and advance imaging. But what about transparency within health care organizations?

Brown and Skelley (2017) say that overcoming the current lack of transparency within hospitals involves much more than revealing the cost of supplies and other resources. Instead, it involves outcomes, different quality initiatives underway in different hospital departments, and the chronic failure and resistance among heath care groups to sharing lessons learned from ongoing quality efforts. These shortcomings are a result of longstanding cultural norms in which quality metrics have been obsessively guarded, as well as the myriad technological challenges inherent in accessing databases that store critical quality data.

In 2015, Ellison identified the major challenges that have hampered the move toward greater transparency in health care. These include the following:

1. *Difficulty locating information*—In numerous surveys, cost conscious consumers who were interested in comparing health care prices reported considerable difficulty locating the essential information. One survey found that 90% of states did not provide adequate pricing information for consumers, while another reported that 45 states failed to meet even a minimum standard for price transparency.

2. *Meaningless prices*—Hospitals that provide prices without the associated quality data are doing a disservice to consumers because widely different prices are meaningless without quality data. Assuming that a highly priced medical service is also a high-quality service is a mistake, said Ellison (2017).

The good news is that changing cultural norms, industry pressures, and advances in technology are beginning to improve transparency in the industry. Brown and Skelley (2017) cite one success story, the Texas Children's Hospital's Department of Pediatric Radiology. Aided by an enterprise data warehouse (EDW) and advanced analytics, the staff of this large pediatric radiology center now has full access to valuable data such as average procedure duration, results turnaround time to providers, anesthesia utilization, patient flow cycle time, and utilization of each piece of equipment. The data have helped the staff members see how their work contributes to the end-to-end process, revealed additional capacity that allowed the staff to maximize utilization and reduce scheduling lags, and helped the entire center reduce variation and costs, which in turn improved both patient and staff satisfaction.

Wetzell (2014) also acknowledges that some progress has been made toward greater transparency, although he concluded that "the gap between what is available and what is needed is significant" (p. 9). Wetzell (2014) anticipates that the federal government will play an expanding role in advancing transparency, although such efforts will encounter considerable resistance and lobbying pressures by industry interest groups; access to clinical data will be less than ideal until the time when electronic medical records are fully introduced; and improvements in cost transparency for health plans and hospitals will need to become a priority in the years ahead (p.9).

The 2014 report of the Healthcare Financial Management Association's Price Transparency Task Force agreed:

> The lack of price transparency in healthcare threatens to erode public trust in our healthcare system, but this erosion can be stopped. Patients are assuming greater financial responsibility for their healthcare needs and in turn need the information that will allow them to make informed healthcare decisions. Price is not the only information needed to make these decisions; as this report has noted, price must be presented in the context of other relevant information on the quality of care. But it is an essential component. The time for price transparency in healthcare is now. (p. 18)

If the time for transparency in health care really is now, DNP nurse executives and their C-Suite collegaues who are truly serious about improving transparency in their hospitals may need to look to Ray Dalio, the sucessful, controversial founder of Bridgewater Associates, the largest hedge fund in the world. In a recent interview (Blodget, 2017), Dalio explained his concept of radical transparency:

> I think the greatest tragedy of mankind is that people have ideas and opinions in their heads but don't have a process for properly examining these ideas to find out what is true. That creates a world of distortions. That's relevant to what we do, and I think it's relevant to all decision making. So when I say I believe in radical truth and radical transparency, all I mean is we take things that ordinary people would hide, and we put them on the table, particularly mistakes, problems, and weaknesses. We put those on the table, and we look at them together. We don't hide them. (p. 1)

According to Gino (2017), scientific evidence confirms Dalio's belief that, as human beings, we tend to assess information with bias. Such *confirmation bias* promotes the natural tendency to focus on confirming evidence rather than searching for contradictory data. This bias weakens our judgments and decisions, said Gino (2017).

> With radical transparency, Dalio built an organizational culture at Bridgewater that was different, a culture in which employees know the importance of challenging others' points of view, regardless of rank, and where they discuss idea and issues openly, even when that means pointing out others' mistakes. Dalio has said that such a culture can be uncomfortable for some who have trouble adjusting to "thoughtful disagreement." But, the end result is a climate in which "employees engage and exchange ideas without creating lasting conflict, even when the ideas were controversial, . . ." (Gino, 2017, p. 1).

Sustainability

Sustainability is also a regular agenda item for today's C-Suite executives and, for many hospitals, sustainability has become part of the core business. According to Mosher (2016), ". . . Integrating sustainability into a company's core business model enables the business to create more value, manage risk, and address today's global environmental, social, and financial challenges," (p.1). Mosher (2016) suggested that "sustainability leads to greater employee engagement, better decision-making, and a more holistic and comprehensive understanding of risks and opportunities. In addition to corporate benefits, bringing sustainability issues into the business model enables a company to contribute to solving today's challenges such as water scarcity, climate change, inequality, and under and over nutrition," (p. 1). The bottom line, according to research by Eccles, Ioannou, and Serafeim (2012), is that "sustainability pays off. Companies that manage their environmental and social performance have superior financial performance and actually create more value for their shareholders. They do this by attracting and keeping better and more committed employees and having more loyal customers" (p. 1).

Like other sectors, the health care industry has been slow to respond to rising consumer pressure for greater corporate responsibility in business. According to Cohen (2016), the CoFounder and President of Healthcare Without Harm and Practice Greenhealth, this pressure has meant that companies must show that their business can help "people, profit, and planet all thrive together," (p. 1). Annual surveys conducted by Practice Greenhealth have shown progress over recent years. "Healthcare has been working behind the scenes to create sustainable, responsible facilities that provide better care that is supportive of local communities and more mission-aligned than ever before. The industry is well-positioned to meet the growing patient and staff demand for sustainable hospitals," said Cohen (p. 1). As shown in Figure 13.1, the longitudinal surveys found that hospitals have focused their decisions in areas that help them deliver health care that is better for patients, local communities, and the planet.

Waste. Practice Greenhealth estimated that 20–30% of the total hospital waste is generated by the operating room (Cohen, 2016). Another study found that operating rooms could decrease medical waste by an average of 65% by simply using reusable products, which the surgical staff actually preferred to disposal items (Conrardy, Hillanbrand, Myers, & Nussbaum, 2010). Artemia (2016) advises hospital clients to reduce their environmen-

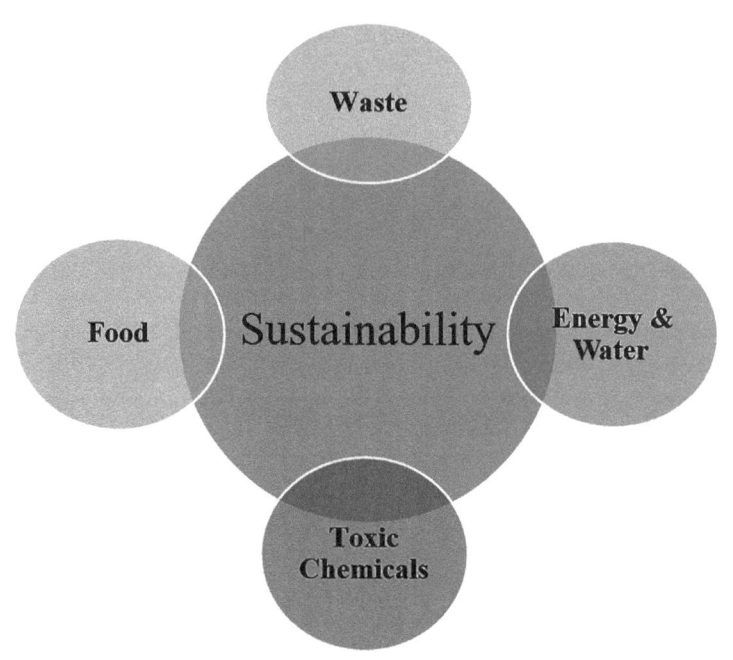

Figure 13.1. *Conscious Decisions in Health Care Sustainability. Source: Cohen, G. (2017, March 10). How healthcare is pushing sustainability ahead of consumer demand. Sustainable Brands. Retrieved from http://www.sustainablebrands.com/news_and_views/organizational_change/ gary_cohen/how_health_care_pushing_sustainability_ahead_consumer.*

tal footprint and waste management costs by using reusable supplies instead of single use items, digital x-ray equipment (instead of film), and washable surgical and isolation gowns, linens, mattress pads, and basins that can be sterilized and reused.

Energy and Water. Project Greenhealth found that a greater number of hospitals today are relying on renewable energy. In 2016, Cohen reported that the percentage of health care facilities that are generating or purchasing renewable energy has increased by 81%. Hospitals have also begun reducing anesthetic gases that escape during surgery, using electric vehicles for fleet transportation, and decreasing food waste. Artemia (2016) reported that some of their client hospitals are installing energy efficient lighting systems, and water conservation projects with low-flow plumbing fixtures.

Biason and Dahl (2016) make a strong business case that "saving energy leads to savings for hospitals," (p.1). They cite the Energy Star® analysis that summarized the effects of the energy cost savings on the financial health of hospitals:

- One dollar saved from energy conservation is approximately $20 in new revenue for hospitals, based on a typical 5% profit margin.
- Assuming a 20% annual energy savings, implementing a $100,000 energy conservation project (and reaping $20,000 in savings) would be the equivalent of generating $400,000 in new revenue per year (for the life of the improvement).

Toxic Chemicals. Assuring good sanitary practices while "going green" is a challenge for hospitals. Important steps forward include removing furniture, fabrics, and building materials which contain toxic chemicals that have negative effects linked to developmental delays, reproductive problems, and cancer; and using green cleaning practices with cleaning tools that use less water and chemicals (Quan, Joseph, & Jelen, 2011). Practice Greenhealth reported that in 2016 that ". . . The percentage of hospitals prioritizing furniture and medical furnishings free of halogenated flame retardants, formaldehyde, perfluorinated compounds, and PVC more than doubled from the previous year, . . ." (Cohen, 2016, p. 1). These efforts, suggested Mosher (2016), reflect the application of "a sustainability lens to products and services" (p.1), which embeds sustainability issues into routine business operations.

Food. Cohen (2016) said that in his work, there is a better understanding that the kind of food a hospital serves really matters—to individual health, to the environment, and to the community. In the surveys conducted by Practice Greenhealth, the majority of hospital respondents viewed sustainable food as an important focus, i.e., 62% had a policy in place, whereas more than 70% of the hospitals reported purchasing locally grown and/or sustainably grown foods. There is also evidence that hospitals are decreasing meat consumption, and prioritizing antibiotic-free meat (Artemia, 2016).

Driving the Demand. Cohen (2016) believes that the business case for sustainability in today's hospitals has gained real traction among hospital executives, and that this attention in the C-Suite represents "a total mind shift" (p. 1). In reporting its exhaustive international research study of sustainable products in health care, health care giant Johnson & Johnson (J&J) (2012b) offered some additional insights about future demand for greater sustainability: ". . . The importance of sustainability has begun to take root all along the healthcare supply chain. But the progress has been slow, because the vast percentage of purchasing decisions are still being made with the environment as a secondary consideration, . . ." (p. 6).

The J&J report (2012b) reiterated a well-known principle of change management; that is, the success of system-wide change initiatives, such as improving sustainability in health care, requires change champions who will "advocate the merits of sustainability, establish the strategy, and secure resources for related initiatives" (p. 6). As shown in Figure 13.2, the J&J survey respondents, all key decision makers in hospitals, indicated that purchasing and materials managers were the group most interested in sustainability and sustainable health products, followed by C-Suite executives and then nurses.

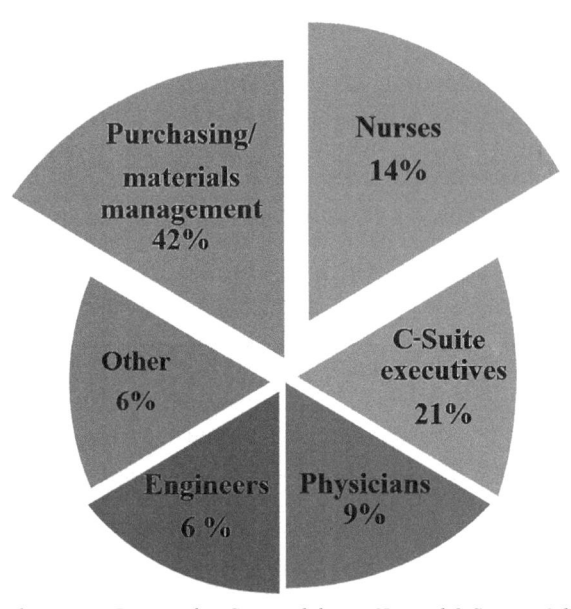

Figure 13.2. *Who is Most Interested in Sustainability in Hospitals? Source: Johnson & Johnson Services, Inc. (2012b). The growing importance of more sustainable products in the global healthcare industry. Retrieved from https://www.jnj.com/_document?id=00000159-6a81-dba3-afdb-7aeba25f0000.*

For nurses who are new to the C-Suite, these data identify a new opportunity for DNP prepared nurse executives who, as patient advocates, have the potential to develop their skills as sustainability experts in their hospitals, experts who work toward assuring that all executive decisions consider environmental, social, and financial value in meaningful ways.

It's the Brand

New nurse executives who bring a traditional perspective about the patient experience to the C-Suite may be surprised to hear so much discussion about their hospital's brand, and to see how their professional background in nursing can contribute to strengthening that brand. No longer the sole province of a hospital's marketing department, branding is an important business concept that reflects the competitive landscape of health care today. According to Koehn (2015), "A brand is usually defined as a name, logo, symbol, words, or combination of these, intended to distinguish a particular company's offerings from those of competitors," (p. 1). Great brands, Koehn (2015) says, command awareness, esteem, and loyalty from consumers, employees and other stakeholders, and they enhance a firm's profitability and influence in the competition within its industry.

Koehn (2015) calls world-class brands "ballasts in turbulent times." (p. 1). In periods of rapid-fire change and proliferating choice, brands serve as guides for consumers who are searching for consistent performers. These, said Koehn (2015), are the institutions that continually deliver on their promises to customers. In moments of economic contraction, trusted brands—especially those that respond to changing consumer priorities—recover quickly and help sustain customer loyalty.

In its 2016 *Hospital and Healthcare Marketing Trends* report, Franklin Street (2015), a Virginia-based consulting company that specializes in health care branding, identified three macro trends in branding that has implications for hospital executives, as follows:

- *Mapping the Patient's Journey*—Franklin Street said that one of the best ways to improve the patient experience is through mapping. According to Gray (2017), perceptual mapping is a 40-year-old marketing technique that diagrams the perceptions, behaviors, and feelings of a customer or potential customer, and identifies potential problem areas that need improvement. The Franklin Street (2015) report recommended mapping the entire patient's journey through the complex hospital system. This might include identifying the patient's feelings and state of mind, their overall awareness of options, the individuals (such as physicians, family and friends) who influenced their decisions, information sources (such as Facebook), their first point-of-contact with the hospital brand, ways in which they received care at different points in the hospi-

tal system, and their experience with matters related to insurance, medications, post-hospital follow-up care and communication.
- *Collecting Critical Marketing Metrics*—Franklin Street (2015) found that an increasing number of hospitals are moving away from "vanity metrics" (such as likes on Facebook) toward tracking activities that reflect new patient acquisition. These activities might include conversions — the step from "clicking on a digital marketing offer to taking a next step to becoming a patient," growth in e-mail lists, calls for physician referral, registrations for hospital-sponsored seminars and events, online requests for medical appointments, and patient downstream revenue.
- *Keeping the Hospital Brand Visible All Year*—Marketing a hospital's brand is no longer a seasonal, campaign-based effort. Instead, Franklin Street (2015) recommends "consistent campaigning," a year-round marketing approach that optimizes content and web channels for search engine optimization, includes seminars and educational events for key services, and leverages the hospital brand locally and nationally as well.

Branding, Better Patient Experience, and the Bottom Line. Writing in the *Harvard Business Review* (2017), Lee—the chief medical officer at Press Ganey Associates, a practicing physician at Brigham and Women's Hospital, and a faculty member at Harvard Medical School—discussed extensive data analytics that add important depth and breadth to a hospital's brand. In their analysis of their data on patient experience and publicly reported data on patient safety and business performance, Lee and colleagues (2017) found that health care organizations with better patient experience also had better safety records and better financial margins. In addition, they affirmed the value of "focused, effective efforts aimed at enhancing the engagement of physicians, nurses, and other personnel...If they believe that the organization cares about quality and safety, and if core values include compassion for patients and teamwork, there is a good chance that better quality and financial performance will follow, ..." (Lee, 2017, p. 1).

Using such performance data to strengthen a hospital's brand is critical, Koehn (2015) suggested the following:

> Changes happening in healthcare today will put a new premium on strong, trusted brands. As payment models shift to fee-for-value service, patients and referring clinicians are increasingly motivated to shop for quality care at the most affordable cost. The government is demanding and patients are expecting new levels of transparency in these areas. Hospitals are advertising their quality rankings and patient satisfaction scores on NPR and in local papers, in an effort to differentiate themselves in competitive markets. (Koehn, 2015, p.1).

In this competitive landscape, Koehn said that the creation and curation of an institution's brand must be central components of the ongoing business strategy.

Buy a Bot

It's highly unlikely that the graduate training of today's hospital executives included a course that taught them how to purchase a robot for their hospital's admissions department. Yet in hospitals today, decisions are being made in the C-Suite every day about purchasing very expensive robots—powered by artificial intelligence (AI) —that can reach into virtually every aspect of patient care and hospital operations.

Arnold and Wilson (2018), reporting for PWC Global, remind us that robots and AI have been used in medicine for more than 30 years. However, as shown in Figure 13.3, recent advances in technology have made them much more sophisticated, more efficient, less costly, and more far-reaching into almost every aspect of our health care system.

According to a recent review by Weintraub (2017) in *US News*, "... hospitals are getting into the game, deploying AI to take on challenges from diagnosing patients more quickly in the emergency room and streamlining communication between doctors to lessening the risk of complications so patients can go home sooner and avoid being readmitted," (p. 1). Weintraub (2017) cites a variety of AI-powered systems that help both patients and providers. There is a software system that uses pattern recognition and predictive analytics to detect a patient's risk of falling and alert nurses who

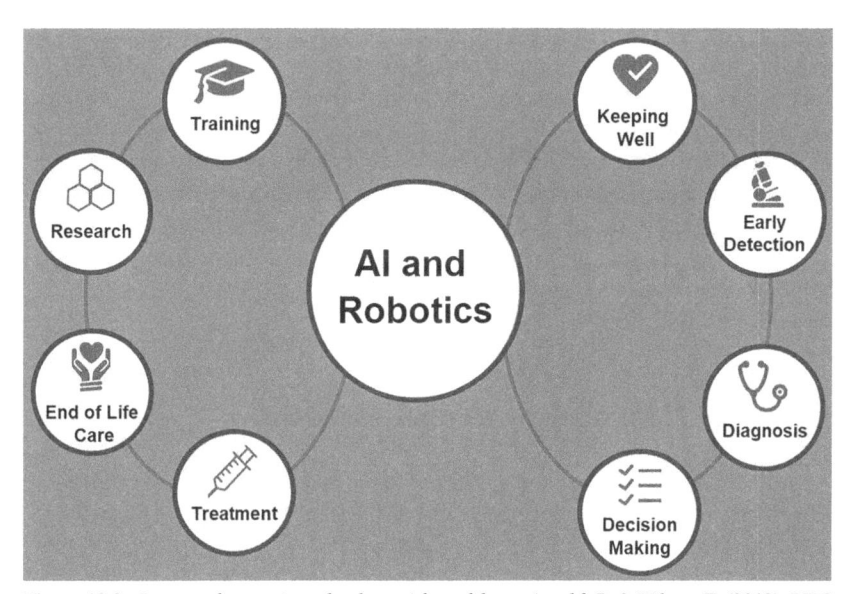

Figure 13.3. *Recent advances in technology. Adapted from: Arnold, D & Wilson, T. (2018). PWC Global. No longer science fiction, AI and robotics are transforming healthcare. Retrieved from https://www.pwc.com/gx/en/industries/healthcare/publications/ai-robotics-new-health/transforming-healthcare.html. Courtesy of Diane B. Stoy.*

can then move the patient and monitor them more closely; diagnostic systems that help oncologists determine the best treatment for a cancer patient; systems that can read CT scans and other medical images more quickly than a human and even offer a possible diagnosis; others that can assist physicians in making an accurate diagnosis in the emergency room; robots that conduct routine tasks in a hospital laboratory; and those that can improve hospital efficiencies in patient care scheduling, as well as staff and supply utilization.

Weintraub (2017) suggested that the explosive use of AI systems in health care is being tempered by financial concerns within the industry—concerns about whether or not expensive investments in AI-powered systems offer hospitals a good return-on-investment. She cited a 2017 survey by HIMSS Analytics and Healthcare IT News, which found that 35% of health care organizations plan to adopt AI within two years, although 15% of respondents said they could not make a business case for doing so. In the survey, more than 20% said they thought the technology was still underdeveloped.

In her assessment of the AI's future in medicine, Norman (2018) said that ". . . From powerful diagnostic algorithms to finely-tuned surgical robots, the technology is making its presence known across medical disciplines. Clearly, AI has a place in medicine; what we don't know yet is its value, . . ." (p. 2). As research and debate continue about the best use of robots and whether robots might even replace humans in health care, financial forecasts suggest that the role of AI in medicine will grow in the years ahead. As a report on AI by Accenture Consulting (Collier, Fu, & Yin, 2018) concluded, AI is a "self-running engine for growth in healthcare," (p. 1). The Accenture report found that "when combined, key clinical health (care) AI applications can potentially create $150 billion in annual savings for the US healthcare economy by 2026," (p. 2). The report also found that the market value of AI in medicine in 2014 was $600 million, and that by 2021, the market value will reach 6.6 billion. For new nurse executives and the other executives in a hospital's C-suite, these figures cannot be ignored. Very difficult decisions lie ahead.

Whitewater, Black Swans, Leadership, and Learning

More than thirty years ago, Vaill (1989), a well-known international consultant and business professor from George Washington University in Washington, DC, used the term *permanent white water* to describe the complex, turbulent, rapidly changing environment of modern life. The metaphor comes from recreational rafting in which adventure seekers attempt to pilot their rafts through the sometimes frightening, always rough, foaming whitecaps of the rapids.

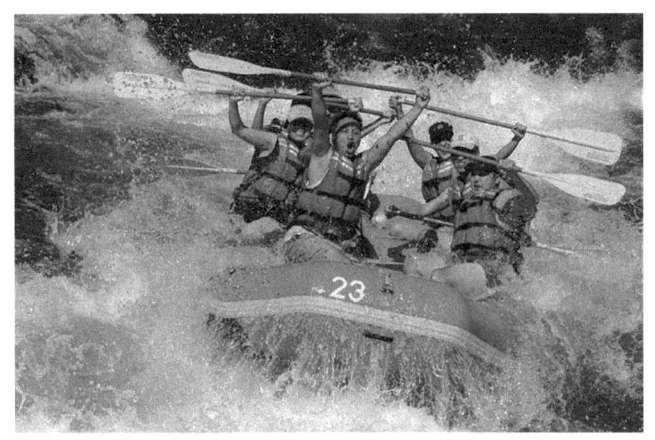

FIGURE 13.4. *White water. Courtesy of Diane B. Stoy.*

Vaill (1996) believes that permanent white water is an apt metaphor for modern life, which has become increasingly complex, fast, technological, and unpredictable. White water, Vaill (1996) suggested, is full of surprises that are not expected to happen, and which produce novel, unanticipated problems that are "messy, unstructured, and costly," (pp. 10–13). He said that "permanent white water means permanent life outside one's comfort zone," (Vaill, 1996, p. 14). Viewed another way, riding through the rapids can be downright frightening, because you cannot see what is ahead of the next curve—you might fall out of your raft at any time, there simply is no turning back, and you are just not sure about how to steer your raft to stay afloat. "Permanent white water puts organizations and their members in the position of continually doing things they have little experience with or have never done before at all," said Vaill (1996, p. 19). With these words, Vaill (1996) captured the essence of work life for today's hospital executive teams.

Fast forward 21 years for a new take on whitewater and living in turbulent times. Taleb (2010) introduced the concept of black swans that describes a highly improbable event—something environmental, economic, political, societal, or technological in nature that (1) is unpredictable and an outlier beyond normal expectations; (2) has a massive, cataclysmic impact; and (3) has retrospective predictability (i.e., the event becomes the basis of an explanation that makes it appear predictable and justified). The metaphor of the black swan was built originally on the historical fallacy that black swans did not exist in nature and was eventually extended to connote any impossibility.

New leaders might wonder why any organization would spend executive time and resources on black swans when they are so unpredictable. According to LeMerle (2011), there's an easy answer. Organizations just

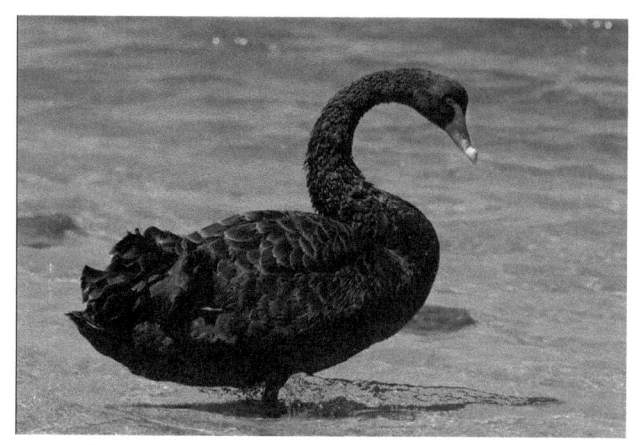

FIGURE 13.4. *Black Swan. Courtesy of Diane B. Stoy.*

cannot afford to ignore black swans because ". . . These events can threaten a company's survival, and boards and senior leaders are responsible for protecting shareholders and other stakeholders. They must ask, What else can go wrong?" (LeMerle, 2011, p.1).

LeMerle (2011) suggested that the solution involves going beyond the limited capacity of typical enterprise risk management (ERM) that identifies potential business disruptions, maps out their most likely effects, and develops mitigation plans and preventive actions that reduce the risk exposures. Given the unpredictability and gravity of black swans, he suggested that organizations use "disruptor analysis," which complements ERM by mapping the shape of the enterprise, determining the breadth of potential disrupters, asking the "what ifs" to determine how severely certain events could stress the enterprise, and then designing contingency plans (LeMerle, 2011, p. 1). According to LeMerle (2011), mapping a company usually includes more than just its geographic footprint. Such a map should include detailing all operations, composition and construction of the company's supply chain, and all internal and external channel partners and customers; creating a disruptor list of all potential disruptors; assessing the relative impact and consequences of any given catastrophe; and generating mitigation options for each possible scenario (2011, p. 1).

Whereas LeMerle (2011) advocated for using disruptive analysis at the organizational level, Cort (2015), writing for the Yale Center for Business and the Environment, offered a global perspective in his warning about the disastrous, unpredictable effects of black swan events on the environment and the world. Cort (2015) said the following:

> Sustainability challenges and Black Swan events go hand in hand. This suggests that sustainability challenges will continue to arise in those places least

expected. The bad news is that these events will be disruptive, costly and sometimes tragic. Lives, well-being, ecosystems, and money will all be lost as sustainability Black Swans continue to rampage. By and large, we will not see them coming (they are Black Swans after all), although we will be able to rationalize them after the fact. (Cort, 2015, p. 2)

Given that black swans are so ominous, both locally and globally, and are impossible to predict, what can hospital executives do to be prepared for the unexpected that may arise in the midst of such unprecedented changes in health care today? For an answer, we return to whitewater and the wise words of Vaill (1996), who wrote in his best-selling book *Learning as a Way of Being*, ". . . Permanent white water has made learning the preeminent requirement of all managerial leadership, beyond all the other characteristics and requisite competencies," (p. 126).

Vaill (1996) makes a strong case that successful leaders are leaders who truly understand that learning on the job is the key to success. In contrast to formal subject-matter, learning approaches that require long-term retention of a large, pre-determined amount of content, "leaderly" learning, says Vaill, means that "managerial leadership is not learned, managerial learning is *learning*, . . ." (p. 126). Today's reality of whitewater and unpredictable, ominous black swans require leaders to develop insights into how they and their employees learn best, and skills in learning what to do.

To do this, Vaill offers some directions for professional development that can help today's leaders who realize that they must become serious about becoming good learners:

- *Self-Directed Learning*. This means that a leader takes the initiative to think through what kind of approaches and timing are likely to work with a particular challenge. According to Vaill (1996), ". . . In permanent white water, the managerial leader not only learns about what to do, and proposes it (or requires it) of others. He or she also leads others in *learning* what needs to be done, that is, takes the lead through leaderly learning," (p. 134).

  Leaders, said Vaill, must experience what they need to know and lead themselves in a learning process relevant to what they have discovered (p. 134).

- *Creative Learning*. In his 1989 book, Vaill wrote that permanent whitewater means that leaders must embrace exploration and discovery, topics that are not typically included in the standard business school curriculum. Today's leaders will find themselves working in "process frontiers," which as the terms suggest, are new areas where there is little precedent and no compendium of best practices that can guide executive actions. As shown throughout this chapter, new nurse executives can expect to find themselves right in the middle of these process frontiers, which might focus on blockchain technology, robots, issues related to sustainability or transparency, and other areas that are just as complex. Vaill reminds us that within these process frontiers, everything is new, and that to be successful, the work simply cannot be managed by old policies, processes, and traditions that will just not work in new whitewater conditions.

- *Expressive Leaderly Learning.* Vaill (1996) suggested that that this type of learning is unique because it is learning in, through, from, and by expressing (p. 136). "Managerial leadership is expressive, and it *is* learning," Vaill said (1996, p. 138). How can this be nurtured in new leaders? Vaill (1996) is assertive about his recommendations. Stop memorizing and regurgitating formulaic lists of managerial abilities. Help them to realize that "information and their latitude to act will be sharply limited by the realities of the situation . . . help them to see that their effectiveness depends on their *personal* expressiveness," (p.139). In the end, Vaill (1996) concluded, "learners of managerial leadership have to try to lead, and those who facilitate their learning must help them take this fateful step," (p. 139).

- *Online Leaderly Learning.* Vaill emphasized the importance of leaders understanding the online environment and the kind of learning that is possible there (p.143). However, his warning would have certainly been much more emphatic had it been written today in the current turbulent media ecosystem of fake news. Recent research conducted by the Pew Research Center and Elon University's Imagining the Internet Center (Anderson & Rainie, 2017) with technologists, scholars, practitioners, and strategic thinkers, found that experts are divided about whether the coming decade will see a reduction in false and misleading online narratives. Some believed that technology improvements will not be able to prevent a future information landscape in which fake information crowds out all the reliable information. According to Anderson and Rainie (2017), the more optimistic experts said that "the rising speed, reach and efficiencies of the Internet, apps, and platforms can be harnessed to rein in fake news and misinformation campaigns," (p. 1). The optimists also believed that "better information literacy among citizens will enable people to judge the veracity of material content and eventually raise the tone of discourse, . . ." (p. 1).

It's doubtful that today's business schools are offering courses focused on information literacy, but perhaps they should, given the growing national concerns about the integrity of our media ecosystem and the professional demands on business executives who must navigate on a daily basis through such a complicated system. However, the issue is being addressed in higher education. For example, Brown University's Leadership Institute is now offering a two-week academic program that "helps students cultivate the knowledge, skills, and attitudes associated with effective and socially responsible leadership," (Brown University,

2018). A course, entitled *Leadership and Media Literacy in The Age of Fake News and Big Data*, challenges students to "pay closer attention to the media they create and consume on a daily basis," by addressing "the changing state of journalism in the age of clickbait and digital advertising, the role social media data and algorithms plays in shaping the news feeds we read, the impact of smart phones on what, where, and how we read about and document the world, and the rhetorical strategies that have proven effective in shaping public discourse in the digital age, . . ." (p. 1)

- *Continual Learning.* Vaill (1996) discusses this in simple terms: "Continual learning is necessary because ongoing change demands it, . . ." (p. 144). Vaill (1996) concluded that "learning as a way of being is the key to personal effectiveness and mental health in permanent white water, . . ." (p. 144). However, as the large literature on the post-doctoral experience suggests, new nurse executives who have finally completed the long, challenging doctoral process may indeed be exhausted. They may also believe that they are finally finished with the learning process now that they have been welcomed into the academy at their school's commencement. However, as defined, commencement is really a beginning and a start rather than an ending, and that means that promotion to an executive role will certainly require learning about a host of new subjects in the C-Suite. As Vaill said, ". . . In permanent white water, we are going to be beginners indefinitely," (1966, p. 81). Although learning in the C-Suite will be structured differently than in graduate school, this means that new nurse executives, in collaboration with their executive peers, can expect to be learning in those process frontiers where all hospital executives today find themselves.
- *Reflexive Leaderly Learning.* Vaill (1996) suggested that reflexive learning is also critical to a leader's success. This involves being conscious of the learning process, being comfortable asking for help, being able to separate self-worth from learning struggles with a specific project, viewing the learning process as continual experimentation, maintaining a sense of humor, and avoiding the desire for a magic bullet, or a fast cookbook approach.

Some leadership development programs have incorporated the seminal work of adult education specialists (Merriam & Caffarella, 1999), who offered two basic, helpful processes that leaders can use to become more reflective: *reflection-on-action*, the conscious act of returning to a situation after it has happened for analysis and identification of new perspectives on experience, behavioral change, and commitment to action, and *reflection-in-action*, which is the conscious attention to the present, the here, and the now (pp. 236–237).

Vaill (1996) suggests that reflection and heightened consciousness about learning has many benefits for the learner, insights about what works well and what does not; new and different ways of learning; better understanding of limitations and barriers to learning; greater enjoyment from learning; and reinforcement for incorporating learning into our essence (pp.84–85).

Chapter Takeaways

1. Understanding today's business climate requires that nurse executives gain sufficient knowledge to engage in developing C-Suite agendas.
2. Blockchain technology is considered a game-changer as current technology fails to meet new and envisioned attributes required of medical records.
3. Transparency in business and health care leadership practices has come of age and addressing the issue requires strong leadership and value reorientation.
4. Integrating sustainability into the health care industry's wheelhouse can invite improve employment participation that can lead to better decision-making and industry success.
5. Branding within the health care industry is rapidly becoming the norm for health care facilities and suggests a trend toward concrete value identification and enhanced transparency.
6. Engaging in white water events and planning for black swans results from leaning about existing environment factors that bring potential risks; learning to deal with potential disruptors marks the leader who fully appreciates that learning on the job equals success.

Chapter Summary

This final chapter has been a short, exciting, and at times, overwhelming journey into a hospital's C-Suite, where new DNP prepared nurse executives with DNP degrees will be joining an executive team that includes diverse, serious, savvy business executives. Members of this team—outfitted with safety helmets, life jackets, and oars—can expect to be riding the rapids of white water each and every day, as they shepherd part of the behemoth that has become the American health care system. A people-oriented place devoted to caring for the sick, hospitals are also research laboratories, educational institutions, major employers, and high-tech big businesses. Inside each hospital is a maze of committees, departments, personnel, services, and information transmission requirements in which a hierarchy of personnel and multiple channels of authority and responsibility are wrapped around the leadership's constant concern about the business bottom line.

According to Thompson (2018), in the last quarter and for the first time in history, "healthcare has surpassed manufacturing and retail, the most significant job engines of the 20th century, to become the largest source of jobs in the U.S. In 2000, there were 7 million more workers in manufacturing than in health care. At the beginning of the Great Recession, there were 2.4 million more workers in retail than health care. In 2017, healthcare surpassed both, . . ." (p. 1). According to the Kaiser Family Foundation (Sawyer & Cox, 2018), as a "high income country, the U.S. spends more per person on health than comparable countries. Health spending per person in the U.S. was $10,348 in 2016—31% higher than Switzerland, the next highest per capita spender," (p. 1). In its characterization of the reach of hospitals, The American Hospital Association (AHA) found that in 2015,

> America's hospitals treated 142 million people in their emergency departments, provided 581 million outpatient visits, performed almost 27 million surgeries and delivered nearly 4 million babies. Every year, hospitals provide vital healthcare services like these to hundreds of millions of people in thousands of communities. However, the importance of hospitals to their communities extends far beyond health care. (p. 1)

The AHA said that the health care sector is an economic mainstay that provides stability in communities—not just in jobs, but also in purchases of nearly $852 billion in goods and services from other businesses. Hospitals support more than $2.8 trillion in economic activity, the AHA found.

Within this complex, billion-dollar mega-business of hospitals, there is an emerging trend. Today's hospital executives will be managing a new type of workforce. Called the "nocollar workforce," human resource experts from Deloitte (Abbatiello, Boehm, Schwartz, & Chand, 2017) predict that ". . . In the near future, human workers and machines will work together seamlessly, each complementing the other's efforts in a single loop of productivity. And, in turn, HR organizations will begin developing new strategies and tools for recruiting, managing, and training a hybrid human-machine workforce, . . ." (p. 1). It will be a workforce, the experts suggest, in which people, robots, and AI work side-by-side.

To help those hybrid teams, hospitals will need to "develop innovative ways of learning and institutionalizing training opportunities that can help workers contribute substantively, creatively, and consistently to transformational efforts, no matter their roles," the experts said (p. 1). Learning, as Vaill has told us, will be the key to leaders' success in these ever-changing uncertain times. The experts from Deloitte agreed that continuous discovery will be needed because ". . . today's clear-cut answers will likely have limited shelf lives."

The bottom line is that old ways of thinking will no longer work for the new nurse executive and the entire hospital executive team that is heading down the rapids, watching out for black swans, struggling to balance all

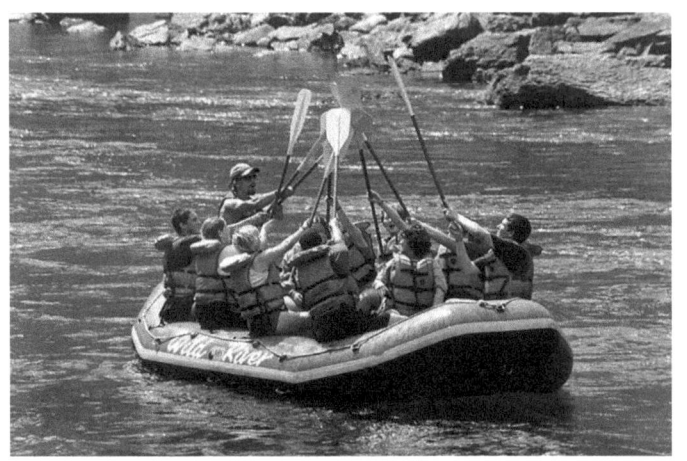

FIGURE 13.4. *Successful journey. Courtesy of Diane B. Stoy.*

the various pressures on the raft, assessing the potential risks that might emerge at each turn, and doing their very best every day for the team and their hospital. As the Deloitte experts concluded ". . . this is more like a promising journey of discovery than a clearly delineated sprint toward a finish line." (p. 1).

Chapter Reflection Questions

1. What business components are most critical to the DNP C-Suite nurse executive's success?
2. In the rapidly changing dynamics of the C-Suite, what key attributes must an executive exhibit in order to succeed among C-Suite peers?
3. How can a C-Suite DNP nurse executive best navigate potential turmoil of whitewater and disasters inherent in black swans?
4. What parameters best enable the C-Suite team to engage in blockchain technology, improving transparency and sustainability?
5. Which types of learning are most valuable for C-Suite executives enabling professional and business success?

Case Study #1: Trial by Technology

Scenario

You have recently graduated with your Doctorate in Nursing Practice and have begun a new job as an executive with your local hospital. You are very excited about this new professional opportunity and you look forward to collaborating with your new colleagues, who you expect to be very interesting and very diverse in terms of their professional backgrounds. But you are also feeling scared and a little uncertain because working as an executive in the C-Suite will certainly be quite different than your previous work as a head nurse. You are hoping that your knowledge and leadership skills meet the expectations of the hospital's senior leaders.

After you finish your orientation, you receive an e-mail with the agenda for the first monthly executive meeting you will be required to attend. Most of the agenda items seem quite routine and straightforward, such as review of hospital admissions, occupancy rates, infection control, and staff retention. However, at the end of the agenda, you notice that there will be a discussion of a proposal on blockchain technology. You start to panic. You have heard bad things about Bitcoin but are not familiar with this type of technology. For many years, you have been an admitted techni-phobe, who dislikes working on any technology related project. In your previous role, you were required to work as the nursing representative on your hospital's electronic medical records (EMR) committee. You found this committee work to be very stressful and not very satisfying, and you were relieved when it ended. Now, it appears that technology might be back on your work agenda.

Case Study Questions

1. What will you do to prepare for the executive meeting?
2. How will you respond if the senior leaders ask you to work on a subcommittee that will be tasked with studying the adoption of blockchain technology at your hospital?
3. Who will you ask to help you prepare for the meeting?
4. What *can* you do? What *will* you do?

Courtesy of J. Johnson, PhD, RN, NEA-BC, FAAN, 2018

Case Study #2: Capturing the Patient's Journey

Scenario

You are a new nurse executive. The senior leadership of your hospital has asked you to work with the hospital's marketing department on a very special project that involves the hospital's large, lucrative maternity service. In the past, the hospital has had a reputation for providing the absolute best, most holistic maternity care in the region. Occupancy rates in the maternity service have traditionally been very high and very stable, and patient satisfaction scores have also been very high. During the last year, however, post-hospitalization customer satisfaction surveys have reported escalating dissatisfaction with maternity care. Since the survey data have not identified specific issues of concern, you and a marketing representative have been asked to conduct a study of the maternity patient's journey, which will involve mapping to diagram the perceptions, behaviors, and feelings of maternity patients, and identify the potential problem service areas in maternity care. You are excited about this new assignment because you have considerable experience with the collection and analysis of qualitative data, your doctoral dissertation included a variety of qualitative data collection methods, you have always been interested in the patient experience, you consider yourself an advocate for patients, and you are eager for a quick win in your new executive role.

Case Study Questions

1. What will you do to prepare for this assignment?
2. How will you decide on the sample for this project? Which maternity patients will be included? How many mothers will you interview?
3. What questions about their hospital experience will you ask the new mothers?
4. What additional types of data will you collect?
5. How will you present your findings to the hospital's executive group?

Courtesy of J. Johnson, PhD, RN, NEA-BC, FAAN, 2018

References

Abbatiello, A., Boehm, T., Schwartz, J., & Chand, S. (2017, December 5). No-collar workforce: Humans and machines in one loop—collaborating in roles and new talent models. *Deloitte Insights*. Retrieved from https://www2.deloitte.com/insights/us/en/focus/tech-trends/2018/no-collar-workforce.html.

American Hospital Association (2018). *Hospitals are economic anchors in their communities*. Retrieved from https://www.aha.org/system/files/content/17/17econcontribution.pdf.

American Organization of Nurse Executives (AONE) (2015). *Nurse executive competencies*. Chicago, IL: AONE. Retrieved from http://www.aone.org/resources/nec.pdf.

Anderson, J. & Rainie, L. (2017, October 19). *The future of truth and misinformation online*. Retrieved from http://www.pewinternet.org/2017/10/19/the-future-of-truth-and-misinformation-online/

Arnold, D & Wilson, T. (2018). PWC Global. *No longer science fiction, AI and robot-*

ics are transforming healthcare. Retrieved from https://www.pwc.com/gx/en/industries/healthcare/publications/ai-robotics-new-health/transforming-healthcare.html.
- Artemia. (2016, June 29). Four trends in hospital and healthcare facility sustainability. Retrieved from http://artemia.com/four-trends-hospital-healthcare-facility-sustainability/
- Biason, K. M. & Dahl. P. (2016, October 13). Strategic steps to sustainability in healthcare. *Healthcare Facilities Today*. Retrieved from https://www.healthcarefacilitiestoday.com/posts/Strategic-steps-to-sustainability-in-healthcare-13629
- Brown, B. & Skelley, L. (2017). The key to overcoming the challenges of transparency in healthcare. *Health Catalyst*. Retrieved from https://www.healthcatalyst.com/Key-Overcoming-Challenges-Transparency-in-Healthcare
- Brown University Leadership Institute. (2018). Leadership and media literacy in the age of fake news and big data. Retrieved from https://precollege.brown.edu/catalog/course.php?course_code=CEMS0922
- CCC Innovation Center. (2017). Winners announced! Papers suggest new uses for blockchain to protect and exchange electronic health information. Retrieved from www.cccinnovationcenter.com/challenges/block-chain-challenge/view-winners
- Center for Medicare and Medicaid Services (2017). *Accountable care organizations*. Retrieved from https://www.cms.gov/Medicare/Medicare-Fee-for-Service-Payment/ACO/.
- Cohen, G. (2017, March 10). How healthcare is pushing sustainability ahead of consumer demand. *Sustainable Brands*. Retrieved from http://www.sustainablebrands.com/news_and_views/organizational_change/gary_cohen/
- Collier, M., Fu, R. & Yin, L. (2018). AI: An engine for growth. Retrieved from https://www.accenture.com/us-en/insight-artificial-intelligence-healthcare how_health_care_pushing_sustainability_ahead_consume
- Conrardy, J., Hillanbrand, M., Myers, S. & Nussbaum, G. F. (2010). Reducing medical waste. *AORN J, 91*(6), 711–721. doi: 10.1016/j.aorn.2009.12.029.
- Cort, T. (2015, August 3). Black swans and sustainability. *Environmental Leader*. Retrieved from https://www.environmentalleader.com/2015/08/black-swans-and-sustainability/
- Das, R. (2017, August 8). Top 5 reasons why every healthcare company should invest in blockchain. Retrieved from https://www.forbes.com/sites/reenitadas/2017/08/08/top-5-reasons-why-every-healthcare-company-should-invest-in-blockchain/3/#6d404fa84c4b
- Eccles, R., Ioannou, I., & Serafeim, G. (2012, January 6). Is sustainability now the key to corporate success? *The Guardian*. Retrieved from https://www.theguardian.com/sustainable-business/sustainability-key-corporate-success
- Ellison, A. (2015, April 8). 3 major challenges of healthcare price transparency. *Becker's Hospital CEO report*. Retrieved from https://www.beckershospitalreview.com/finance/3-major-challenges-of-healthcare-price-transparency.html
- Franklin Street. (2015, December 8). Hospital brand trends for 2016. Retrieved from http://www.franklinstreet.com/hospital-brand-trends-for-2016
- Funston, F., Wagner, S., & Ristuccia, H. (2010). Risk intelligent decision-making: Ten essential skills for surviving and thriving in uncertainty. *Deloitte Review* (7). Retrieved from https://www2.deloitte.com/content/dam/insights/us/articles/risk-

intelligent-decision-making/US_deloittereview_Risk_Intelligent_Decision_Making_Jul10.pdf

Gino, F. (2017, October 10). Radical transparency can reduce bias but only if it is done right. *Harvard Business Review*. Retrieved from https://hbr.org/2017/10/radical-transparency-can-reduce-bias-but-only-if-its-done-right

Gordon, W., Wright, A., & Landman, A. (2017, February 9). Blockchain in health care: Decoding the hype. *NEJM Catalyst*. Retrieved from https://catalyst.nejm.org/decoding-blockchain-technology-health/

Gray, K. (2017, January 5). What is perceptual mapping? Retrieved from https://www.thedigitaltransformationpeople.com/channels/analytics/what-is-perceptual-mapping/

Healthcare Financial Management Association. (2014). Price transparency in health care: Report from the HFMA Price Transparency Task Force. Westchester, IL: Healthcare Financial Management Association. Retrieved from file:///C:/Users/Diane/Downloads/Price%20Transparency%20Report.pdf

Johnson & Johnson Services, Inc. (2012b). The growing importance of more sustainable products in the global healthcare industry. Retrieved from https://www.jnj.com/_document?id=00000159-6a81-dba3-afdb-7aeba25f0000

Johnson & Johnson Services, Inc. (2012a). Appreciating the value of sustainability in health care. Retrieved from https://www.jnj.com/_document?id=00000159-6a81-dba3-afdb-7aeba25f0000

Lee, T. H. (2017, May 31). How U.S healthcare got safer by focusing on the patient experience. *Harvard Business Review*. Retrieved from https://hbr.org/2017/05/how-u-s-health-care-got-safer-by-focusing-on-the-patient-experience

LeMerle, M. (2011, August 23). How to prepare for a black swan. *Strategy & Leadership, 64*. Retrieved from https://www.strategy-business.com/article/11303?gko=e5fac.

Koehn, N. (2015, January 9). Why brand matters in health care. Retrieved from https://www.athenahealth.com/blog/2015/01/09/why-brand-matters-in-health-care

Merriam, S.B. & Caffarella, R.S. (1999). *Learning in adulthood: A comprehensive guide*. (2nd ed.) San Francisco: Jossey-Bass Publishers.

Miliard, M. (2017, April 13). How does blockchain actually work for healthcare? *Healthcare IT News*. Retrieved from http://www.healthcareitnews.com/news/how-does-blockchain-actually-work-healthcare

Mosher, M. (2016, Febuary 11). *Sustainability incorporated: Embedding sustainability into a company's core business strategies*. Retrieved from http://www.csrwire.com/blog/posts/1701-sustainability-incorporated-embedding-sustainability-into-a-companys-core-business-strategies

Norman, A, (2018, January 2018). Your future doctor may be human. This is the rise of AI in medicine. Retrieved from https://futurism.com/ai-medicine-doctor/

Office of the National Coordinator. (2016). ONC announces blockchain challenge winners. Department of Health and Human Services, Office of National Coordinator. Retrieved from https://wayback.archive-it.org/3926/20170127190114/https://www.hhs.gov/about/news/2016/08/29/onc-announces-blockchain-challenge-winners.html

Peters, A.W., Till, B.M., Meara, J.G., & Afshar, S. (2017, December 6). Blockchain technology in health care: A primer for surgeons. *Bulletin of the American College of Surgeons*. Retrieved from http://bulletin.facs.org/2017/12/blockchain-technology-in-health-care-a-primer-for-surgeons/#.Wn4H6qinG1s

Quan, X., Joseph, A. & Jelen, M. (2011). Green cleaning in healthcare: Current practices and questions for future research. Retrieved from https://www.healthdesign.org/chd/knowledge-repository/green-cleaning-healthcare-current-practices-and-questions-future-research

Sawyer, B. & Cox, C. (2018, February 13). How does health spending in the U.S. compare to other countries? Retrieved from https://www.healthsystemtracker.org/chart-collection/health-spending-u-s-compare-countries/#item-relative-size-wealth-u-s-spends-disproportionate-amount-health

Sharma, U. (2017, October 30). Blockchain in healthcare: Patient benefits and more. IBM Blockchain Blog. Retrieved from https://www.ibm.com/blogs/blockchain/2017/10/blockchain-in-healthcare-patient-benefits-and-more/

Taleb, N. N. (2010). *The black swan: The impact of the highly improbable*. 2nd ed. New York, NY: Random House.

Thompson, D. (2018, January 9). Healthcare just became the U.S.'s largest employer. Retrieved from https://www.theatlantic.com/business/archive/2018/01/health-care-america-jobs/550079/

Vaill, P. B. (1996). *Learning as a way of being: Strategies for survival in a world of permanent white water*. San Francisco, CA: Jossey-Bass Publishers.

Vaill, P, B. (1989). *Managing as a performing art: New ideas for a world of chaotic change*. San Francisco, CA: Jossey-Bass Publishers.

Weintraub, A, (2017, October 31). Hospitals utilize artificial intelligence to treat patients. *US News*. Retrieved from https://www.usnews.com/news/healthcare-of-tomorrow/articles/2017-10-31/hospitals-utilize-artificial-intelligence-to-treat-patients

Wetzell, S. (2014, March). Transparency: A needed step towards healthcare affordability. Washington, DC: The American Health Policy Institute. Retrieved from http://www.americanhealthpolicy.org/Content/documents/resources/Transparency%20Study%201%20-%20The%20Need%20for%20Health%20Care%20Transparency.pdf

Index

10-point writing improvement plan, 332
  begin well, 330
  careful choice of words, 331
  choice of words, 331
  fundamentals right, 327
  pledge to grow as a writer, 324
  read as a writer, 326
  second opinion, 332
  so-what question, 329
  writers block, 331
  writing as a process, 325
  writing improvement plan, 332

AACN DNP essentials, 5, 6, 8–10
AACN Essential IV, 289
Advanced Practice Nursing (APN) role transformation, 75, 76, 78–88
Academic-practice collaborative research, 130, 132, 154
Accelerate model, 22, 38
Accountable care organization, 18, 36
Achievement and improvement points, 126, 127, 130, 135, 139
Active and passive voice, 327
Adaptive leadership, 24, 38
Adoption rate, 252
  compatibility, 252
  complexity, 252
  measuring marketing strategy spend rate, 253
  observability, 252
  relative advantage, 252
  trialability, 252

Advocate, 108
Affordable Care Act (ACA), 75, 87
Affordable Care Act (ACA) update, 163–165, 169, 170, 177, 178, 181, 185, 187, 188, 194
Agency for Healthcare Research and Quality (AHRQ) 133, 135, 136, 141–143, 149
  home and community-based, 142
  inpatient quality, 142
  patient safety, 134, 138, 142, 146
  pediatric quality, 142
Aging population, 75, 81
Aiken study, 50
Alternative criterion matrix, 159, 188
Altmann societal influences, 50, 51
American Association of Colleges of Nursing (AACN), 46–48, 53–55
American Nurses Association (ANA), 46, 48
American Nurses Credentialing Center (ANCC), 47, 49, 126
American Organization for Nursing Leadership (AONL) (formerly the American Organization of Nurse Executives), 1, 5, 7–9, 13, 18, 46, 48, 54, 55, 94, 160, 163, 164, 176, 180, 185, 187, 243, 289, 291, 293, 309, 316, 322, 323, 339–341, 343, 345, 352, 365
AONL Nurse Executive competencies, 1, 5, 7–9, 13

395

APN-DNP transition, 75, 76, 82, 84
Argumentation, 176–178
Artificial intelligence (AI), 379, 380, 387
Assisted living, 82, 83, 88
Authorizing environment, 178, 188, 194, 195, 206

Banner health, 297
Best-fit policy option, 159, 175
Big data and analytics, 301
Big data key principles, 302
Black swan, 380, 382
Blockchain technology, 366–368, 386
Blockchain Technology
  anonymity, 368
  immutability, 367
  transparency, 365, 367, 370, 371
Bot, 379
Branding, 377, 378, 386
Brand visibility, 377, 378
  marketing metrics, 378
  patient journey mapping, 377, 390
Brand visibility, 377, 378, 386
Budget variance, 235
Burnout signs, 98, 105, 120
Business acumen, 241, 243, 244
Business plan framework, 241, 245
Business plan key elements, 245
Business planning, 241, 245, 253, 283
Business plan packaging, 282
Business plan pitfalls, 282
  complicated terminology, 282
  excessive length, 282
Business risk, 226, 227, 228, 229
Business writing, 315, 316
Busyness, 31

Care coordination, 79, 86–88
Care trajectory, 119
Catheterassociated bloodstream infection (CLABSI), 103, 104, 110, 112
Case review, 110, 112
  intervention, 110
  prevention project charter, 111
  process measures, 112, 113
Catheterassociated urinary tract infection (CAUTI) Intervention, 103, 104, 109
Catheterassociated urinary tract infection (CAUTI) Prevention, 103, 104, 109
CCNE accreditation, 13
Centers for Medicare and Medicaid Services (CMS), 98, 99, 102–104, 134, 136, 138–140, 146, 148
Centers for Medicare and Medicaid Services (CMS) cost reduction initiative, 82, 86, 87
Charisma, 343, 344, 358
Chronic disease management, 80, 86
Clinical data shoring, 368, 372
Clinical evaluation parameters, 296
Clinical functionality parameters, 295, 296
Clinical nurse champions, 131
CMS hospital value-based performance measures, 138, 139
CMS value-based purchasing, 138, 139
CNIO role, responsibilities 291–293
Collaborative practice 28, 29
Collaborative research, DNP and PhD 130, 132, 154
Commerce clause of Constitution 221, 222
Competencies, 288, 289, 290
Composition, 317, 318, 320, 321, 324–326, 330, 332–334
Consequences of policy, 159, 168, 181
Contemporary HIT essential skill set, 290
Continuous learning, 95, 96
Coordination, 328
Core competencies nurses as leaders, 108
  data stewardship, 98, 100–103, 109, 110, 112
  engagement, 93, 104, 119
  role model, 93, 97, 101, 113, 118
Core competency, 242, 252
Core competency domains, 28
Core functions IT crosswalk, 293
Core mindsets, 351

Cost-benefit analysis, 159, 168, 174, 193, 196, 231, 235, 236
Criteria selecting and weighting, 171, 174, 175, 196
Crossing the Quality Chasm, 126
C-Suite, 370
C-Suite DNP nurse, 54, 65, 68
C-Suite performance expectations, 17, 18, 21, 28, 29, 34, 38
Culture of health, 17, 18, 26, 27, 30, 38

Dashboards, 125, 148
Data dashboards, 303–305
Data display, 303, 304, 310
Defining and measuring outcomes, 125, 127–130, 132–134, 136, 142, 146–150, 152
Description of the business, 246
Designing effective interventions, 17, 24, 25
Development of APN specialties, 76, 77, 87
  clinical Nurse Specialist (CNS), 76, 79
  midwife, 76, 87
  nurse anesthetist, 76, 78, 87
  nurse practitioner, 76, 87
Development plan and schedule, 250
Disruptive innovation, 22
Disruptive technology, 352
Diverse healthcare population, 80, 81
DNP curriculum, 1, 9, 10, 15
DNP evolution, 65, 69
DNP leadership self-assessment, 18, 20, 31, 32, 38
DNP nurse executive role, 287–292, 294, 295, 298–307
DNP & PhD/DNS/DNS differences, 1, 3
DNP program growth, 45, 66, 69
DNP programs, current state, 2, 5
DNP role development, 78
DNP role integration, 78, 79
Doctoral education evolution, 3
Doctoral graduate growth, 3, 4
Doctoral writing skills, 315
Doctorate in Nursing Practice (DNP), 241–243

Domain 1—Safety, 103, 104, 106, 109, 110
Domain 2—Infections, 103, 109, 110
Donabedian theory, 93

Educational requirements for nurse leaders, 43, 47, 53, 54, 56, 66, 68
Effective written communication, 316
eHealth, 307, 308, 310
EHR interoperability, 297
Electronic medical records, 223
Emerging technologies, 303, 310
Emotional intelligence, 31
Employee-sponsored healthcare, 161
Enterprise governance structure, 301
Enterprise risk management (ERM), 382
Entrepreneurial thinking, 244
Entrepreneurship, 241
Essential HIT skill set evolution, 289
Evaluation design development, 168, 184, 185, 188
Evidenced-based analysis, 169
Evidenced-based practice, 121
Executive summary, 256, 282
Executive summary components, 241

Failure Mode and Effects Analysis (FMEA), 149, 150
Federal government, 217, 218, 222, 225
Federal health care programs, 136
Financial performance tools, 232
  asset management, 233, 235
  liquidity, 233, 235
  long-term solvency, 233, 235
  profitability, 232, 233, 235
Financial plan, 253–255
Financial risk, 217, 225–229, 232, 234–236
Financial strategy, 217, 235
Framework for safe, reliable, effective care, 94, 95, 120
  culture, 94–96, 98, 107, 118, 120
  learning systems, 95
Free market principles, 218, 219, 223, 234

Gantt chart, 181, 182
Generation diversity, 337, 354–357
Government policy concerns, 159–173, 178, 180
Government role in healthcare, 159–173, 178, 180

Health care ecosystem, 289, 290, 294
Healthcare Effectiveness Data and Information Set (HEDIS), 138, 141
Health care Information Technology, (HIT), 287–295, 297–303, 305–309
Healthcare stakeholders, 219–221, 225, 226, 238, 239
  consumer, 218–220, 223
  insurer, 219, 220, 223, 225
  provider, 219–224, 234
  regulator, 220, 225
Healthcare transformation, 20, 30
Health policy, 160, 164
Health Savings Account (HSA), 219, 220, 224
Hidden assumptions, 159, 169, 170, 197, 206
Higher order thinking, 315
HIMSS CNO-CNIO vendor roundtable, 291, 302
HITECH Act, 305
Home care, 86–88
Hospital acquired conditions (HAC), 139
Hospital Acquired Conditions (HAC), score calculation, 103, 104
Hospital Acquired Conditions (HAC) Reduction Program ,102–104
Hospital Consumer Assessment of Healthcare Providers and Systems (HCAHPS), 139, 141
Hospital C-Suite, 365, 366, 372, 373, 376, 377, 379, 380, 385, 386
Hospital Readmission Reduction Program, 104
Human factors, 292, 293, 298

Implementation barriers, 291, 292, 294, 295, 297–300

Implementation planning, 181
Imposter syndrome, 43, 67, 68
  diligence and hard work, 67
  masking behavior, 67
  using charm or perceptiveness to gain approval, 67
Improvement and measurement, 97
Income statement, 254
  balance sheet, 253, 254
  cashflow statement, 253, 254
  income statement, 254
Influence, 93, 99, 107–109, 120
informatics, 306
Informatics, 287–292, 295, 297, 301, 303, 305, 306
Information asymmetry, 220
Information source subsets, 159
Institute of Medicine (IOM), 126, 129, 133–135, 291, 292, 297, 305, 309
Institute of Medicine (IOM) advanced nursing education, 46, 47, 51, 69
Integrated technology model, 298
Interdisciplinary teams, 26, 28
Interpreting arguments, 177
IOM Future of Nursing Campaign indicator, 3
IOM Recommendations, 18, 25

JCAHO accreditation, 222
Joint Commission on the Accreditation of Hospitals and Healthcare Organizations (JCAHO), 223

Key HIT implementation milestones, 299
Kingdon policy stream model, 167, 169

Leadership assessment tools, 31, 32
Leadership mindset, 65
Leadership soft skills, 337–343, 352, 357
Learning, 365, 366, 380, 383, 384, 385
  continual learning, 385
  creative learning, 383
  expressive leaderly learning, 384
  on-line leaderly learning, 383, 384

Reflexive leaderly learning 385
Self-directed learning 383
Legislation ad EHRs, 305, 306, 309, 311
Lippitt's planned change theory, 44
Long-term care, 75, 81, 82, 87

MACRA, 20
Macrofinancing, 217
Macro-level finance principles, 218, 225, 226
Magnet status, 126, 127
Market and competition analysis, 247
Market complexity, 217–220, 222–224, 230, 234, 235
Marketing metrics, 378
Marketing plan, 251
Marketplace transparency, 370
Medicare, 218, 222–225, 237
Medicare waiver, 87
Merit-based Incentive Payment System (MIPS), 20, 21
Microfinancial business risk, 217, 218, 225–227, 236
Microfinancing, 217
Mobile health, 307, 310
Mobile Nursing Information Systems (m-NIS), 307, 308
Monitoring strategies, 217, 225, 237
Monitoring system design process, 181, 208
Multiple perspectives, 168, 188

National Committee for Quality Assurance, 140
National Data Base of Nursing Quality Indicators (NDNQI), 109
National Healthcare Quality and Disparities Report, 143
National League for Nursing (NLN), 46, 49
National Quality Forum (NQF), 139, 143
National Quality Forum Serious Reportable Events, 145
  care management, 145
  environmental events, 145
  patient protection events, 145
  potential criminal event, 145
  product or device event, 145
  radiologic event, 145
  surgical or invasive procedure event, 145
National Quality Measures Clearinghouse domain framework, 143, 144
  health care delivery measures, 143
  population health measures, 143
National Quality Measures Clearinghouse (NQMC), 143
National quality strategy levers, 137
National Quality Strategy (NQS) 135, 136
National Quality Strategy, six priorities, 135
National Strategy for Quality Improvement (NQS), 100, 101
Normalization of deviance, 106, 107
Nurse Executive Competencies, 7, 13
Nurse leader policy responsibilities, 187
Nurse-managed clinics, 84–86
Nurse manager role, 44, 47, 52, 54, 55, 65, 66
Nursing degree progression, 45, 49
Nursing informatics, 287, 288, 291, 295, 297, 308, 310
Nursing's social contract, 186

Operational budget planning, 217, 218, 221, 231–235
Operational financial management, 217, 218, 225–227, 229, 230, 232
Operational plan, 242, 247, 255
Organization chart, 251
Organizational readiness assessment, 299

Parallelism, 327
Pareto charts, 181–183
Patient and Family-Centered Care (IPFCC), 93, 113
Patient-centered medical home, 21
  accessible Services, 19
  comprehensive Care, 19
  coordinated care, 20

coordinated care, 19
patient-centered care, 19, 28
quality and safety, 19, 30
Patient journey mapping, 365–377
Personal assessment, 32
PERT chart, 181, 182
PhD & DNP, number of graduates, 2–4
PhD & DNP program differences, 1, 3
Polarity thinking, 289
Policy actions and outcomes, 184
Policy agendas, 163, 187, 188
Policy analysis, 159, 160, 166–171, 173, 175, 181, 185–188
Policy analyst types and role, 159, 167, 168, 169, 172–174, 177, 178, 189
Policy argumentation, 177, 178
Policy evaluation, 159, 185
Policy implementation, 159, 179–181, 184, 188
Policy options, 159, 167, 173, 174, 188
Policy outcome monitoring, 184, 208
Policy recommendation process, 168, 170
Political influence, 163
Population level data, 224, 227
Practice barriers, 75, 80, 84, 88
Practice deviation, 97
Practice doctorate position statement, 1, 2, 5
Practice Environment Scale of the Nursing Work Index (PES-NWI), 51
Pre-existing conditions, 219
Primary care, 80–84, 86
Problem identification, 171, 173
Professional practice environment, 27
Public/private payer mix, 219–227, 230

Quadruple aim, 98, 105, 107, 120
Quality and Safety Education for Nurses (QSEN), 133
Quality improvement, 125, 126, 132–136, 144, 146, 148–150, 153
Quality improvement methods, 153
 failure mode and effects analysis (FMEA), 149, 150
 just-in-time, 152, 153
 lean approach, 150, 152
 plan-do-study-act cycle, 150
 root cause analysis, 149
 six sigma, 152
Quality metrics, 126, 153, 154
Quality payment program, 20
Quantitative finance, 217

Readmission reduction program, 80, 82, 86, 87
Reduction of autonomy, 97
Regulatory environment, 217, 221, 223, 226
Regulatory strategies, 219, 223
Remote patient monitoring (RPM), 290
Research process knowledge, 125, 128, 154
Research programs, grounded in practice, 132
Responsibility assignment matrix, 181–183
Revenue analysis, 221
Revenue planning, 221, 223, 230
Rhetoric, 315, 317–321, 323
Rhetorical triangle, 320, 324, 333
Rhetorical situation, 319, 322, 324, 334
 the audience 319, 321, 324
 type of document, 324
 your position, 321
Robotics, 365, 379, 380, 383, 387
Role of nursing in policy advocacy, 159, 160, 166–171
Role of nursing in policy analysis, 159, 160, 167–171, 175, 181, 186
Role of nursing in policy formation, 160, 187
Role of policy analysis, 167
Role of the policy analyst, 159, 167
RWJ Future of Nursing campaign, 3

Sample business description, 247
Sample executive summary, 257
Sample marketing plan, 251
Sample SWOT analysis, 248
 Opportunities, 248
 Strengths, 248
 Threats, 248
 Weaknesses, 249

Simplification, 97
Small Business Administration (SBA), 251, 252, 253
  affordability, 252
  fit, 252
  media mix, 252
  repetition extent, 252
Smart tools, 303, 304, 310
Social compact, 161, 162, 221, 222, 234, 235, 236
Social policy statement, 186
Stakeholder management strategies, 226
Stakeholder mapping, 223, 225, 235, 238, 239
Stakeholders, 159, 170, 171, 173, 177, 178, 184, 188
Standardization, 97
State Medicaid programs, 218, 222–224
Statistical methods, descriptive and inferential analyses, 152
Storytelling, 344, 345, 358
Strategic agility, 17, 18, 21, 38
Strategic financial management tools, 217, 229
  cost management, 230
  revenue management, 221, 229
Strategic planning and management budgeting, 218, 225, 231
Strategic planning, 337, 352
Subject-verb agreement, 328
Subordination, 328
Sustainability, 365, 373, 375– 377, 382, 383
  energy, 375
  food, 375
  toxic chemicals, 375
  waste, 374, 375
  water, 373, 375
SWOT analysis, 173, 174
System life cycle, 294, 295, 297

Technical writing, 315, 316, 319
Technical writing basics, 319
Technological growth, 287, 308, 309
Technology
  adoption models, 298
  life cycle 292, 295, 297
  selection 292, 294, 295
  trends 287, 295, 309
Technology of writing, 317, 325
Telehealth, 307, 308, 309, 310
The Joint Commission (TJC), 134, 144, 146, 148, 149
  core measures, 144, 146
  hospital-related sentinel events, 147
  national patient safety goals, 146
TIGER concepts, 289
TIGER Institute, 288, 298, 308
Transformational care delivery methods, 30
Transformational leadership theory, 288, 289, 291
Transparency, 95, 96, 98, 159, 169, 173
Triple aim, 98–100, 105
  experience of care, 98–100
  per capita cost, 98, 99
  population health, 98, 99
Triple aim transition to Quadruple aim, 98, 105
Trusted advisor, 337, 346–351, 353, 356, 358
  accountability, 341, 351, 356
  candor, 351
  generosity, 351
  vulnerability, 351
Trustworthiness formula, 338, 350, 351
  credibility, 350, 351, 358
  intimacy, 350, 351
  limit self-orientation, 350, 351
  reliability, 350, 351, 358

Urgent care, 84, 85, 87, 88

Value-based care, 17, 18
Value-based performance domains, 138, 139
  clinical care, 141
  efficiency and cost reduction, 141
  person and community engagement, 141
  safety, 141

402 Index

Value-based purchasing, 99
Value-based purchasing domains, 102
  culture, 99
  learning systems, 95
Variance analysis, 231, 232, 235

Weak verbs, 329
What writing is, 317

White water, 380, 381, 383, 385, 386
Workflow maps, 299
Writer-text-reader triad, 321
  arrangement ,325
  invention, 317, 325
  style, 325, 326, 331, 332
Writing process 318, 326, 333
Writing proficiency 315

Donemere's Music

Thy Path Begins

(Book One in the Series)